Evidence-Based Manual Medicine

A Problem-Oriented Approach

Evidence-Based Manual Medicine

A Problem-Oriented Approach

Michael A. Seffinger, DO, FAAFP
Associate Professor
Department of Osteopathic Manipulative Medicine
College of Osteopathic Medicine of the Pacific
Western University of Health Sciences
Pomona, California

Raymond J. Hruby, DO, FAAO, MS
Professor and Chair
Department of Osteopathic Manipulative Medicine
College of Osteopathic Medicine of the Pacific
Western University of Health Sciences
Pomona, California

Illustrator:
William A. Kuchera, DO, FAAO
Professor Emeritus
Kirksville College of Osteopathic Medicine
A.T. Still University
Kirksville, Missouri

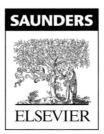

SAUNDERS

ELSEVIER

SAUNDERS
ELSEVIER

1600 John F. Kennedy Blvd.
Ste 1800
Philadelphia, PA 19103-2899

EVIDENCE-BASED MANUAL MEDICINE:
A PROBLEM-ORIENTED APPROACH

ISBN-13: 978-1-4160-2384-5

Copyright © 2007 by Saunders, an imprint of Elsevier Inc.

Library of Congress Cataloging-in-Publication Data
Seffinger, Michael A.
    Evidence-based manual medicine : a problem-oriented approach/Michael A. Seffinger, Raymond J. Hruby; illustrator, William A. Kuchera. – 1st ed.
        p. ; cm.
    Includes bibliographical references and index.
    ISBN 978-1-4160-2384-5
    1. Evidence-based medicine–Handbooks, manuals, etc. 2. Musculoskeletal system–Diseases–Handbooks, manuals, etc. I. Hruby, Raymond J. II. Title.
    [DNLM: 1. Musculoskeletal Diseases–therapy. 2. Evidence-Based Medicine–methods. 3. Manipulation, Orthopedic–methods. 4. Pain–therapy. 5. Sprains and Strains–therapy. WE 140 S453e 2007]
RC55.S426 2007
616–dc22   2007004481

Acquisitions Editor: Rolla Couchman
Project Manager: Bryan Hayward
Design Director: Steve Stave

Printed in United States of America

Last digit is the print number: 9 8 7 6 5 4 3 2 1

Foreword

Professional organizations, government agencies, insurance companies, and the general public now demand that clinical decision making by health care providers should rely as much as possible on evidence that has been derived from research. The comprehensive approach to clinical problem-solving and therapeutic planning set forth in this book offers physical/manual medicine practitioners therapeutic choices *based on,* or that are *informed by,* evidence.

The description of detailed approaches to clinical problem solving is a major feature of this book. This feature provides physical/manual medicine practitioners with an excellent resource to meet standards requiring evidence-informed reasoning and planning. The therapeutic decision-making processes necessary to meet these requirements may involve overcoming a number of obstacles, such as evaluating apparently conflicting evidence and judging the efficacy of long-used procedures of assessment and treatment.

For the health care provider, the old adage that "lack of evidence of efficacy does not equal evidence of lack of efficacy," can be comforting. The reality of clinical practice and decision-making involves uniting and integrating sound research evidence—where it exists—with clinical experience. The human dimension in all this is also an essential part of the equation, with the patient's condition, fears, ideals and wishes all forming integral features of the process involved in evolving safe and effective treatment strategies.

These considerations are summarized by Sackett's (1996) observation that, "evidence-based medicine is the conscientious, explicit, and judicious use of current best evidence in making decisions about the care of the individual patient. The practice of evidence-based medicine means integrating individual clinical expertise with the best available external clinical evidence from systematic research."[1]

At the very least, when there is unequivocal evidence of lack of benefit relating to a particular treatment procedure or approach, or overwhelming evidence of the unreliability of a specific assessment method, this should inform clinical choices. Using evidence in this way should help to weed out the use of inappropriate or ineffectual methods and modalities. However, research evidence alone is unlikely to offer firm direction for choosing which manual or other method should be employed in any given case. Examples abound of modalities where research studies offer conflicting evidence, either because of flawed research or built-in variables that make comparisons between conflicting outcomes confusing and possibly unreliable. What 'evidence' is the practitioner to choose then, other than that based on clinical experience?

Even when evidence is unchallenged, numerous therapeutic choices still remain. For example, the type of training (osteopathic, chiropractic, physical therapy, etc.), as well as the skill and experience of the practitioner, together with the condition and preferences of the patient, all factor in the determination whether a restricted spinal segment should be treated with a high velocity low amplitude (HVLA) thrust, or by means of soft tissue techniques, or exercise, or by means of some other modality altogether.

The reality is that different procedures, modalities, and techniques have all been shown to result in therapeutic benefit when delivered to appropriately identified and categorized conditions.[2]

Additionally the therapeutic objectives in any given case can leave a wide range of choices available. Information gathered from the individual's history, presenting symptoms, as well as observation, assessment, palpation, and where appropriate, evidence from scans and other tests, filtered through clinical experience, should inform the practitioner as to what needs to be achieved in order to enhance endogenous self-regulatory processes. Such objectives may include reduction of pain, increased range of motion, greater stability, or a modification of some other feature of the patient's condition.

When it comes to application of manual modalities, combinations of modes of the loading of tissues (shear force, translation, compression, etc.), varied by the degree of force employed (light, moderate, heavy, etc.), direction of force (direct towards the restriction barrier, or indirect involving disengagement from the barrier, or alternating combinations of these), as well as the amount of time involved in force application (continuous, rhythmic, brief, lengthy, etc.), the rate at which loads are applied (rapidly, slowly, variably), the number of repetitions, whether the method is passive, active, or involves a combination of patient and practitioner effort, as well as which tissues are involved (muscle, fascia, scar tissue, joint, etc.), and their properties (inflamed, flaccid, fibrosed, etc.), along with practitioner intent, creates a huge range of variables that make up the orchestral variety of the many therapeutic options open to the practitioner.[3,4]

Some, but by no means all, of these variables have been researched to the degree that evidence can inform therapeutic choices. However, all have been studied clinically for generations, and so can contribute to expert opinions that form the basis for research inquiries. Thus, successful clinical experience, passed on from one generation to the next offers valuable and often employed 'evidence'.

Fortunately, both forms of evidence—that derived from research and that emerging from expert opinion—are provided in this book, making it a resource that can aid both the student and the experienced clinician towards the formulation of informed clinical decisions and therapeutic strategies.

Systematic reviews and meta-analyses are often used to culminate the results from several clinical trials in order for experts to formulate practice guidelines. Although useful, these practice guidelines cannot become strict protocols, since the clinical trials and systematic reviews upon which they are based are not perfect representations of clinical practice where patients often present to practitioners with co-morbidities and complex multifactorial etiologies of their musculoskeletal complaints.

As Herbert (2007) points out:

"Clinical trials would be a simpler enterprise if patients presented with homogenous clinical presentations to which we could assign simple diagnoses, if therapists uniformly applied standardised therapies using mechanistic decision rules based on objective and universally accepted criteria, and if patients responded in more or less uniform ways to intervention. Unfortunately, the clinical presentations for each diagnosis are varied, diagnosis can be difficult, therapists choose to intervene very differently for the same condition or presentation, and patients' outcomes often appear hard to predict. For almost any clinical problem, clinical presentations, diagnoses, interventions and outcomes are heterogenous. This makes clinical trials difficult. Clinical research is a messy business."[5]

Fortunately the authors of this text, while referring to the results of systematic reviews, also include references from other clinical trials, outcome studies, and expert panel opinions in their recommendations. Shortcomings of the research and guidelines are pointed out in each chapter, by identifying the research that needs to be done next in order to clarify clinical decision algorithms and practice recommendations.

The epidemiological sections in each problem-oriented chapter are valuable in that they portray key aspects and characteristics of those patients who tend to develop particular patterns of musculoskeletal dysfunction. It is axiomatic that each individual needs to be evaluated by means of a comprehensive history and careful physical examination of their present illness, in order to delineate all the factors at play in their presenting condition. The differential diagnosis is considered for each problem, alerting the practitioner to the fact that each type of potential etiology must be considered and discounted *en route* to determining precise causes of the problem. It is only then that specific manual treatment can be selected and delivered with confidence of securing functional improvement, pain reduction, and ideally, resolution of the problem.

For example, two seemingly similar sets of symptoms ('low back pain') might have completely different etiological and aggravating features. These might be determined to be likely to benefit from quite different therapeutic and rehabilitation strategies—one possibly requiring deactivation of myofascial trigger points followed by postural re-education, with the other calling

for joint mobilization achieved by high velocity thrust methodology, supported by appropriate soft tissue normalization, possibly involving stretching and/or core stability training. Treatment should always be individualized and patient-centered.

Peters (2006) has summarized a part of the way forward as we seek evidence to inform therapeutic choices: "The notion that osteopaths offer non-specific treatment for nonspecific mechanical back pain is less tenable now that good research has shown how more precise diagnosis is often possible, and that treatments differentiated accordingly lead to good outcomes.[6] The contrary assumption—that manipulative technique effects are nonspecific, and that most back pain has no specific cause—if applied to medical research would be the equivalent of researching the effect of a randomly chosen drug on an undiagnosed symptom! The ADTO (Assessment/Diagnosis–Treatment/Outcome) approach recommended by Donelson (2004) will be crucial to evolving back pain research methods that are genuinely fit for purpose."[8]

This book has been successfully compiled to meet the need for evidence-based therapeutic approaches that are 'fit for purpose'. It offers detailed, comprehensive, problem-solving clinical descriptions, more than ably supported by excellent illustrations, photos, and by DVD sequences of assessment and treatment methods. In doing so it focuses on a wide range of conditions providing a resource of immense value. As a result, evidence-informed manual medicine practice becomes more readily achievable to the benefit of patients and practitioners alike.

Leon Chaitow, ND, DO
School of Integrated Health
University of Westminser
London, United Kingdom

REFERENCES

1. Sackett D, Rosenberg W, et al. Evidence based medicine: What it is and what it isn't—It's about integrating individual clinical expertise and the best external evidence. British Medical Journal 312(7023):71-72, 1996.
2. Scott-Dawkins C. Comparative effectiveness of adjustments versus mobilizations in chronic mechanical neck pain. Proceedings of the Scientific Symposium. World Chiropractic Congress, Tokyo, June 1997.
3. Lederman E. Science and practice of manual therapy, 2nd ed. Edinburgh, Churchill Livingstone, pp 87-224, 2005.
4. Mehling WE, Hamel KA, et al. Randomized, Controlled Trial of Breath Therapy for Patients With Chronic Low-Back Pain Altern Ther Health Med 11(4):44-52, 2005.
5. Herbert R. Dealing with heterogeneity in clinical trials. Manual Therapy 12(1):1-2, 2007.
6. Niemier K, Seidel W, et al. Introduction and Evaluation of a Multiprofessional Assessment System for the Differential Diagnosis of Chronic Musculoskeletal Pain Syndromes. J Osteopath Med (27):71-80, 2005.
7. Donelson R. Evidence-based low back pain classification. Improving care at its foundation. Eura Medicophys. 40(1):37-44, 2004.
8. Peters D. Letter to the Editor. Journal of Bodywork and Movement Therapies 10(4):314, 2006.

Foreword

There are two issues confronting today's primary care physicians, one new and one old. The new issue is the 21st century emphasis on "evidence-based medicine" and the old one is the prevalence of patients with musculoskeletal conditions presenting for care. This volume deals well with both issues. Its focus is on manual medicine, one of the oldest forms of health care, predating Hippocrates. Found within this work is a problem-oriented approach to the most common musculoskeletal system problems that confront the primary care practitioner. Within each problem area are references to the most current literature about the field of manual medicine. In all probability, the role of manual medicine in mechanical low back pain has been one of the most widely researched of the non-operative interventions for this condition. The author also identifies pertinent research questions still awaiting attention.

This volume begins with easily readable, current, and well illustrated basic information on the mechanisms of somatic dysfunction (the manipulable lesion), manual diagnostic procedures, and manual treatment procedures. This material provides the neophyte, as well as the experienced practitioner, with an up to date snapshot of the field. The common problems then follow with a format that provides the reader with a consistent and comprehensive diagnostic and therapeutic approach to the problem. Of particular interest is the inclusion of education and exercise to assist the patient in taking charge of their health problems and become less dependent upon the practitioner. The current "state of the art" in evidence-based medicine is included. Like many other disciplines in medicine, manual medicine has a long history of dependence upon experience and anecdotal information. In the 21st century this is no longer acceptable and fortunately there is a burgeoning body of research literature that supports this historical background.

With an ever-increasing interest in manual medicine in the medical community that has not had the educational opportunities to study the field, this book is a welcome addition to one's library bringing assistance to both the old and new challenges to the primary care practitioner. This book is one that is easily readable with lots of current information and will not just sit on the shelf. Read and enjoy.

Philip E. Greenman, DO, FAAO
Emeritus Professor,
Department of Osteopathic
Manipulative Medicine
Emeritus Professor, Department of Physical
Medicine and Rehabilitation
Michigan State University College
of Osteopathic Medicine

Acknowledgments

The authors would like to thank the many people who have supported this team effort. First and foremost, we owe a debt of gratitude to our loving and supportive wives and families who endured our indulgence in this project over many nights and weekends during "family time."

William A. Kuchera, DO, FAAO, Professor Emeritus at the A.T. Still University Kirksville College of Osteopathic Medicine was amazingly attentive and devoted to the artwork production and review of the material on a daily basis for over a year and a half. He spent several hours each day perfecting his incredible drawings, which clearly depict the concepts proposed.

David Redding, DO, Associate Professor of Family Medicine and Osteopathic Manipulative Medicine in the Department of Osteopathic Manipulative Medicine at Western University of Health Sciences College of Osteopathic Medicine of the Pacific (COMP) in Pomona, California, is a true inspiration at 60 years young, fit as a fiddle, which he plays adeptly by the way. His exercise photos will help keep patients in good shape and flexible as well. We are grateful for his participation in this project.

The professionalism and talent of Jess Lopatynski, photographer extraordinaire, and Joe Marilo, wizard videographer and editor, both at Western University of Health Sciences, are exemplary and much appreciated. The models for the photographs and videos were tireless, tolerant, and exhibited great poise. We are very grateful for their work. They are Miyako Seffinger, Stephen Dechter, Susan Yu, Rebecca Render, Kathryn Stroup, and Aiko Seffinger. Astute perspectives and assistance with the literature reviews and applications to primary care practice for some of the chapters were appreciated from Khanh X. Nguyen, DO, MPH. Editorial critique, organization and formatting assistance was adeptly provided by Mai Kim Ho and Micah Wittler, DO. Their guidance in the early renditions of the book was crucial as we laid the foundation. Courtney Mizuhara Cheng, DO, painstakingly placed the tenderpoints on the photos in their precise locations. Her attention to detail was much appreciated. Sayuri Seffinger labored untiringly to enter the references in uniform format into the computer, made seemingly endless editorial corrections, formatted the photos and their captions into spreadsheets for us, and entered editorial corrections of the manuscript as the chapters evolved over several months. Without her assistance this project would never have been completed.

Eric Hurwitz, DC, PhD, Associate Professor, Public Health Sciences and Epidemiology, John A. Burns School of Medicine, University of Hawaii in Manoa, Hawaii, and H. James Jones, DO, Associate Professor of Neurology and Osteopathic Manipulative Medicine, Department of Osteopathic Manipulative Medicine, College of Osteopathic Medicine of the Pacific, Western University of Health Sciences in Pomona, California and William A. Kuchera, DO, FAAO, performed peer review of the chapters and provided excellent recommendations.

Rolla Couchman at Elsevier was instrumental in guiding the development and production of this book. We owe a debt of gratitude for his patient and gentle encouragement to finish the manuscript, chapter by chapter, until it was finally completed.

Philip Greenman, DO, FAAO, stands out amongst many as both a mentor and role model for the authors. His clarity of vision and methods of instruction, the organization of his courses and standard textbook on the *Principles of Manual Medicine*, and his passion for the science and art of manual medicine are truly inspirational. We both had the privilege of learning from and teaching with him in his post graduate courses at Michigan State University and are honored that he has agreed to write a foreword to this book.

Leon Chaitow, DO, ND, is an educational pioneer in osteopathic and manual medicine. His lectures, journal and numerous books are renowned for their clear, thoughtful and thorough presentation of manual medicine for students of all levels. We are honored he has also agreed to write a foreword for this book.

Dr. Seffinger would like to acknowledge his mentors from which much of the manual medicine approach used in this book was derived: Robert C. Ward, DO, FAAO, William L. Johnston, DO, FAAO, Fred L. Mitchell, Jr., DO, FAAO, John P. Goodridge, DO, FAAO, and Viola M. Frymann, DO, FAAO, FCA. Support and encouragement from Sandy Shelton, CME, Production Manager and her staff and supervisors at the American Academy of Family Physicians in developing the evidence-based manipulative medicine courses are greatly appreciated. The advice, support and guidance provided by Harry D. Friedman, DO, FAAO, COL R. Todd Dombroski, DO, Dennis Cardone, DO, and Carl Steele, DO, MS, PT was critical in developing the problem oriented manual medicine approaches for the low back, neck, cervicogenic headache, and shoulder dysfunctions. Support and encouragement from past Presidents of the American Osteopathic Association, Donald J. Krpan, DO, and George Thomas, DO, is much appreciated. Finally, he would like to express his appreciation to his co-author for agreeing to embark on this endeavor with full commitment and passion. Raymond J. Hruby, DO, FAAO, MS, a 1973 graduate of Des Moines College of Osteopathic Medicine and Surgery, has been a Department Chair of Osteopathic Manipulative Medicine for 12 years, first at Michigan State University College of Osteopathic Medicine from 1995-1999, then at Western University of Health Sciences College of Osteopathic Medicine of the Pacific from 1999 until the present. He is a past-President of the American Academy of Osteopathy (AAO), past

Executive Editor of the AAO Journal, and is currently serving as Chair of the AAO Publications Committee. He was an Associate Editor and is currently an author of the Foundations for Osteopathic Medicine textbook. He has brought his expertise in manual medicine literature and 30 years of expert teaching and practice experience to the project.

In addition to those noted in the previous paragraph, Dr. Hruby would like to acknowledge the following people who also served as teachers, mentors, and guides in the development of his career in manual medicine: Edward G. Stiles, DO, FAAO, Anthony G. Chila, DO, FAAO, Lawrence H. Jones, DO, FAAO, Stephen D. Blood, DO, FAAO, William E. Wyatt, DO, Paul E. Kimberly, DO, FAAO, George W. Northup, DO, FAAO, Alan R. Becker, DO, FAAO, Frank H. Willard, PhD, and Irvin M. Korr, PhD. Of critical importance is the inspiration and encouragement of his many Undergraduate Osteopathic Manipulative Medicine Teaching Fellows, who give him his biggest reason to go to work every day. He would like to give a special acknowledgement to his parents, John J. Hruby, Jr., and Helen M. Hruby. Finally he would like to especially acknowledge his co-author for giving him the honor and opportunity to participate in this project. Michael A. Seffinger, DO, FAAFP is a 1988 graduate of the Michigan State University College of Osteopathic Medicine and is an Associate Professor of Family Medicine and Osteopathic Manipulative Medicine at the Western University of Health Sciences College of Osteopathic Medicine of the Pacific. He is board certified in Family Medicine and Osteopathic Manipulative Treatment, and Neuromusculoskeletal Medicine and Osteopathic Manipulative Medicine. He is vice-Chair of the American Osteopathic Association Bureau of Osteopathic Clinical Education and Research and Chair of the American Academy of Osteopathy Louisa Burns Osteopathic Research Committee. Dr. Seffinger is an Associate Editor and author of the Foundations for Osteopathic Medicine textbook and Managing Editor of the California DO Journal of the Osteopathic Physicians and Surgeons of California. He brings to this writing nearly 20 years of clinical experience, his passion for research, and his ability to keep Dr. Hruby focused on the fact that some things, in order to be perfect, sometimes take just a little more time.

The authors would like to offer their sincere gratitude to Western University of Health Sciences for their support and production of the photos and videos used in this book and accompanying dvd.

The authors offer this humble endeavor to help promote the growth, development, and practice of manual medicine. If we have assisted even one practitioner to more fully combine both the art and science of manual medicine into practice then we have more than accomplished our goal.

Contents

Chapter 1: Overview 1

Chapter 2: Somatic Dysfunction Mechanisms 3

Chapter 3: Manual Diagnostic Procedures Overview 35

Chapter 4: Treatment Procedures Overview 59

Chapter 5: Mechanical Low Back Pain 71

Chapter 6: Mechanical Neck and Upper Back Pain 129

Chapter 7: Cervicogenic Headache 189

Chapter 8: Temporomandibular Joint Dysfunction 207

Chapter 9: Shoulder Pain and Dysfunction 221

Chapter 10: Carpal Tunnel Syndrome 273

Chapter 11: Ankle Sprain 291

Chapter 12: Manual Medicine Coding 313

Index 317

CHAPTER 1

Overview

Primary care practitioners worldwide encounter common problems in their daily clinical practice that often respond to manual treatment. The patients and conditions that respond best and most consistently are those with identifiable mechanical (musculoskeletal) components to their problems. Using a problem-oriented format, this book and accompanying video clips can guide the primary care practitioner through basic palpatory diagnostic and manual treatment procedures useful in treating a wide variety of illnesses. Recent evidence-based research literature regarding these procedures is presented along with patient management guidelines. This book promises to be a valuable resource to all primary care practitioners regardless of where they practice.

BACKGROUND

Awareness and respect for manual approaches to common health care problems has increased over the past century since the development of the osteopathic, chiropractic, and physical therapy professions and the medical disciplines of orthopedic surgery and medicine, physical medicine and rehabilitation, occupational medicine, and sports medicine. In 1994, the U.S. Department of Health Care Policy and Research (now called the U.S. Department of Healthcare Research and Quality) recommended spinal manipulation for Americans with acute mechanical low back pain.[1] The national guidelines on low back pain treatment in the United Kingdom, Switzerland, Sweden, New Zealand, Germany, and Denmark also recommend spinal manipulation as an option in the initial weeks of an acute mechanical back pain episode.[2] However, primary care practitioners usually are not well trained to provide this recommended care.

Systematic reviews and meta-analyses of clinical trials evaluating the efficacy and effectiveness of spinal manual treatments for back pain have indicated that this approach is beneficial.[3] Spinal manipulation is as effective as conventional nonmanual approaches and is a viable option for patients. Compared with acupuncture, manual treatment for low back pain has produced better outcomes.[4]

There are no international or national standards on manual evaluation and treatment procedures. Although traditionally different professional groups who promote manual therapies have not interacted much in developing standard methods of manual evaluation or treatment, the three major professional associations that promote manual treatments for the treatment of back pain in the United Kingdom have agreed on a manual treatment protocol for use in clinical research.[5] In the United States, the osteopathic profession has standardized its terminology and manual evaluation and treatment methods, but other professions are lagging in that process.[6] There is no formal interaction between professions on these issues in the United States.

Although nonphysician osteopaths, chiropractors, physical therapists, naturopaths, massage therapists, and unregulated, nonprofessional individuals use manual treatments, medical doctors other than American-trained osteopathic physicians are not educated or trained in these methods of manual treatment as part of their standard medical training. Specialty societies of physicians, such as the American Society of Orthopedic Medicine, American Academy of Physical Medicine and Rehabilitation, American Academy of Neurology, and American Academy of Family Physicians, do offer limited introductory courses in manual medicine for medical doctors. Extensive programs designed to train American physicians in manual medicine are offered by the American Academy of Osteopathy and some osteopathic medical schools, such as Michigan State University. Europe has several physician societies of manual medicine that sponsor introductory and extensive programs in manual medicine. The International Federation of Manual Medicine consists of physicians worldwide who use and research manual medicine. They hold committee meetings annually and sponsor an international conference once every 3 years.

In 1992 at the annual scientific assembly, the American Academy of Family Physicians (AAFP) asked Ray Hruby, DO, FAAO, to introduce their physician members to osteopathic manual approaches to the treatment of common musculoskeletal conditions seen by family physicians. COL R. Todd Dombroski, DO (1993-present), Harry D. Friedman, DO, FAAO (1994-2000), Michael Seffinger, DO, FAAFP (1995-present), Dennis Cardone, DO, FAAFP (1995-present), and Carl Steele, DO, MS, PT (1998-present) have expanded the AAFP offerings to its members over the years to include several procedure workshops in manual treatment of a variety of common problems, including upper back and neck pain, upper extremity musculoskeletal dysfunctions, respiratory problems, headache, and sports injuries. These workshops have been well rated and appreciated by participants annually. Since they are evidence based medicine (EBM) courses, participants are rewarded with two continuing medical education credit hours for every one hour of participation. This textbook has evolved from these courses.

Health care professionals who use manipulative treatments employ visual and palpation tests to determine whether manipulative treatments are indicated. These tests assess symmetry of bony landmarks, quantity and quality of regional and segmental motion, paraspinal soft tissue abnormalities, and tenderness on provocation. The decision to use manipulation and decisions about the effectiveness of manipulative treatments rely on the skill and training of the practitioner and on an accurate diagnosis. The ability to arrive at an accurate diagnosis depends on the education and training of the individual practitioner. This textbook and DVD are meant to be a personal instructional guide to supplement formal training and education in a regulated health care discipline. They are not meant to replace professional training, formal education, or board certification in manual methods of diagnosis and treatment. However, the clinical effectiveness of a practitioner already trained in manual methods of diagnosis and treatment of musculoskeletal dysfunction will likely improve with practice of the principles and techniques included herein.

During the past 10 years, myriad textbooks on manual treatments have been written by physical therapists, chiropractors, osteopaths, orthopedic surgeons, physical medicine and rehabilitation specialists, and sports medicine specialists, and massage therapists. There has not been, however, a text for the primary care practitioner on this topic. Previous books have been written for the manual therapist specialist, not the time-pressured primary care practitioner. These books have provided instruction on manual therapy for the various body regions or a particular technique applied to all body regions. None has been structured in the problem-oriented format. Primary care practitioners are not sure which techniques to apply, when to apply them, and how many to apply per patient per visit for each condition.

There are also abundant texts on what is called integrative medicine or complementary and alternative medicine, which are in problem-based formats but merely list the variety of treatments available for patients with each condition. Although manual treatment is mentioned, which techniques, how to apply them, and when to use them are not included in these books.

This textbook seeks to remedy this situation by giving the primary care practitioner a handle on the field of manual treatment for common musculoskeletal problems or conditions with musculoskeletal components that are amenable to manual treatment. Each chapter provides the rationale for application of these methods for each clinical condition. The somatic dysfunction mechanisms chapter and the anatomy and pathophysiology sections within each chapter provide the basic science foundation for the treatments. Epidemiology, history, and physical findings to look for and differential diagnoses to consider provide the context in which manual treatment is indicated. Contraindications to treatment are also given.

The evidence-based medicine literature reviews on the efficacy and effectiveness of manual treatment for each problem provide additional rationale and support for the use and reimbursement of these procedures in primary care. Recommendations for clinical application of manual treatments are provided for each problem using the latest literature sources. The highest level of evidence that supports the recommendation is presented using the following definitions:

> Grade A: Based on randomized clinical trials, systematic reviews or meta-analyses
> Grade B: Based on case-control or cohort studies, retrospective studies, and certain uncontrolled studies
> Grade C: Based on concensus statements, expert guidelines, usual practice, and opinion

The pictures and clear descriptions of the manual diagnostic and treatment procedures and a DVD with techniques demonstrated and explained in real time should aid the clinician in acquiring the skills needed to successfully apply these techniques. Adjunct treatments, patient education, and exercise sections for each problem are intended to help the practitioner form appropriate management plans for each patient. The exercises are included as handouts for patients on the accompanying DVD.

Controversies and further research suggestions are included at the end of each problem-oriented chapter to stimulate further discussion, and they indicate the need and direction for growth and development of these hands-on approaches to patient care. References and recommended reading lists are provided for those interested in pursuing further information on the manual approach to each problem. There are many more references available. The sources given are not comprehensive; they come from the authors' personal accumulation of articles over the years.

Practitioners who desire to use manual diagnosis and treatment procedures in patient care should obtain the appropriate and necessary skills and training from accredited educational sources and institutions. This textbook should serve as a guide and resource to licensed health care practitioners. It is not intended as a stand-alone self-instruction manual for the lay public.

REFERENCES

1. Bigos SJ, Bowyer OR, Braen GR, et al: Acute Low Back Problems in Adults: Assessment and Treatment. Clinical practice guideline number 14. Publication no. 95-0643. Rockville, MD, U.S. Department of Health and Human Services, Public health Services, Agency for Health Care Policy and Research, December, 1994.
2. Koes B, vanTulder M, Ostelo R, et al: Clinical guidelines for the management of low back pain in primary care: An international comparison. Spine 26:2504-2514, 2001.
3. Assendelft WJJ, Morton SC, Yu EI, et al: Spinal manipulative therapy for low back pain. A meta-analysis of effectiveness to other therapies. Ann Intern Med 138:871-881, 2003.
4. Cherkin DC, Sherman KJ, Deyo RA, Shekelle PG: A review of the evidence for the effectiveness, safety, and cost of acupuncture, massage therapy, and spinal manipulation for back pain. Ann Intern Med 138:898-906, 2003.
5. Harvey E, Burton AK, Moffett JK, Breen A: Spinal manipulation for low-back pain: A treatment package agreed by the UK chiropractic, osteopathy and physiotherapy professional associations. Manual Ther 8:46-51, 2003.
6. Ward RC (ex. ed.): Foundations for Osteopathic Medicine, 2nd ed. Philadelphia: Lippincott Williams & Wilkins, 2003.

CHAPTER 2

Somatic Dysfunction Mechanisms

PATHOPHYSIOLOGY

Definition of Somatic Dysfunction

- Somatic dysfunction is defined as "impaired or altered function of related components of the somatic (body framework) system: skeletal, arthrodial, and myofascial structures and related vascular, lymphatic, and neural elements."[1]
- It is a dysfunction that can be corrected or improved by manual treatments such as those described in this textbook.
- The most common precipitating cause of somatic dysfunction is overuse injury from repetitive activities that strain and induce microtrauma in the soft tissues of the musculoskeletal system.
- Macrotrauma from injuries, inflammation from a variety of causes, and poor postural mechanics are other causes.
- The ultimate manifestation is identifiable by physical examination using visual and palpatory assessment. Asymmetry of structural landmarks, altered range and quality of regional and segmental joint motion, abnormal localized tissue texture, tenderness, and temperature changes (ART or TART) are the cardinal findings indicating the presence of somatic dysfunction (Table 2.1).

Characteristics of Somatic-Neural Reflexes

Somatic Motor and Sensory Systems
- Neural control of the somatic motor system involves complex feedback mechanisms between the brain, spinal cord, peripheral nerves, and musculoskeletal structures.
- Each component is functionally and structurally capable of adaptation and modulation to maintain as much efficiency as possible.
- The motor system continually adapts to injuries and somatic dysfunctions, but each adaptation is less efficient than its predecessor. *Manual treatments are designed to alleviate somatic dysfunction to help the motor system improve its efficiency.*
- Afferent nerve impulses travel from the peripheral muscle or joint structures to the spinal cord, conveying information about pain, temperature, and position.

- The afferent information from the muscles and joints is transmitted to the dorsal root ganglion (DRG) and then to the dorsal horn of the spinal cord.
- Vibratory sensation or proprioception is transmitted superiorly to the ipsilateral side of the brain, and other information, such as pain and temperature, is transmitted across the cord to the spinothalamic tract before being transmitted to the contralateral side of the brain (Fig. 2.1A).
- Somatic afferent impulses may also be transmitted to somatic efferent cell bodies in the ventral horn, which send axons back to the muscles to regulate muscle length and tone, completing the somatosomatic reflex (see Fig. 2.1B).
- Afferent impulses may travel to one or several levels of the spinal cord before the information is sent out of the cord to the brain or to the periphery.
- At every level, there is modulation and processing of the information with other afferent stimuli.
- After the central nervous system processes and integrates the information it receives from the peripheral structures, it sends out commands for action or inhibition of action to achieve a desired result.

The Myotatic Reflex
- Muscle tension is regulated by the Golgi tendon apparatus, which responds to the forces of muscle stretch and contraction (Fig. 2.2).
  1. Alpha motor neurons are efferent nerves from the ventral horn of the spinal cord that stimulate the extrafusal muscle fibers to contract in response to central nervous system (i.e., brain and spinal cord) demands.
  2. The Golgi tendon apparatus reports to the central nervous system the effect of the efferent stimulus from the alpha motor neuron and enables refinement and further modulation for controlled and appropriate activity.
- Muscle length is regulated by spinal nerves that innervate the muscle spindle in the belly of the muscle (see Fig. 2.2).
- The spindle is innervated by gamma afferents and efferents and regulates intrafusal muscle fiber length in response to extrafusal muscle fiber length.
- There are annulospiral and flower spray–type nerve endings within the muscle spindle that work in tandem.

Table 2.1   Criteria for diagnosis of somatic dysfunction

Designation	Diagnostic Criteria
T	Tissue texture abnormalities
A	Asymmetry of bony landmarks
R	Range or quality of motion abnormalities
T	Tenderness or temperature variations

- The muscle spindle reports the changes of muscle length and the rate of change in response to alpha and gamma motor neuron activity and enables appropriate adjustment by the central nervous system to regulate muscle length.

Reciprocal Inhibition

- Opposing muscle groups work together to control precise joint motion.
- To control joint movements, when one group is activated, its opposing group is simultaneously inhibited.
  1. Flexor muscle contraction is accompanied by reflex inhibition of the extensor muscle groups acting on the same joint and by contralateral flexor muscle group inhibition. The reverse is also true for extensor muscle contraction.

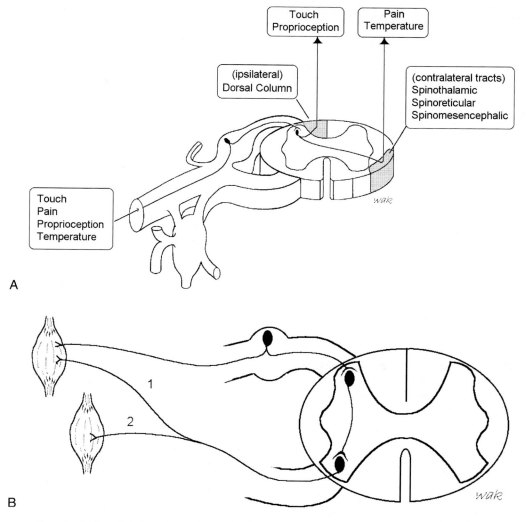

Figure 2.1   A, Sensory afferent spinal cord pathways: communicating with the brain. Touch and proprioception sensations ascend ipsilaterally within the spinal cord, whereas pain and temperature sensations ascend contralateral to the side of the stimulus. **B,** sensory afferent spinal cord pathways: somatosomatic reflex. Efferents stimulate the same muscle (1) that generated the afferent discharge from muscle contraction, sustaining its hypertonicity. Efferents stimulate agonist muscles (2) that were not part of the initial afferent discharge, causing them to contract or at least to increase in tone.

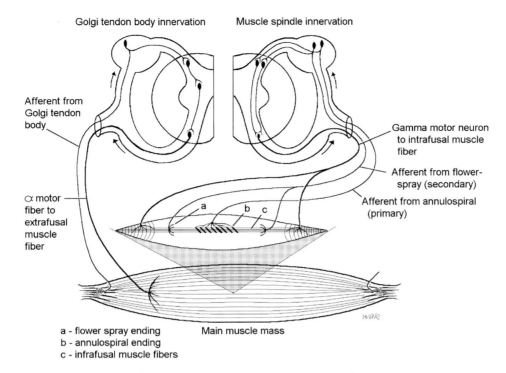

Golgi tendon body innervation   Muscle spindle innervation

Afferent from
Golgi tendon
body

Gamma motor neuron
to intrafusal muscle
fiber

Afferent from flower-
spray (secondary)

Afferent from annulospiral
(primary)

α motor
fiber to
extrafusal
muscle
fiber

a   b   c

wak

a - flower spray ending
b - annulospiral ending
c - infrafusal muscle fibers

Main muscle mass

Figure 2.2 Myotatic reflex. Muscle tone and length is controlled by spinal cord reflexes through afferents from and efferents to muscle spindles and Golgi tendon organs.

2. If a muscle is held in a sustained contractual state, as in muscle spasm, or somatic dysfunction, its opposing muscle groups will be reciprocally inhibited.

Neuroimmune Pathophysiology

Strain injury or trauma causes peripheral stimulation of proinflammatory compounds (e.g., bradykinin, histamine, cytokines, prostaglandins), which extravasate fluids and irritate primary afferent nerves[2] (Fig. 2.3).

- Primary afferent nociceptors are small nerve fibers that transmit impulses to the spinal cord from peripheral structures such as muscles and joints in response to noxious stimuli.
- They have little or no myelin and are classified as C-fibers.
- Their excitation often causes the perception of pain, but they can be stimulated without eliciting a pain sensation.
- They are capable of promoting pain and of inhibiting pain.
- The peripheral nerves become sensitized, lowering their threshold of activation and increasing their rate of firing.[2]
- Although sensory nerve fibers used to be considered only capable of sending impulses and transmitting action potentials from the periphery to the spinal cord and releasing neurotransmitter peptides at their spinal cord synapses, it is now understood that they can be stimulated from reflex activity by interneurons within the spinal cord's dorsal horn and through the dorsal root ganglia (i.e., dorsal root reflexes). Transmission of neuropeptides to peripheral tissues through afferent nerves from spinal cord stimulation is called *antidromic transmission*.

- At low levels of intensity, nociceptors can inhibit pain sensation, but at higher intensity, they can generate a series of spinal cord reflexes that increase the sensitivity of the peripheral tissues, increasing pain sensation to lesser stimuli and facilitating further inflammatory response.
- The nociceptors that are stimulated also release substance P, calcitonin gene–related peptide (CGRP) and somatostatin antidromically, which also mediate vasodilation, spread the inflammatory response, and contribute to hyperalgesia of the inflamed area.
- Increased peripheral nervous system C-fiber afferent activity leads to increased release of glutamates from the dorsal horn. The process, called *windup*, occurs when the DRGs become sensitized to afferent input, which in effect amplifies the nociceptive message. This hyperexcitability also affects spinal cord neurons and results in central sensitization or facilitation (see Fig. 2.3).
- This neurogenic inflammation is mediated from spinal neurotransmitters such as γ-aminobutyric acid (GABA).
- Sympathetic efferents from the spinal cord can modulate this neurogenic inflammation.
- Enhanced sympathetic output from the hypersensitive spinal cord segments induces palpable alterations in local temperature and hydration of the soft tissues (Fig. 2.4).
- Increased blood flow, heat, and moisture in the acute stage of injury and inflammation under the influence of local vasoactive peptides and nitric oxide (NO) can be modulated by sympathetic tone and decreased blood flow, coolness, and dryness in the chronic stage (Table 2.2).

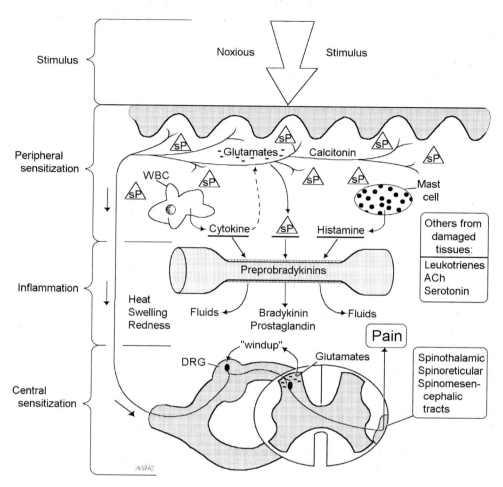

Figure 2.3 Neurogenic inflammation. A cascade of biochemical events involving neurotransmitters and proinflammatory peptides in response to peripheral noxious stimuli causes peripheral inflammation and leads to peripheral and central sensitization, also called *facilitation*. Ach, acetylcholine; Calcitonin, calcitonin gene–related peptide; sP, substance P; WBC, white blood cells.

- This leads to the palpable abnormal tissue texture (i.e., edema) and hyperalgesia (i.e., sensitivity to touch) characteristics of somatic dysfunction.

Central-Peripheral Nervous System Sensitization

- Beta afferent nerve stimulation (i.e., nociception) alters patterns of neural activity in the dorsal and ventral horns of the spinal cord.
- Persistent spinal cord stimulation leads to hypersensitivity and adaptation of the spinal cord at the segments affected.[2-4]
- Spinal facilitation (i.e., central sensitization) also causes sensitization in related sensory receptive regions of the brain.
- Dorsal root reflexes can be generated by descending activity from the brain.
  1. Stimulation of the midbrain periaqueductal gray (PAG) increases serotonin release from descending fibers originating in the raphe magnus nucleus in the brain stem and GABA release from spinal interneurons.

  2. PAG stimulation is influenced by higher centers, such as the prefrontal cortex and amygdala, which are associated with emotions.
  3. Emotional processes likely modulate spinal cord and peripheral nerve activity and influence muscle and joint responses to strains, damage, or trauma.
- The result of this sensitization is a sustained hypertonicity of muscles innervated by the facilitated spinal cord segments and hypotonicity of antagonistic muscles (Fig. 2.5).
  1. It is hypothesized that muscle spindles are influenced by neurogenic antidromic stimulation as well as the familiar effect of ventral horn alpha motor neuron and gamma efferent modulation as part of the myotatic reflex.
  2. Sustained muscle hypertonicity as found in muscle spasm and somatic dysfunction is thought to be the result of a combination of peripheral and central neuronal reflex activity that involves prodromic and antidromic neurotransmission.[2]
- This reaction produces visible anatomic asymmetry of easily identified bony landmarks and measurable abnormal quality and quantity of related joint motion.

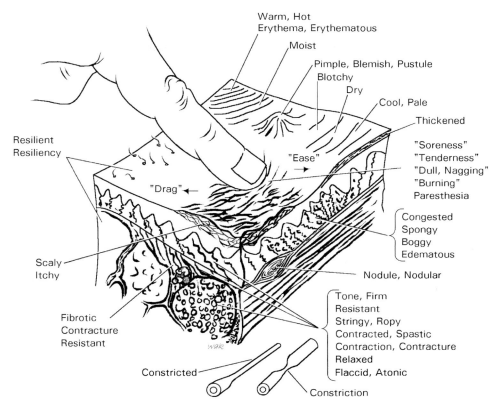

Figure 2.4 Palpable soft tissue changes occur because of differences in fluid content of the subcutaneous tissues. These alterations can be acute or chronic in nature. They are caused by neurologic and circulatory events, and they are modified by sympathetic tone. From Kuchera WA, Kuchera ML, Osteopathic Principles in Practice, Second Edition Revised, Greydon Press, Columbus, OH, 1994:510. Used with permission.

Myofascial Adaptations

- Myofascial connective tissue matrix adaptations accompany the articular and periarticular motion restrictions and muscle imbalance.
- Joint immobilization or prolonged periods of decreased motion enable the formation of an increased amount of collagen crosslinks that cause myofascial connective tissue stiffness.[5]
- The fluid content and contractile elements within these connective tissues adapt to modify tensions and maintain biomechanical integrity and efficiency of the region.[5,6]
  1. Glycosaminoglycans (GAGs) are generated from fibrocytes in response to motion.

  2. GAGs are the linear polymers of repeating disaccharide units that make up the ground substance in the connective tissues throughout the body.
  3. GAGs form the milieu in which the fibrous collagenous fibers provide the form and stiffness of the connective tissue.

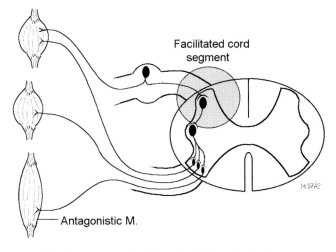

Figure 2.5 Somatosomatic reflexes in facilitated spinal cord segments create sustained muscle hypertonicity and antagonist inhibition. M, muscle.

Table 2.2   Palpable skin changes from altered blood flow due to somatic dysfunction

Acute Phase (hours to days)	Chronic Phase (weeks to months)
Hyperemic	Ischemic
Boggy or edematous	Firm or flat
Warm	Cool
Moist	Dry
Sticky	Slippery

4. GAGs are hydrophilic, and the amount of GAGs present determines the relative fluid content of the connective tissue.
5. The more GAGs there are, the more water binds to them, forcing the collagen fibers to be farther apart and less able to form crosslinks.
6. The fewer GAGs there are in the ground substance, the stiffer and more noncompliant is the connective tissue.

- Myofascial structures respond to sustained stress forces (e.g., muscle spasms) by undergoing deformation to accommodate the load (i.e., creep). After the load is released, the myofascial structures return toward their initial state, but they never regain their exact preload structure (i.e., hysteresis).
- Axoplasmic flow of nutrients within peripheral nerves can be impeded by the compressive affect of myofascial tissues.[5]

Neuropathic Pain

- When there is trauma or damage to peripheral nerve endings, neuropathic pain can develop. This is characterized by abnormal sensations of hypersensitivity, hyperalgesia, or allodynia.
  1. *Hypersensitivity* is defined as altered perception of pain. For example, a small amount of pressure causes pain out of proportion to the stimulus, but there is a normal response in adjacent areas.
  2. *Hyperalgesia* is defined as an enhanced pain sensation to a noxious stimulus. For example, a pin prick elicits severe pain.
  3. *Allodynia* is defined as abnormal sensation of pain to previously non-noxious stimuli. For example, light touch causes shooting pain or a burning sensation.
- The body's response to peripheral nerve injury entails altered neuronal connections and central sensitization or facilitation[7] (Fig. 2.6A and B). The following anatomic and pathophysiologic changes can occur after a peripheral nerve crush injury (numbers correlate with the illustration in Figure 2.6B):
  1. A peripheral crush injury initiates the neuropathic pain process.
  2. Peripheral nerve fibers are damaged.
  3. There is proliferation of α-adrenergic receptors on primary sensory afferent endings and primary sensory cell bodies in the DRG.
  4. There is sprouting of C-fibers in the spinal cord.
  5. A lowered threshold for firing of C-fibers (i.e., hyperesthesia) and A-delta fibers (i.e., allodynia) create a facilitated spinal cord segment.
  6. There is glutamate excitotoxic cell death of inhibitory neurons (i.e., glutamate storms) within the spinal cord that leads to inability of the brain to control the pain cycle process.
  7. There is an inadequacy of central descending serotonin, norepinephrine, and opioid peptide pathways to control nociception.
  8. Hyperactivity of "wide dynamic range" interneurons in the spinal cord at the same anatomic level of activity continually stimulates sympathetic cell bodies in the lateral horn of the spinal cord.
  9. This leads to sprouting of sympathetic postganglionic nerve fibers on primary afferent nerve endings.
  10. Ephaptic afferent activation can occur.
  11. Sprouting of sympathetic postganglionic nerve fibers on primary sensory cell bodies in the DRG can also occur.
  12. Immobilization by pain decreases gating of nociceptive input (ability to override the slower C-fiber nociceptive input by more rapidly conducting A-delta sensory pathways), limiting the ability of physical or manual therapy to initiate gating.

Local and Distant Effects of Somatic Dysfunction

- Blood flow and lymph flow become sluggish, and congestion ensues because of the lack of mobility in the area of somatic dysfunction.[8]
- There are potential systemic consequences of brain sensitization after the hypothalamus becomes involved.[4]
  1. The hypothalamus integrates peripheral nociception (afferent pain) information with limbic or emotional stimuli and input from the visceral organs.
  2. The hypothalamus activates the pituitary and brainstem, along with the autonomic nervous system, endocrine system, and immune system.
  3. Together, these stimuli elicit the general adaptive response (i.e., increased level of cortisol and norepinephrine).

Associated Pathophysiology

- Other pathophysiologic processes interact with and affect the biochemical and mechanical manifestations of somatic dysfunction.
  1. Visceral diseases, especially inflammatory conditions, create palpable somatic changes in the paraspinal soft tissues that are similar to those found with primary muscle strain or trauma-related somatic changes, including tissue texture abnormalities, restriction of motion, asymmetry of landmarks, and tenderness and temperature alterations. The practitioner must learn to differentiate viscerally generated somatic changes from mechanical somatic dysfunction.
  2. Viscerosomatic reflexes are generated from inflammatory organ disease conditions, such as asthma, coronary artery disease, duodenal ulcer disease, hepatitis, pancreatitis, inflammatory bowel disease, and cholecystitis (Fig. 2.7).
- Structural congenital or acquired deformities, such as scoliosis and short-leg syndrome, distort symmetry, motion, and the feel of the tissues and must be considered in the interpretation of physical findings.
- Neurologic reflexes from central, peripheral, and autonomic nervous system adaptations and diseases can further distort local somatosomatic reflexes.
- Circulatory dysfunctions, such as ischemia, edema (i.e., congestion), and respiratory diseases or dysfunctions have wide range of effects on the soft tissues.
- Metabolic processes (i.e., nutritional, immunologic, and endocrine processes; medications; toxins, and exercise) can

A. Normal nociceptive reflex pattern

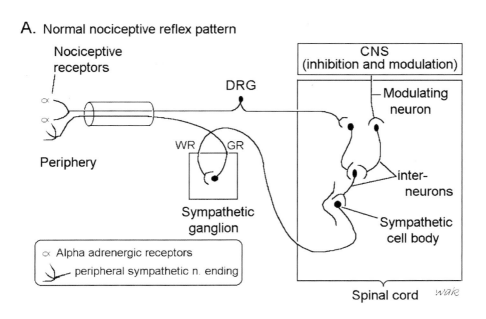

B. Neuropathic pain sympathetically maintained

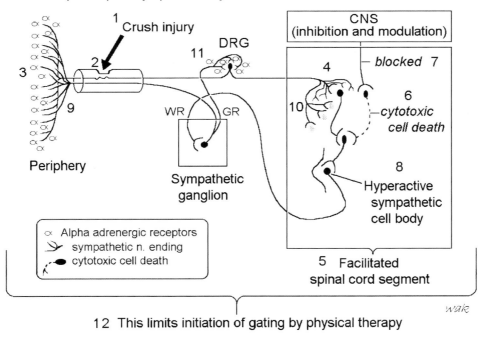

12 This limits initiation of gating by physical therapy

Figure 2.6 Normal pain versus neuropathic pain pathways. **A,** Nociceptors stimulated in the periphery send afferents to the dorsal root ganglia (DRG) en route to the spinal cord gray matter. Interneurons in the intermediolateral cell column of the spinal cord, modulated by neurons descending from the brain (CNS), modulate the pain information en route to sympathetic cell bodies in the lateral horn. Sympathetic efferents transmit information to the sympathetic ganglion by means of white rami (WR) communicans neurons. Gray rami (GR) communicans neurons carry the efferent information from the sympathetic ganglion to the peripheral tissues to alter blood flow and sweat gland activity. **B,** Neuropathic pain is maintained by altered anatomy and pathophysiology of the peripheral and central nervous systems. The sequence of events is numbered.

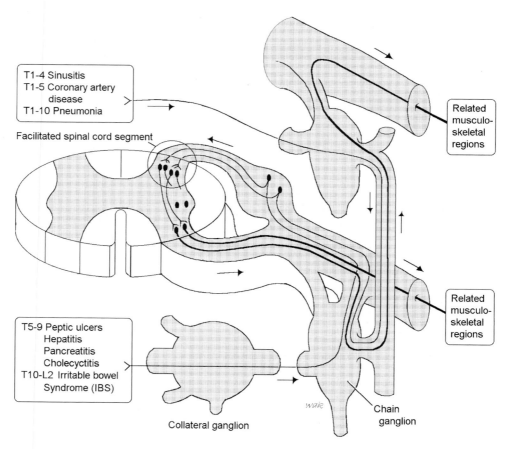

Figure 2.7 Viscerosomatic reflexes are generated most commonly from inflamed organs, and they cause hypertonicity in segmentally related musculature and paraspinal soft tissues.

cause electrolyte imbalance, tissue atrophy, and toxicity to nerve and muscle function, and they can affect bony structure and function.

- Behavioral issues such as obesity, smoking, emotional stress, alcohol and drug abuse, social isolation and loneliness, depression, and anxiety play significant roles in musculoskeletal disability and rehabilitation.

Reversal of the Pathophysiology

Manual treatment is designed to do the following:[2,3,5,8]
- Alleviate somatic dysfunction
- Restore normal neuromusculoskeletal structural and functional relationships
- Decrease the stimulation of nociceptors, mechanoreceptors, and proprioceptors; *the hypalgesic (pain-relieving) effect of manipulation is mediated by serotonin and adrenergic neurotransmitters at the spinal cord dorsal horn level.*[9]
- Improve joint mobility
- Reduce congestion of fluids
- Arrest the previously described cascade of effects

Clinical Characteristics of Somatic Dysfunction

- Somatic dysfunction affects people of all ages.
- Somatic dysfunction is three times more common in female than male patients.[10]
- The incidence of somatic dysfunction has been assessed using a validated and standardized medical record, developed by the American Academy of Osteopathy for the American Osteopathic Association.[10] Sleszynski and Glonek analyzed 3908 medical records of patients seen over 17 months by 206 osteopathic physicians and 2 osteopathic manipulative medicine research fellows. The diagnosis of somatic dysfunction requires at least 1 of the four cardinal signs of tissue texture changes, asymmetry of anatomic landmarks, range of motion abnormalities, and tenderness (TART). TART changes were found in all patients, but more so in some body regions than in others. The greatest incidence per body region of one or more TART changes according to the outcomes study derived from the use of the standardized medical record are as follows:
1. Cervical: 72.3%
2. Thoracic, T1-T4: 70.9%

3. Upper left extremity (26.8%) (the lowest incidence of at least one TART change[10])
- Patients that have three or four of the cardinal signs of TART are considered to have a higher severity of somatic dysfunction than those that have only one or two findings at any particular spinal segment. The incidence of highest severity level of TART changes (i.e., all four TART changes found) per anatomic region are as follows:[10]
  1. Cervical: 24.2%
  2. Lumbar: 23.2%
  3. Head: 22.1%
  4. Thoracic, T1 to T4: 20.5%
  5. Thoracic, T5 to T9: 16.9%
- Physical examination findings vary.
  1. Asymptomatic
     Poor posture
     Poor, inefficient body mechanics
     Occult visceral or musculoskeletal dysfunction or disease
  2. Symptomatic
     Visceral disease or illness
     Musculoskeletal tenderness on palpation or movement
     Decreased movement
     Fatigue
     Depression
  3. Somatic dysfunction (microscopic findings after trauma)
     Acutely (hours to days)
        Hyperemia
        Congestion and dilation
        Minute hemorrhages and thrombosis
     Chronic (weeks to months)
        Organization
        Fibrosis
        Local ischemia
        Atrophy and sclerosis
  4. Somatic dysfunction (macroscopic findings after trauma)
     Erythema
     Swelling
     Temperature changes
     Tenderness
     Altered range and quality of motion
     Asymmetric landmarks
- Laboratory and radiologic findings
  1. Findings may be nonspecific.
  2. Usually, no neuromusculoskeletal disease is apparent.
  3. Laboratory tests and radiography may be used to rule out organic disease that may be related to the somatic dysfunction.

BIOMECHANICS

Nomenclature of Spinal Motion

When performing a spinal structural examination to evaluate for the presence of spinal somatic dysfunction, the practitioner must be thoroughly familiar with the biomechanical principles governing spinal motion. Although recent research indicates that spinal motion may not always strictly adhere to these principles, they still provide the practitioner with an efficient means of describing physiologic and dysfunctional motions that occur in the spine.

Standard Terminology

Before proceeding to discussion of principles of spinal motion and spinal somatic dysfunction, it is helpful to review the standard terminology for intervertebral motion.
- The *anatomic position* is the reference position for naming and describing motion or position. It is the position of a person who is person standing, arms at the sides, palms of the hands facing anteriorly, and toes pointing forward.
- Motion is described as occurring around the axes of the body and within or along the planes of the body (Fig. 2.8).
- The anterior surface of the vertebral body is the point of reference for describing vertebral motion.
- The primary spinal motions are flexion, extension, rotation, and sidebending.
- Neutral is described as the range of motion, large or small, within the sagittal plane that occurs between the extremes of hyperflexion and hyperextension.

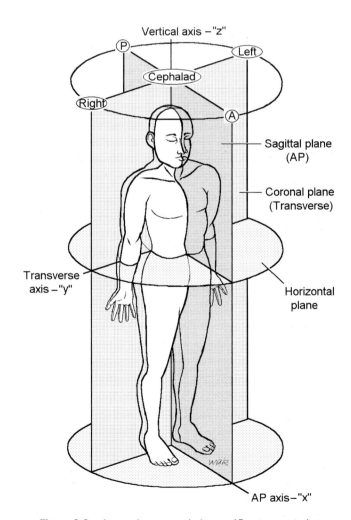

Figure 2.8 Anatomic axes and planes. AP, anteroposterior.

- Other motions, such as translation, distraction, or compression, can also occur in the spinal area. However, the movements of flexion, extension, rotation and sidebending are the ones that will be of primary focus in the ensuing discussion.
- These principal spinal motions are applied during segmental examination and form the basis for formulating a diagnosis and manual treatment, especially when using articulatory and muscle energy procedures.

Principal Motions

- *Flexion* is forward or anterior bending of the superior segment of a vertebral on the one below it or that of a group of vertebrae in a region of the spine in the sagittal plane around a transverse axis (Fig. 2.9).
- *Extension* is backward or posterior bending of the superior segment of a vertebral unit on the one below it or that of a group of vertebrae in a region of the spine in the sagittal plane around a transverse axis (Fig. 2.10).
- *Rotation* is turning of the superior segment of a vertebral unit in relation its inferior segment or that of a group of vertebrae

in a region of the spine around a vertical axis. Rotation describes motion in the transverse (horizontal) plane of a midline located on the anterior surface of a vertebra. Notice that a right-rotated vertebra's spinous process is to the left of midline (Fig. 2.11).

- *Sidebending* (i.e., lateral flexion) is motion occurring in a coronal plane around an anteroposterior axis or an axis described by the intersection of the transverse and sagittal planes. Sidebending of the superior vertebra in a unit in relation to the one below is described as left or right sidebending depending on which direction the moving segment bends in the coronal plane (Fig. 2.12).

Describing Vertebral Position, Motion, and Motion Restriction

- When a position of a vertebra is described, the suffix *-ed* is used (i.e., flexed, extended, rotated, or sidebent).
- When motion restriction is found, the direction toward which motion is restricted is described using the suffix *-ion* (i.e., flexion or extension). A vertebra can be flexed and resist extension,

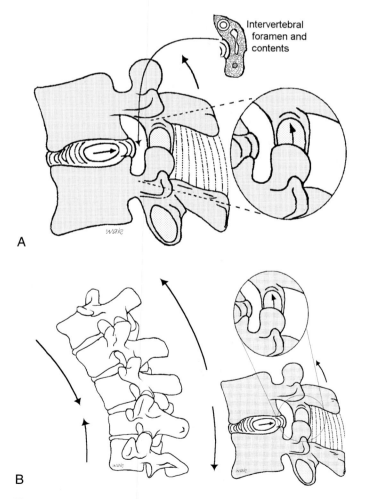

Figure 2.9   A, Flexion of a vertebral unit. Notice that the zygapophyseal joints, also called *intervertebral facets,* open in flexion. **B,** Flexion of a spinal region compared with flexion of a vertebral unit.

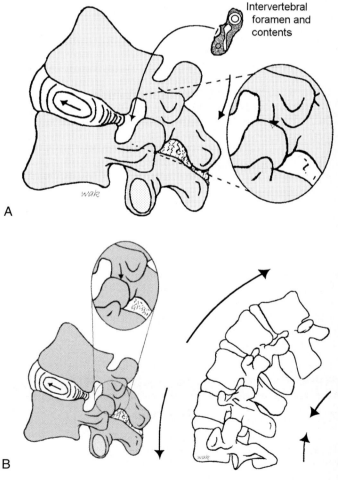

Figure 2.10   A, Extension of a vertebral unit. Notice that the facets close in extension. **B,** Extension of a spinal region compared with extension of a vertebral unit.

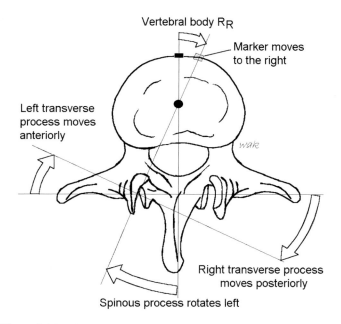

Figure 2.11   Vertebral rotation. Notice that the anterior vertebral body is the reference point for naming the direction of rotation.

be extended and resist flexion, rotated right and resist rotation left, or sidebent right and resist sidebending left.

- The structural foundation of the vertebral unit consists of two vertebrae and their intervertebral disc (Fig. 2.13). Soft tissue components include the associated arthrodial, ligamentous, muscular, vascular, lymphatic, and neural elements.

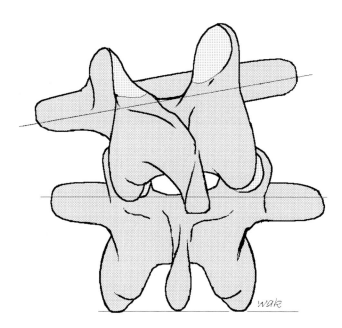

Figure 2.12   Vertebral sidebending. Notice that the facet closes on the side to which the superior vertebra bends and opens on the opposite side.

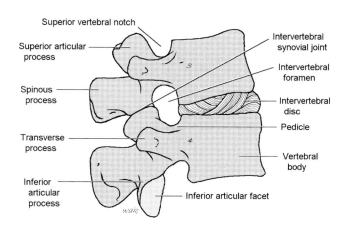

Figure 2.13   A vertebral unit consisted of two vertebrae and their intervertebral disc.

- Vertebral facet motion is described as occurring between the inferior articular facets of the superior vertebra as it moves on the superior articular facets of the inferior vertebra of the unit (Fig. 2.14).
- A flexed vertebra has its inferior articular facets in an open position (see Fig. 2.14B), and an extended vertebra has its inferior articular facets in a closed position (see Fig. 2.14C).

Facet Orientations

- Spinal motions are governed by the orientation of the zygapophyseal joints (i.e., intervertebral facets) and the intervertebral discs, costal cage, and muscular and ligamentous attachments.
- The superior articular facets in the cervical, thoracic, and lumbar spine vary (Fig. 2.15).
  1. Typical cervical (C2 to C7) facets face posteriorly and superiorly at a 45-degree angle;
  2. The thoracic facets face posteriorly and laterally in the vertical plane.
  3. The lumbar facets face medially at 45 degrees to the sagittal plane.

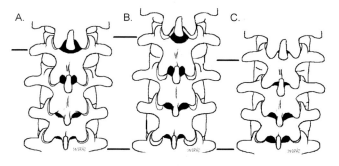

Figure 2.14   Flexed versus extended vertebral units. **A,** Vertebrae in the easy normal or resting position have slightly open facets. **B,** Flexed vertebrae have open facets. **C,** Extended vertebrae have closed facets.

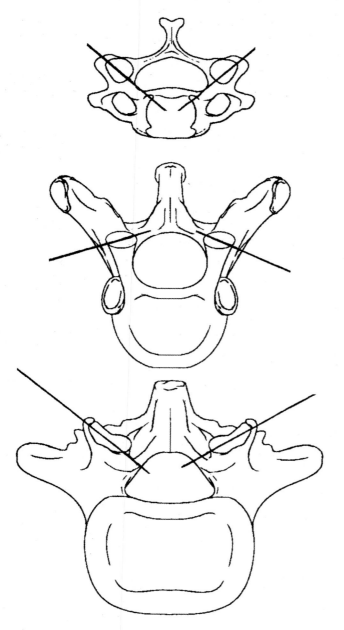

Figure 2.15 Facet orientation: a typical cervical vertebra (top), a thoracic vertebra (middle), and a lumbar vertebra (bottom). The facet orientation differs in each spinal region and is the determining factor in vertebral motion mechanics.

- Asymmetry of facet orientation (i.e., facet trophism) may play a significant role in the production of faulty postural mechanics during activities of daily living and at work and may facilitate the creation and persistence of mechanical back and neck pain[11] (Fig. 2.16).
- In evaluating asymmetry of vertebral structure and motion, the practitioner should keep in mind that not all people are constructed symmetrically and that morphologic asymmetries are not expected to become symmetric through manual medicine procedures.

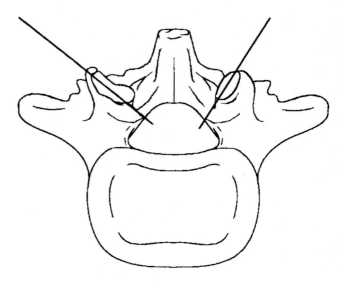

Figure 2.16 Facet trophism. Facets can be asymmetric and create altered motion mechanics and persistent or recurrent somatic dysfunctions.

Principles of Spinal Motion

- Each vertebral unit can move singly or as a group into flexion, extension, rotation, and sidebending.
- Rotation and sidebending are coupled motions that occur simultaneously as a result of the unique vertebral unit anatomic structure and the ligaments and muscles attached to it and acting on it.
- The position of a vertebral unit at rest can be described as neutral (N), flexed (F), or extended (E) and as rotated (R) and sidebent (S) to the right or left.
- In the neutral position, the facet joints are neither fully open nor fully closed.
- When the spine is in the fully flexed position, the facets are fully open.
- When they are in the fully extended position, the facets are closed and in apposition.
- In the closed position, the surface of the facets of each single vertebra must follow the contour of the surface of the facet to which it is articulating. This exerts a guiding influence on the coupled motions of sidebending and rotation.
- Three basic principles of spinal motion are helpful in guiding the practitioner to a diagnosis and treatment plan when signs of spinal somatic dysfunction are found (Table 2.3).
  1. The first two of the three principles help to understand and describe how F/E, R, and S movements combine to produce primary thoracic and lumbar spinal motions.
  2. Originally proposed by Harrison H. Fryette, DO, and C.R. Nelson, DO, in 1948, the osteopathic profession has adopted them as key principles in standardizing the terminology used to describe spinal motion and naming spinal somatic dysfunction.[1]
- The cervical spine and the sacrum have special motion characteristics, which are delineated later in this chapter.

Table 2.3 Principles of spinal motion

Principle	Description and Characteristics
I	When the thoracic or lumbar spine is in neutral position (easy, normal), the coupled motions of sidebending and rotation for a group of vertebrae are such that sidebending and rotation occur in opposite directions, with rotation toward the convexity.
II	When the thoracic or lumbar spin is bent sufficiently forward or backward (non-neutral), the coupled motions of sidebending and rotation in a single vertebral unit occur in the same direction.
III	Initiating motion of a vertebral segment in any plane of motion modifies the movement of that segment in other planes of motion.

Principle I

When the thoracic or lumbar spine is in neutral position (easy normal), the coupled motions of sidebending and rotation for a group of vertebrae are such that sidebending and rotation occur in opposite directions, with rotation occurring toward the convexity of the curvature (Fig. 2.17).

- For the thoracic and lumbar spine in the neutral position, sidebending creates a concave curve to the side of the sidebending and a convex curve to the opposite side. For example, sidebending to the right creates a concave curve of the spine to the right and a convex curve to the left.

- It may be stated that in the neutral position, the response of the thoracic or lumbar spine to sidebending will be a rotation of the vertebral bodies *toward the convexity* of the sidebending curvature.
- More commonly used is this expression: In neutral thoracic and lumbar spinal mechanics, sidebending and rotation are coupled to opposite sides.
- This specific motion complex is referred to as *type I motion mechanics*, and it occurs in a group of successive vertebral units, not in only a single vertebral unit.
- A somatic dysfunction that displays these motion mechanics is called a *type I dysfunction* (see "Somatic Dysfunction").

Principle II

When the thoracic or lumbar spine is sufficiently forward or backward bent (non-neutral), the coupled motions of sidebending and rotation in a single vertebral unit occur in the same direction (Fig. 2.18).

- The second principle applies to a single vertebral unit (i.e., one vertebral unit).
- When simultaneous rotation and sidebending are introduced during spinal hyperflexion or hyperextension, localization or isolation of forces can occur at a single vertebral unit (i.e., one vertebra moving on the one below it).
- For the thoracic and lumbar spine in the hyperflexed or hyperextended position, sidebending of a single vertebral unit in one direction results in rotation of the body of the superior vertebra in the same direction as the intended sidebending (i.e. rotation and sidebending occur to the same side).
- In the hyperextended position, the facet surfaces are together, and for the superior vertebra to sidebend on the inferior one, the superior vertebra's facet surfaces must follow the contour

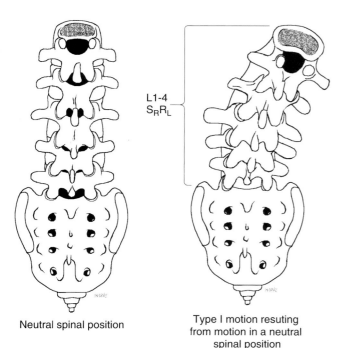

Neutral spinal position

L1-4
$S_R R_L$

Type I motion resuting from motion in a neutral spinal position

Figure 2.17 Principle I spinal motion. In neutral position, the spine rotates and sidebends to opposite directions.

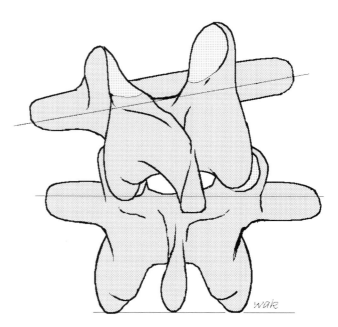

Figure 2.18 Principle II spinal motion. In flexion or extension, rotation and sidebending occur to the same side.

of the inferior vertebra's opposing articular facet, producing rotation and then sidebending.

- This motion complex is referred to as *type II motion mechanics*.
- A somatic dysfunction that displays these motion mechanics is called a *type II dysfunction* (see "Somatic Dysfunction").

Principle III

The third principle explains effects on multiplanar motion of a spinal region when motion is first introduced into one of the planes. This principle is helpful for localizing forces at a particular vertebral segment and maintaining patient balance during the manipulative procedure. The third principles states that initiating motion of a vertebral segment in any plane of motion will modify the movement of that segment in other planes of motion.

- When motion of a vertebral joint in any spinal region is introduced in one plane, the amount of available motion in other planes is inhibited or decreased. For example, during flexion from a neutral position, the segments that are flexed automatically have a decreased amount of sidebending and rotation (Fig. 2.19).
- A cervical vertebra has a certain amount of rotation when the cervical spine is in the neutral (N, upright) position (see Fig. 2.19B1). The amount of rotation permitted when the cervical spine is in the flexed (i.e., chin to chest position) or extended position is limited (see Fig.2.19B2 and B3).
- This principle is important when performing motion tests or manipulative treatment techniques.
  1. For example, if the practitioner is testing for motion or performing a manipulative procedure with the patient in the neutral position but consciously or unconsciously introduces flexion into the spine before introducing rotation or sidebending, there will be an automatic reduction in the range of rotation and sidebending compared with that

which would have been present if flexion had not been initially introduced.
  2. This third principle also facilitates localizing and reduces the amount of force necessary to treat a single dysfunctional joint. It is also used to maintain the patient's balance and comfort while on the treatment table.

Somatic Dysfunction

Somatic dysfunction is suspected in a spinal region by paraspinal soft tissue changes, asymmetric vertebral landmarks, altered range and quality of vertebral motion, tenderness on palpation, and altered skin temperature and moisture.

- Abnormal motion mechanics in the spine is diagnosed most commonly when the practitioner finds restriction to the normal motions in the cardinal planes (i.e., flexion, extension, rotation, and sidebending).
- In general, a dysfunction is said to exist when the spine is placed in the neutral position, and a spinal segment or group of segments is found to not be in neutral.
- The position of the dysfunctional segment and its motion restrictions are defined by the results of segmental active or passive motion tests.
- Vertebral segmental somatic dysfunction is described as flexed or extended, rotated, and sidebent in one direction or the other (i.e., F/E, $R_{R \text{ or } L}$ and $S_{R \text{ or } L}$, in which F stands for flexed, E stands for extended, subscripted R stands for right, and subscripted L stands for left).
- Because the movements of the spine generally adhere to physiologic principles I and II, dysfunctions of spinal motion are referred to as *type I dysfunctions* and *type II dysfunctions*.

Spinal segmental motion somatic dysfunction refers to motion restriction that occurs within a joint's normal range of motion and that is not caused by an irreversible pathologic condition. These types of motion restriction may be removed with manipulative treatment of the joint directly or indirectly by treatment of its soft tissues.

There are two basic types of spinal somatic dysfunction based on the first two principles of spinal motion. They are delineated as type I and type II dysfunctions (Table 2.4).

Type I Dysfunction

- In type I dysfunction, there is restricted motion in a group of vertebrae.
- This motion is characteristic of a group of three or more vertebra and is maintained by the hypertonicity of long, multisegmental, sidebending muscles located on the side of the concavity and by hypotonicity of the sidebending muscles on the side of the convexity (Fig. 2.20).
- Sidebending is considered to be the primary motion restriction, with rotation a secondary or adaptive component of the type I dysfunction.
- This type of dysfunction produces a group curve that is convex to one side and concave to the other side.
- The curve is diagnosed by observing the asymmetry of the paraspinal soft tissues and transverse processes that are rotated posteriorly in a group during neutral mechanics.

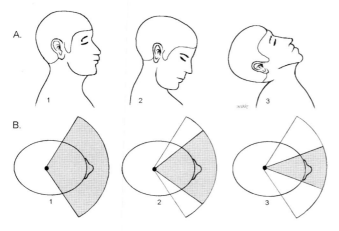

Figure 2.19   Principle III spinal motion. Motion in one plane limits the motion available in other planes. **A,** Cervical spine motion in the sagittal plane around a transverse axis: neutral (1), flexed (2), and extended (3). **B,** The range of cervical spine rotation in the horizontal plane around a vertical axis that is available when the neck is neutral (1), flexed (2), and extended (3). Notice how there is decreased range of cervical rotation available when the neck is flexed or extended compared with when it is in the neutral position.

Table 2.4   Basic types of vertebral somatic dysfunctions

Feature	Type I	Type II
Number of involved vertebrae	3 or more	2
Hypertonicity maintained by	Long sidebending muscles that traverse several vertebral segments on the side of the concavity	Intersegmental paraspinal muscles (i.e., rotatores, multifidi, intertransversarii)
Coupling of rotation and sidebending	All are rotated in the same direction. They do not become symmetric in flexed or extended positions.	Asymmetric transverse processes in the coronal plane become symmetric in flexed or extended positions.
Nomenclature	Ease is in the neutral (N) position, with S(x) and R(y) (i.e., S and R are to opposite sides). Motion is resisted in flexion and extension, with S(y) and R(x).	Ease is in the flexed (F) or extended (E) position, with R(x) and S(x), in which x is the side to which the vertebra is rotated and sidebent (i.e., it is sidebent and rotated to the same side).
Facets	They are partially open, not able to fully open or close on either side.	In flexed somatic dysfunctions, one facet is open and cannot close during extension. In extended somatic dysfunctions, one facet is closed and cannot open during flexion.

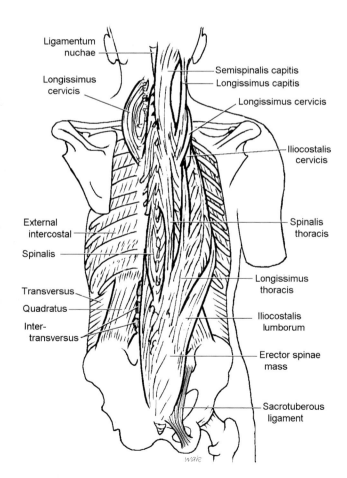

Figure 2.20   Multisegmental spinal muscles. Their unilateral hypertonicity or hypotonicity creates and maintains group (type I) somatic dysfunctions.

- The transverse processes of this dysfunctional group of vertebrae do not become symmetric in flexed or extended positions (i.e., they maintain their dysfunctional orientation throughout the range of sagittal plane motion about a transverse axis).
- The apex of the group curve is identified by finding the most rotated segment or the most posterior fullness of paraspinal soft tissues overlying the transverse process that is most rotated into the convexity.
- A spinal somatic dysfunction that is type I is therefore in stuck, or at ease, in the neutral position, described by the letter N, with S(x) and R(y) (i.e., S and R are to opposite sides). It resists motion in flexion and extension, S(y) and R(x).

Type II Dysfunction
- A type II dysfunction occurs when a vertebral unit loses the ability to open or close on one side.
- This is typically a result of hypertonic intersegmental paraspinal muscles, such as the multifidi, rotatores, or intertransversarii, on one side and hypotonic intersegmental muscles on the contralateral side (Fig. 2.21).
- In the situation in which a facet cannot fully close on one side, that particular spinal segment cannot function properly in extension.
  1. When that segment is extended, the facet that cannot close, causing that segment to move asymmetrically into extension.
  2. Because the facet on the contralateral side can close, the vertebra is tilted or sidebent and rotated to that side.
- A spinal dysfunction that is type II is therefore described as F or E, R(x) S(x), in which x is the side to which the vertebra is rotated and sidebent. It is sidebent and rotated to the same side.
- The transverse process on the side of the facet that can close is more posterior than the one on the contralateral side.
- The posterior transverse process is a vertebral landmark used to determine to which direction a vertebra is rotated. Figure 2.22 contrasts type II and type I somatic dysfunctions.
  1. For example, L3 FR left S left means that the third lumbar vertebra is flexed, rotated left, and sidebent left (FR_LS_L) (see Fig. 2.22B).

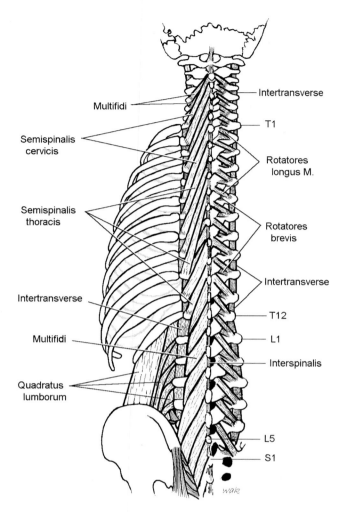

Multifidi

Semispinalis cervicis

Semispinalis thoracis

Intertransverse

Multifidi

Quadratus lumborum

Intertransverse

T1

Rotatores longus M.

Rotatores brevis

Intertransverse

T12

L1

Interspinalis

L5

S1

Figure 2.21 Intersegmental spinal muscles. Their hypertonicity or hypotonicity creates and maintains segmental (type II) somatic dysfunctions. With permission from Gray's Anatomy 35th British Edition, Saunders Co., Philadelphia, 1973:510.

2. In this example, the right inferior facet of L3 cannot close when the vertebra is extended on the right superior articular facet of L4.

3. The left inferior facet of L3 can close on the left superior articular facet of L4. When L3 is extended, only its left inferior facet can approximate to its counterpart, and L3 rotates to the left and tilts or sidebends to the left.

4. The L3 left transverse process is more posterior than the right one.

• If one facet cannot open properly, motion restriction becomes evident when the spine is hyperflexed (see Fig. 2.22C).

1. As a result, there is sidebending and rotation of the vertebral segment toward the side of the closed facet.

2. If the dysfunctional facet is the left inferior articular one, the somatic dysfunction would be named ER_LS_L (Fig. 2.23, see Fig. 2.22C).

Cervical Spine Mechanics

The spinal motion of the cervical region differs somewhat from that of the remainder of the spine.

The Occipitoatlantal Joint

• The primary motions of the occipitoatlantal (OA) joint is flexion and extension, which constitute a nodding-type motion and which are also referred to as *nutation* and *counternutation*, respectively (Fig. 2.24).

• The OA joint has minimal but clinically significant sidebending and rotation motion available. Normal range of motion in each direction is approximately 5 degrees.

• Because of its unique concave-convex and anteriorly convergent facets, OA joint sidebending is coupled with rotation in opposite directions. If the head (i.e., occiput) sidebends to the left on the atlas, it will simultaneously rotate to the right, and vice versa.

• Sidebending and rotation occur in opposite directions whether the OA is in flexion, extension, or neutral.

• Dysfunctions of the OA joint are flexed or extended somatic dysfunctions with rotation and sidebending coupled to opposite sides, such as F or E R(x) S(y).

The Atlantoaxial Joint

• The atlantoaxial (AA) joint has motion that is almost purely rotational in character, and functionally, the predominant motion considered is rotation. The dens and its attachments permit more rotation than is possible for any other cervical joints (45% to more than 50% of the total of 90 degrees of normal head rotation to each side).

• Rotation is the primary motion of the AA joint, which is also the primary rotating joint for the head.

• AA restriction to motion is in rotation left or right in the neutral position.

1. Flexion, extension, and sidebending occur only to a smaller, nonclinical degree.

2. There are no flexion, extension, or sidebending restrictions about which to be concerned.

Typical Cervical Joints

• The area from C2 to C7 does not have a physiologic neutral position. The normal curve of the cervical spine is called *lordotic*, which is concave posteriorly, and is the same as the lumbar spine. The position when the facets are not closely approximated (as when extended) nor maximally separated (as when flexed) can be considered as neutral.

• Because of the angulation of the facet structure and the joints of Luschka, rotation and sidebending occur in the same direction whether these typical spinal vertebral units are in flexion, extension, or neutral (Fig. 2.25). If C5 sidebends left on C6, it simultaneously rotates left.

• If there are limitations to motion in this region of the cervical spine, they are typically in flexion or extension, with sidebending and rotation coupled to the same side.

1. Motion with the cervical spine in the neutral position may be restricted in sidebending and rotation, but these motions are still coupled in the same direction.

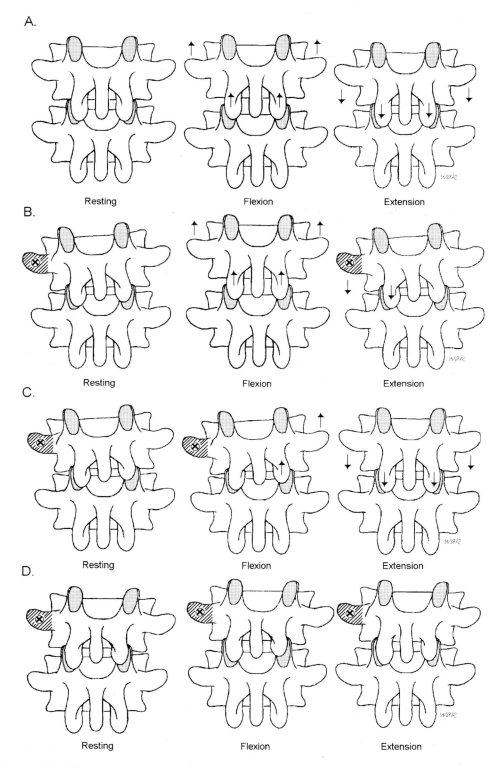

Figure 2.22   FRS, ERS, and NSR differentiation with posterior transverse process palpated on the left. **A,** normal. **B,** FR$_L$S$_L$. **C,** ER$_L$S$_L$. **D,** NS$_L$R$_R$.
E, extended; F, flexed; N, neutral; R, rotated; S, sidebent; subscripted L and R, left and right sides.

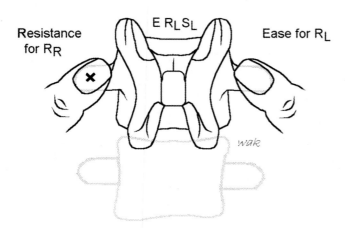

Resistance for R_R

ER_LS_L

Ease for R_L

Figure 2.23 ER_LS_L palpation of left posterior transverse process. E, extended; R, rotated; S, sidebent; subscripted L and R, left and right sides.

2. There is no opposite coupling of sidebending and rotation in the cervical spine between C2 and C7.
3. Type II dysfunction, but not type I dysfunction, can exist in the cervical spine between C2 and C7.

Costal Cage Mechanics

- During inhalation, the anterior aspects of the upper ribs (i.e., ribs 1 to 6) move more anteriorly and superiorly along with the sternum.
  1. This movement increases the anteroposterior diameter of the thorax (Fig. 2.26).

  2. The motion of the upper ribs is commonly described as pump-handle motion, with the rib shaft considered to be the handle of an old-fashioned pump and costovertebral and costotransverse articulations considered to be the pivot.
- During inhalation, the lower ribs (i.e., ribs 7 to 10) move in what is referred to as bucket-handle motion (Fig. 2.27).
  1. This motion of the lower ribs results in the lateral aspects of the rib shafts moving superiorly, increasing the transverse diameter of the thorax.
  2. The rib shaft is considered to be the handle of the bucket and the vertebral column and costochondral or costosternal junctions constitute the pivot points.

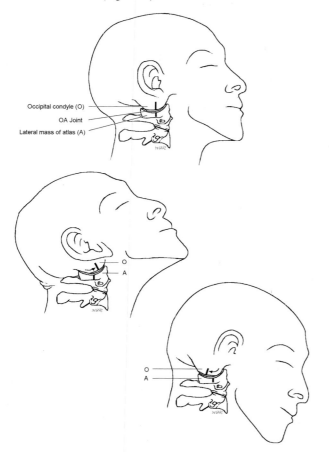

Occipital condyle (O)
OA Joint
Lateral mass of atlas (A)

Figure 2.24 Occipitoatlantal (OA) motion is primarily a nodding type of flexion and extension, also called *nutation* and *counternutation*.

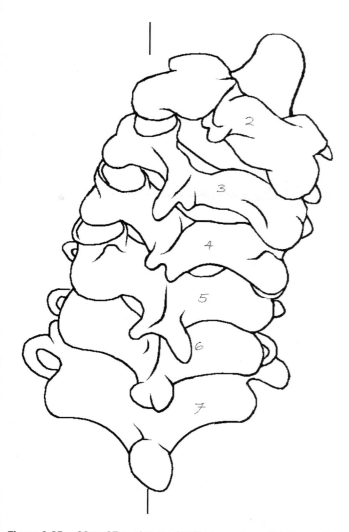

Figure 2.25 C2 to C7 motion mechanics are unique. Rotation and sidebending are to the same side in neutral, flexion, and extension. There are no type I group somatic dysfunctions between C2 and C7.

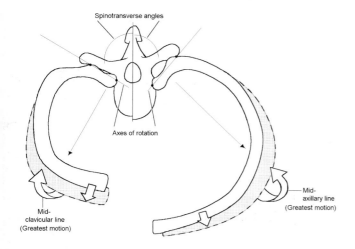

Figure 2.26 Rib motion. Notice the increased anterior motion of the upper ribs compared with the increased lateral motion in the lower ribs.

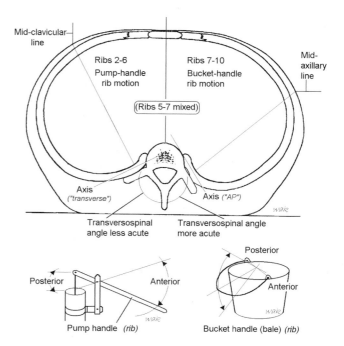

Figure 2.27 Rib motion. Pump-handle–type motion predominates in the upper ribs; bucket-bail–type motion predominates in the lower ribs.

- Ribs 11 and 12 do not attach to the sternum or the chondral mass. These two atypical ribs are described as having a pincer-type movement, commonly referred to as *caliper motion* (Fig. 2.28).

Pelvic Mechanics

Innominates

The movements available to the innominate bones (also referred to as iliosacral motion because the innominate is often considered as part of the lower extremity) may be classified as physiologic and nonphysiologic. Somatic dysfunction can be related to each.

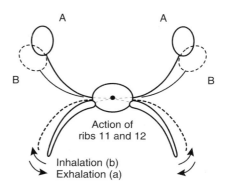

Figure 2.28 Rib motions of the 11th and 12th ribs are like calipers or pincers, with predominately posterior motion in the horizontal plane around a vertical axis.

- Physiologic innominate somatic dysfunction
  1. The physiologic movement of the innominate bone is anterior or posterior rotation about an inferior transverse axis that runs through the inferior arm of the innominate facet as it articulates with the sacrum.
  2. This rotation is considered to be a somatic dysfunction when the motion is restricted (i.e., unable to move further in a certain direction) in its anterior or posterior range of movement but can move in its opposite direction.
- Anterior and posterior innominate rotations
  1. With anterior rotation of the innominate, the innominate moves more easily into anterior rotation, and it is restricted in its ability to rotate posteriorly (Fig. 2.29A).
  2. With posterior rotation of the innominate, the innominate moves more easily into posterior rotation, and it is restricted in its ability to rotate anteriorly (see Fig 2.29B).
- Nonphysiologic innominate somatic dysfunctions
  1. Nonphysiologic movements create somatic dysfunctions because they are shears or twists of the innominates that do not allow normal physiologic rotation to occur. They are,

however, correctable by manual treatments, including the following:
Superior and inferior innominate shears
Inflare and outflare somatic dysfunctions
Pubic symphyseal dysfunctions
  2. Nonphysiologic motions of the innominate occur in the presence of unusual sacroiliac joint surfaces, with laxity of sacroiliac ligaments, or after trauma.
  3. The absence of the usual bevel change that occurs in a sacroiliac joint at about the level of S2 creates an unusual facet that can more easily allow a superior or inferior shear.
  4. Inflare and outflare dysfunctions are more likely to occur when the sacral articular surface is convex and the innominate articular surface is concave, allowing the medial or lateral movement characteristic of this dysfunction.
- A *superior innominate shear* occurs when the innominate slides superiorly on the sacrum and is restricted in gliding inferiorly (Fig. 2.30).
- An *inferior innominate shear* involves sliding of the innominate in an inferior direction on the sacrum and restriction of the innominate in gliding superiorly (Fig. 2.31).

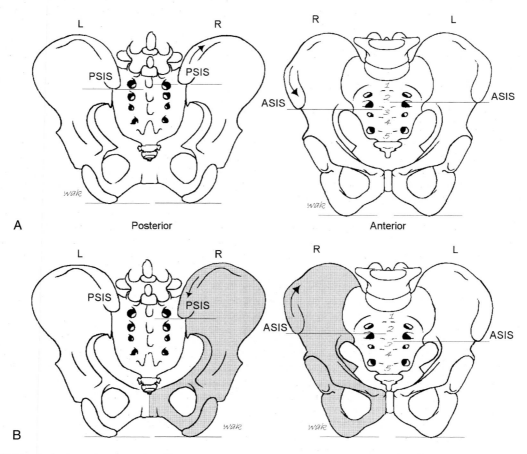

Figure 2.29 **A,** Right anterior innominate rotation. The right posterior superior iliac spine (PSIS) is superior, and the right anterior superior iliac spine (ASIS) is inferior compared with those on the contralateral side. **B,** Right posterior innominate rotation. The right PSIS is inferior, and the right ASIS is superior compared with those on the contralateral side.

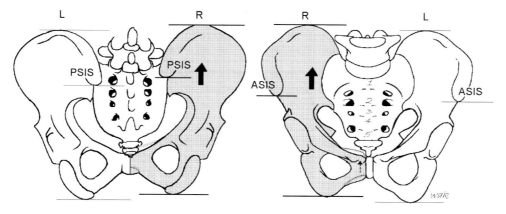

Figure 2.30   Right superior innominate shear. The right posterior superior iliac spine (PSIS) and right anterior superior iliac spine (ASIS) anatomic landmarks are superior to those on the contralateral side.

- *An inflare somatic dysfunction* of the innominate occurs when the innominate glides medially over the facet of the sacrum and subsequently becomes restricted in this position (Fig. 2.32).
- The *outflare dysfunction* involves a lateral glide of the innominate over the facet of the sacrum at the sacroiliac joint (Fig. 2.33).

Pubic Symphysis
- Non-physiologic motions of the pubic symphysis can occur.
- These involve shearing of the symphysis pubis in a vertical direction, so that the symphysis on one side of the pelvis is more superior or more inferior than its counterpart, and is maintained in its respective position (Fig. 2.34).
- The dysfunction is described as a *superior or inferior pubic symphysis shear*, depending on the specific motion restriction being noted.
- *Anterior or posterior shears* are also possible, but these occur rarely, and when seen, they are usually the result of severe trauma.

Sacrum
- Movements of the sacrum are described in relation to L5 superiorly or the innominates bilaterally.

- The sacroiliac joint is a passive joint, with no muscles acting on it to directly move it.
- Motions about this joint occur because of the resultant forces on the sacrum and each innominate, the restrictive ligaments, and myofascial attachments.

Sacral Axes of Motion
Several functional axes of the sacrum have been described to help explain the palpatory and motion testing results found in sacral somatic dysfunctions.
- The *superior sacral axis* is the hypothetical transverse axis about which the sacrum rocks, moving the sacral base anteriorly and posteriorly during the respiratory cycle. It passes transversely through the articular processes posterior to the attachment of the dura at the level of the second sacral segment (S2) (Fig. 2.35).
- The *middle transverse axis* is the hypothetical functional axis of the sacrum for flexion and extension in the standing position. It passes transversely through the anterior aspect of the sacrum at the level of the second sacral segment (S2) (Fig. 2.36).

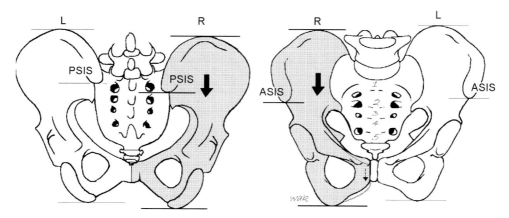

Figure 2.31   Right inferior innominate shear. The right posterior superior iliac spine (PSIS) and right anterior superior iliac spine (ASIS) anatomic landmarks are inferior to those on the contralateral side.

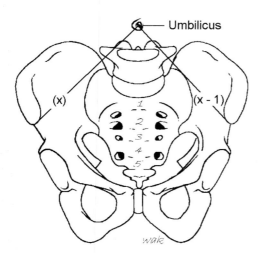

Figure 2.32   Left inflare innominate dysfunction. The left anterior superior iliac spine (ASIS) is closer to the umbilicus than the ASIS on the contralateral side.

- The *inferior transverse axis* is a hypothetical axis that passes transversely on a line through the inferior auricular surface of the sacrum and represents the axis for movement of the innominates on the sacrum (Fig. 2.37).
- *Left and right oblique axes*
  1. Each of the two oblique axes runs between the superior pole of the sacroiliac joint on one side and diagonally across the sacrum to the inferior pole of the sacroiliac joint on the contralateral side.
  2. The direction of the axis is named by the side of its superior pole.
  3. The *left oblique axis* is a hypothetical axis from the left superior sacroiliac articulation to the right inferior sacroiliac articulation (Fig. 2.38).
  4. The *right oblique axis* is a hypothetical axis from the right superior sacroiliac articulation to the left inferior sacroiliac articulation (Fig. 2.39).

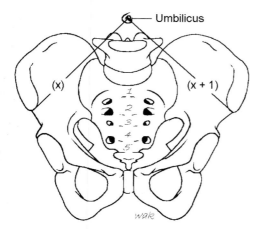

Figure 2.33   Outflare innominate dysfunction. The left anterior superior iliac spine (ASIS) is farther from the umbilicus than the ASIS on the contralateral side.

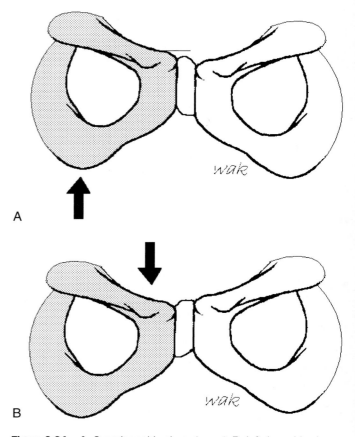

Figure 2.34   **A,** Superior pubic shear *(arrow).* **B,** Inferior pubic shear *(arrow).*

Sacral Motions

Sacral motions consist of flexion (i.e., nutation), extension (i.e., counternutation), rotation, and sidebending.

- Sacral flexion and extension
  1. Motion in the sagittal plane about a transverse axis is commonly referred to as flexion or extension (i.e., nutation or counternutation, respectively).
  2. Flexion and extension nomenclature is used by many manual practitioners to designate voluntary sacral motion; however, those who practice "osteopathy in the cranial field" or its derivatives based on the primary respiratory mechanism and cranial-sacral relationships use *flexion* and *extension* to designate nonvoluntary sacral motions; *nutation* and *counternutation* also are used inversely. To avoid confusion, this textbook uses the two sets of terms together with the understanding that the main idea is sacral base motion around a transverse axis.
  3. Flexion or nutation involves a nodding motion of the sacrum in which the sacral base moves anteriorly and slightly inferiorly and the sacral apex moves posteriorly and superiorly about a transverse axis (Fig. 2.40).
  4. Extension or counternutation involves the opposite motion, with the sacral base moving posteriorly and superiorly and the apex moving anteriorly and inferiorly (Fig. 2.41).

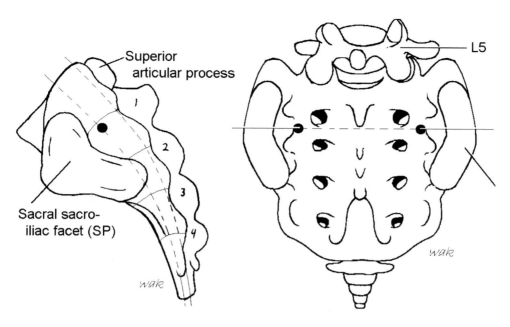

Figure 2.35   Superior sacral axis.

5. The axis around which these motions occur has been the subject of much investigation, and is thought to be at the junction of the upper and lower limbs of the sacroiliac joint at the level of S2.
6. The sacral base flexes when the lumbar spine flexes and extends when the lumbar spine extends.
7. If L5 is hyperflexed, the sacral base accommodates this situation and moves into an extended or counternutated position. When L5 is hyperextended, the sacral base flexes or nutates (Fig. 2.42).
8. The transverse axis is hypothesized to shift from the middle to the superior transverse axis in this instance.[12]

• Sacral rotation and sidebending
1. Because of the limitations placed on the sacrum by its position between the innominate bones, the sacrum is not able to completely rotate around a vertical axis or to

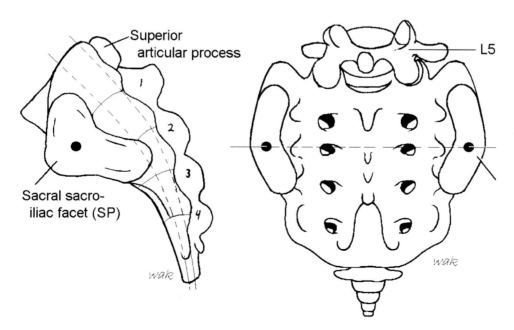

Figure 2.36   Middle sacral axis.

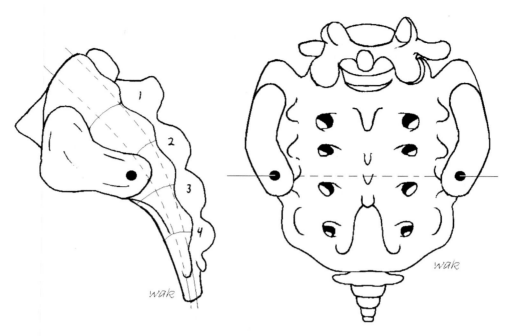

Figure 2.37   Inferior sacral axis.

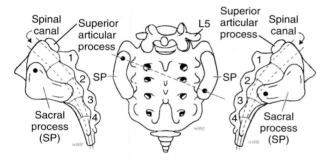

Spinal canal

Superior articular process

Superior articular process

Spinal canal

L5

SP

SP

Sacral process (SP)

Sacral process (SP)

Figure 2.38   Left oblique axis.

sidebend completely about an anteroposterior axis. However, the sacrum moves into positions as if moving about an oblique axis—a combined motion of the antero-posterior and transverse axes.

2. The sacral motions related to the oblique axis are described as occurring between L5 and the sacral base.

3. The primary motion is thought to be rotation, with sidebending coupled to the opposite direction, and it occurs in response to and affects L5 and lumbar motion mechanics.

4. With the lumbosacral spine in the neutral range, the sacrum normally rotates left around a left oblique axis or right around a right oblique axis. These are forward (anterior)

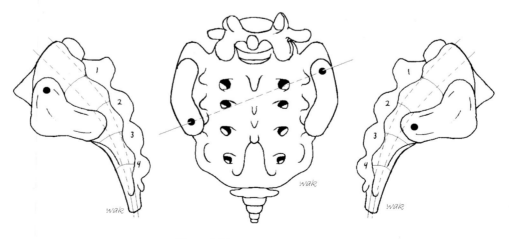

Figure 2.39   Right oblique axis.

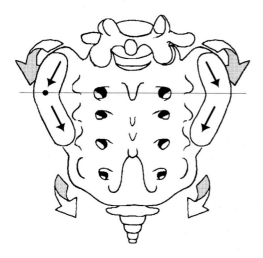

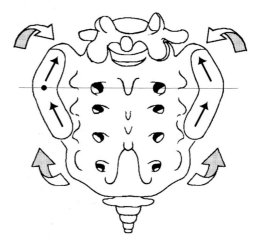

Figure 2.40 Sacral nutation.

Figure 2.41 Sacral counternutation.

motions of one side of the sacrum with coupled sidebending to the opposite side.

If the lumbar spine is in a neutral upright stance posture, and L5 is NS_RR_L, the sacrum will rotate to the right on a right oblique axis and sidebend left. (When the sacrum rotates to the right, the left sacral base moves forward or anteriorly.)

If L5 in NS_LR_R, the sacrum will rotate left on a left oblique axis and sidebend right.

- Forward and backward sacral torsions
  1. In the normal walking cycle, the sacrum appears to move in the following fashion:
     Left torsion on the left oblique axis (left rotation and right sidebending)

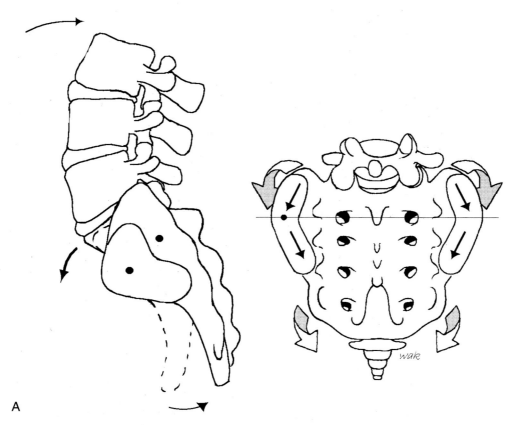

Figure 2.42 **A,** Sacral nutation induced by lumbar hyperextension.

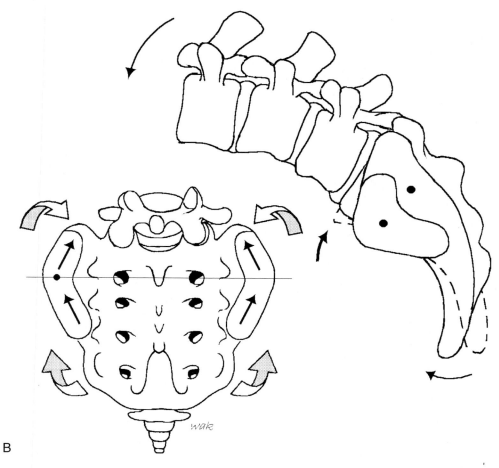

Figure 2.42, cont'd   B, Sacral counternutation induced by lumbar hyperflexion.

Return to neutral
Right torsion on the right oblique axis (right rotation and
left sidebending)
Return to neutral

2. With the normal walking cycle, the left and right torsional movements are anterior only. The sacrum moves anteriorly on one side, back to neutral, then anterior on the other side, and back to neutral. There is no rotation of the sacrum posteriorly past neutral in the normal walking cycle.

3. During the normal walking cycle, as the sacrum sidebends right and rotates left, L5 rotates right and sidebends left (there is a torsion between the L5 rotation and the sacral rotation). The opposite movements occurs on the right.

4. During structural evaluation, the sacrum is commonly found in a forward torsion position on one side or the other, but because this is a common pattern of the walking cycle, it is usually asymptomatic.

If the sacrum cannot resume its normal motions, a somatic dysfunction is created, and this is referred to as a *forward sacral torsion* (Fig. 2.43, upper portion).

With the lumbosacral region in neutral position but sidebent to the right, L5 is NS_RR_L, and the sacrum rotates to the

right about a right oblique axis and sidebends to the left (i.e., the anterior aspect of the left sacral base moves forward toward the right and tilts or sidebends to the left).

The torsion that occurs between the rotation of L5 and the rotation of the sacrum can be held by the various mechanical forces working on the sacrum, pelvis, and lumbar spine in this position.

• Posterior motion of the sacral base past the neutral resting position occurs when the lumbar spine is hyperflexed or when L5 exhibits type II mechanics.

1. The sacrum again would counternutate if L5 hyperflexed, but when L5 rotates and sidebends at the same time, the sacrum must adapt and rotate as well. The sacrum rotates opposite L5 such that if L5 rotates and sidebends left while flexed, the sacrum extends on the right side as it rotated to the right about a left oblique axis and sidebends left to accommodate the left sidebending of L5.

2. If the sacrum was held in this position by the various fascial and ligamentous tension forces on it and could not return to its neutral position after that action was accomplished, these multiplanar movements become a somatic dysfunction of the sacrum, called a *backward sacral torsion* (see Fig. 2.43, lower part).

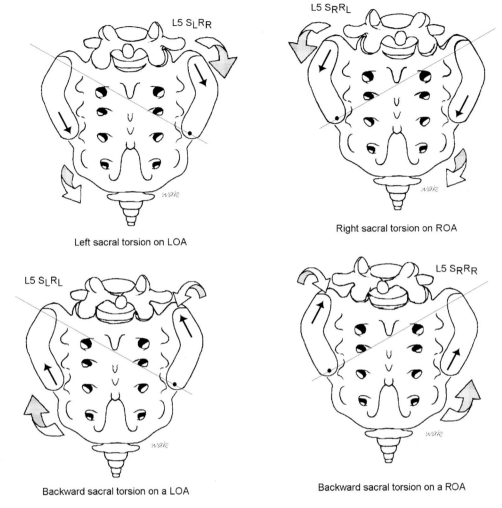

Figure 2.43 Contrasting sacral torsions. **Top,** Forward sacral torsions. **Bottom,** Backward sacral torsions. LOA, left oblique axis; ROA, right oblique axis.

3. This is typically a symptomatic (painful) condition, and it is found in most patients who seek manual treatment for low back pain.

4. Commonly, the patient cannot extend the lumbar spine and walks into the office bent slightly forward. Restoration of normal lumbosacral mechanics with manual treatment has led to the phrase "the old man walked in, and the young one walked out," meaning the patient could stand erect again after the treatment.

Motion Barrier Concept

- Identifying somatic dysfunction entails finding joints whose range or quality of motion is abnormal due to reversible functional factors.

- When a joint is observed to actively or passively move less or not as smoothly as expected, it is said to be *restricted*, meaning it is not being allowed to move normally for some reason.

- The concept of a barrier sense has helped communicate this feeling of restriction when palpating the resistance met during passive joint motion testing.

- The term *restrictive motion barrier* also has been applied to the feel of myofascial drag or resistance on soft tissue motion testing.

- The goal of manual treatments that are directed at improving joint or myofascial motion is to remove the restrictive barrier and enable restoration of normal quality and physiologic range and quality of motion.

- The *physiologic range of motion* is the range in which a normal, healthy joint can be actively moved; the *anatomic range* is the limits of passive motion beyond which there is loss of joint integrity, as when a ligament is severed. Static (i.e., joint structural changes) and dynamic (i.e., muscle tension) factors can be involved in restricting a joint's range of motion.

- In assessing joint motion, the normal physiologic barrier to motion is springy; it has *compliance* (Fig. 2.44).

- Each joint has its own physiologic range. If a joint's motion is restricted, the physiologic range is limited, and on passive

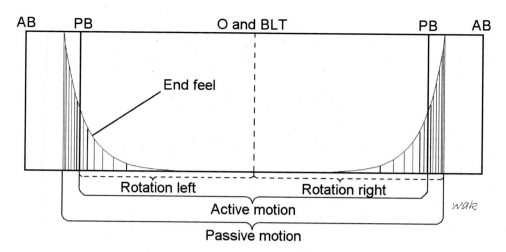

Figure 2.44 Normal motion barriers. The patient's active motion has a physiologic barrier. The practitioner can passively move a joint past the physiologic range, but resistance increases as the physiologic and anatomic barriers are approached. AB, anatomic barrier; BLT, balanced ligamentous tension; O, original tension level at rest; PB, physiologic barrier.

motion testing, there is a distinct barrier sense (i.e., end feel), a hard end-point sensation, which is felt sooner in the range of motion arc than would be expected with normal physiologic motion (Fig. 2.45).

1. The sensation feels as if the joint is being tethered or tied down and is unable to move freely within its range.
2. Typically, this is most notable in one direction more so than in the opposite direction, especially when unilateral hypertonic muscles are the cause, although bilateral motion restriction is also possible.

3. There is increasing resistance when approaching this barrier and decreasing resistance or compliance when moving the joint away from this barrier.

Physiologic Barrier
- The physiologic barrier (see Fig. 2.44) represents the functional limits within the anatomic range of motion.
- It is caused by the soft tissue tension accumulation, which limits the active motion of an articulation.
- Further motion toward the anatomic barrier can be induced passively.

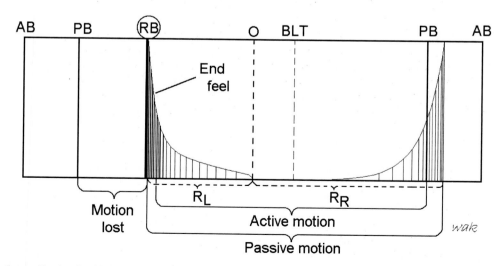

Figure 2.45 Restrictive motion barrier. Notice how tension increases as the restrictive barrier (RB) is approached. The practitioner can move the restricted joint past the restrictive barrier, although with increasing tension. The physiologic barrier (PB) can also be exceeded by passive motion. The point of balanced ligamentous tension (BLT), which is in the middle of a joint's range of motion, shifts to the new midline created by the unilateral restrictive barrier. AB, anatomic barrier; O, original tension level at rest; R_L, rotation to the left; R_R, rotation to the right.

Anatomic Barrier

- The anatomic barrier (see Fig. 2.44) represents the limits of motion imposed by the structure of the body.
- It is caused by the bony contours and soft tissue end points, especially ligamentous, that serve as the final limit to motion in an articulation. Beyond this barrier, tissue damage and joint disruption occurs.
- At the end point, the anatomic barrier has a hard, rigid feel.

Restrictive Barrier

- The restrictive barrier (see Fig. 2.45) represents an impediment or obstacle to movement within the physiologic limits of an articulation that reduces the active motion range.
- Restrictive elements include the skin, fascia, muscles, ligaments, joint capsule, and joint surfaces, and they can include arthritic changes, joint mice (i.e., osteocartilaginous bodies within joints), and other pathologic changes.
- The barrier may or may not be associated with somatic dysfunction.
  1. Somatic dysfunction refers to a reversible, functional disorder that is amenable to manual manipulation procedures. However, restricted motion can be caused by pathologic processes that are not readily reversible.
  2. Edema is sensed as a hard end feel, but it fades with persistent force because the fluid can be dispersed and suppressed by mechanical compressive and pumping actions during motion testing or manual treatments.
  3. Muscle spasm that is reactive, as in "guarding," is found in patients with fractures, herniations, subluxations, or infections. It has increased elasticity on applying stretch, but the spasm often returns, and the restrictive barrier remains. Muscle spasms react erratically to motion testing.
  4. Fibrosis has an abrupt, hard, sudden end feel without elasticity.

Ease and Bind

When there is somatic dysfunction, palpation with the finger pads lightly placed on the soft tissues around the affected joint can pick up a sense of binding or grabbing, because they resist even the slightest passive motion induced by the practitioner from another body region.

- If, for example, T4 has TART changes and the examining fingers monitor the soft paraspinal tissues while the practitioner's other hand passively induces head and neck sidebending in one direction, the tissues will bind or grab in resistance to this motion.
- When head or neck passive motion is induced in the opposite direction, the monitored paraspinal soft tissues around T4 can be felt to be at ease, compliant, and loose. This response of the soft tissues surrounding a dysfunctional joint likely results from facilitation or sensitization of the peripheral and central nervous structures involved with the dysfunction.
- The concept of ease and bind differs significantly from the barrier motion concept in that the range or quality of motion of a dysfunctional joint is not in question. Central nervous system integrative activity is being tested by monitoring the soft tissue response to a passive motion induced from a distant area.

- This concept also differs from myofascial assessment of restriction because the soft tissues being monitored are not being moved, stretched, or tested for range, quality, or restriction to direct contact passive motion.
- The dysfunctional spinal cord segment responds to motion demands by binding the paraspinal soft tissues or relaxing them.
- This reaction is immediate and felt just as the practitioner begins to passively move a peripheral joint (Fig. 2.46).

CONTROVERSIES

There are many concepts and theories about the pathophysiology of somatic dysfunction. There is no consensus about the complete mechanisms underlying the development, maintenance, resolution, and recurrence of the dysfunction, nor is there universal agreement about its existence, importance to health and well-being, necessity of treatment, or effectiveness of manual therapies to resolve it. This lack of consensus among professionals and academicians across the globe makes this an exciting area for research. The many unanswered questions regarding the biology of manual therapy spawned a national conference sponsored by the U.S. National Institutes of Health (NIH) and the Canadian Institutes of Health Research (CIHR).

RESEARCH OPPORTUNITIES

A Conference on the Biology of Manual Therapies was held on June 9-10, 2005, at the National Institutes of Health in Bethesda, Maryland. The conference covered the underlying biology of manual therapies. Experts from the NIH and CIHR joined academic, patient advocacy, and professional organizations to assess current knowledge and identify opportunities for further research.

Key questions were addressed during the sessions and breakout groups:

- What is the validity of the research suggesting manual therapies can impact the nervous system, immune system, or endocrine system?
- Within these scientific disciplines, what additional research would add most to our understanding of the biology of manual therapies?
- How do manual therapies impact the biomechanics of the body?
- What biomechanics underlie the therapies themselves?
- What additional research on biomechanics would add most to our understanding of the biology of manual therapies?
- What type of study designs would facilitate research on the underlying biology of manual therapies?
- What would be the key outcome measures?
- Are there objective measures that are able to capture changes in structure or function hypothesized to underlie these therapies?
- What state-of-the-art methods in neuroscience, immunology, endocrinology, biomechanics, and imaging can be applied to studies of the biology of manual therapies?
- What are the three to five most critical research questions (or needs) to help us understand the biology of manual therapies?

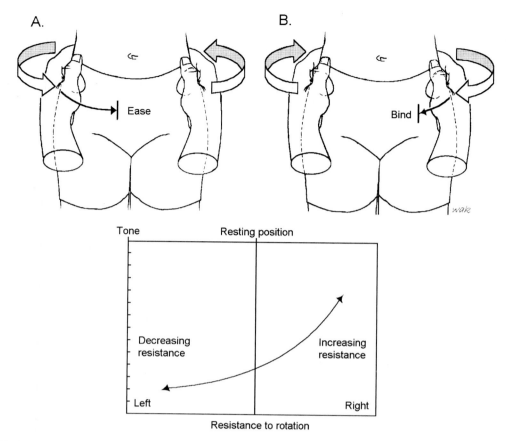

Figure 2.46   Ease-bind concept. **A,** Passive left hip rotation occurs without resistance and is easy. **B,** Passive right hip rotation is increasingly resistant. This gives the examiner a sense of binding as the hips are moved away from resting position toward the right.

The conference summary for research in the biology of manual therapies can be found on the National Institutes of Health web site.[13]

General Questions about Mechanisms of Action for Manual Therapy

- Determine the effects of manual therapy in normal experimental animals and in animal models of tissue injury, including
  1. Behavioral responses to painful stimuli
  2. Fibroblast response
  3. Gene expression
- Does applying very superficial manual therapies, such a light massage, that mainly activate skin afferents produce different effects on the nervous system, immune system, and endocrine system compared with manual therapies that also involve activation of muscle afferents?
- Does paraspinal tissue have any unique physiology compared with appendicular tissues? Is this related to the reported clinical efficacy of manual therapies?
- Do manual therapies produce long-lasting changes in the biomechanics of the spine, torso, or limbs? Are these changes associated with altered activity in the nervous system, immune system, or endocrine system?
- Can valid, reliable biomechanical measures (e.g., posture, kinematics, kinetics, functional imaging) be identified to do the following?
  1. Distinguish between healthy and unhealthy tissues
  2. Subcategorize patients or clients with musculoskeletal disorders
- Can imaging techniques be developed that can be used to capture dynamic in vivo responses to biomechanical signals in healthy and unhealthy tissues?

Questions about Peripheral Mechanisms of Action for Manual Therapy

- Determine and compare the discharge characteristics (i.e., the pattern or frequency of action potentials) of primary sensory neurons in response to various types of manual therapies (e.g., high-velocity loading compared with slower loading rates). Is there any correlation with reported efficacy?
- How do various manual therapies affect peripheral nerve biomechanics?

- What path of mechanical load transmission do various manual therapies take through the body?

Questions about Central Mechanisms of Action for Manual Therapy

- How do different types of manual therapies affect the signaling properties of neurons in the central nervous system or autonomic nervous system? Do they produce long-lasting changes?
- Do different types of manual therapies evoke different patterns of neural activity in the central nervous system or autonomic nervous system?
- What are the effects of peripheral mechanical stimuli (e.g., manual therapies) on spinal cord gating mechanisms and synaptic plasticity?
- How can human models of experimental pain be developed and used to determine the role of the nervous system, if any, in explaining how manual therapies work? Specific areas of investigation can include the following:
  1. Effects of temporal summation
  2. Effect of manual therapies on windup
  3. Quantitative sensory testing
- Non-neural outcomes may include the following:
  1. Heart rate and heart rate variability
  2. Laser Doppler blood flow and blood pressure changes
  3. Respiratory frequency
  4. Carbon dioxide levels
  5. Catecholamine levels
  6. Circulating cells (e.g., numbers, subsets, response)
  7. Cytokines
  8. Vaccine response (i.e., immunoglobulin response)
  9. Contact hypersensitivity or delayed-type hypersensitivity

10. High sensitivity C-reactive protein
11. Lymphatic flow

REFERENCES

1. Glossary of osteopathic terminology. In Ward RC (ed): Foundations for Osteopathic Medicine, 2nd ed. Philadelphia, Lippincott Williams & Wilkins, 2003.
2. Howell JN, Willard F: Nociception: New understandings and their possible relation to somatic dysfunction and its treatment. Ohio Res Clin Rev 15:12-15, 2005.
3. Patterson MM, Wurster RD: Neurophysiologic mechanisms of integration and disintegration. In Ward RC (ed): Foundations for Osteopathic Medicine, 2nd ed. Philadelphia, Lippincott Williams & Wilkins, 2003, pp 120-136.
4. Willard FW. Nociception, the neuroendocrine immune system, and osteopathic medicine. In Ward RC (ed): Foundations for Osteopathic Medicine, 2nd ed. Philadelphia, Lippincott Williams & Wilkins, 2003, pp 137-156.
5. Jones HJ: Somatic dysfunction. In Ward RC (ed): Foundations for Osteopathic Medicine, 2nd ed. Philadelphia, Lippincott Williams & Wilkins, 2003, pp 1153-1161.
6. Schleip R, Klingler W, Lehmann-Horn F: Active fascial contractility: Fascia may be able to contract in a smooth muscle–like manner and thereby influence musculoskeletal dynamics. Med Hypotheses 65:273-277, 2005.
7. Felton DL, Józefowicz R: Netter's Atlas of Human Neuroscience. Figure III.6: Mechanisms of neuropathic pain and sympathetically maintained pain. Teterboro, NJ, Icon Learning Systems, 2003.
8. Pickar JG: Neurophysiological effects of spinal manipulation. Spine J 2:357-371, 2002.
9. Skyba DA, Radhakrishnan R, Rohlwing JJ, et al: Joint manipulation reduces hyperalgesia by activation of monoamine receptors but not opioid or GABA receptors in the spinal cord. Pain 106:159-168, 2003.
10. Sleszynski SL, Glonek T: Outpatient osteopathic SOAP note form: Preliminary results in osteopathic outcomes-based research. J Am Osteopath Assoc 105:181-201, 2005.
11. Al-Eisa E, Egan D, Wassersug R: Fluctuating asymmetry and low back pain. Evol Hum Behav 25:31-37, 2004.
12. Mitchell FL Jr, Mitchell KG: The Muscle Energy Manual, vol 3. Evaluation and Treatment of the Pelvis and Sacrum. East Lansing, MI: MET Press, 1999.
13. National Institutes of Health: Conference on the Biology of Manual Therapies. Bethesda, MD, 2005. Available at http://nccam.nih.gov/news/upcomingmeetings/final_recommendations.htm/ Accessed September 25, 2005.

CHAPTER 3

Manual Diagnostic Procedures Overview

DIAGNOSING SOMATIC DYSFUNCTION

The musculoskeletal examination consists of a series of tests that assess the structure and function of the joints and soft tissues. It enables the practitioner to make an accurate diagnosis of somatic dysfunction and apply an appropriate and specific manual treatment to resolve it. This examination is often performed as part of a standard history and physical examination. It may be done as part of a complete history and physical examination, as is typically performed on the initial patient visit, or as part of a focused, problem-oriented history and physical examination. This text is organized in a problem-oriented manner, and the authors assume that an initial complete history and physical examination have already taken place and that the practitioner knows the patient's health status.

The findings from the musculoskeletal examination are interpreted in the context of the findings from the rest of the history and physical examination. For example, the standard neurologic examination portion of the physical examination, which includes assessment of cognitive, motor, sensory, reflex, and cerebellar functions, may provide evidence of central nervous system pathology, such as a cerebral vascular accident (i.e., stroke). This would alter the interpretation of findings of asymmetric decreased range of joint motion on the musculoskeletal examination. With an intact nervous system, asymmetric decreased range of joint motion may indicate somatic dysfunction, but when there is evidence of central or even peripheral nervous system pathology, these same findings maybe interpreted as being caused by the nervous system deficit. It is also possible that in the face of a central nervous system problem, the patient may be unable to understand the practitioner's questions and commands. Similarly, the findings from the musculoskeletal examination need to be interpreted in the context of any metabolic, circulatory, respiratory, or other diseases that affect musculoskeletal structure and function.

This chapter focuses on the visual and palpatory tests used to diagnose somatic dysfunction. The practitioner should already know the status of the patient's nervous system and any underlying diseases that may have a bearing on the structure and function of the joints being examined. Tests specific for joint and ligament integrity that are often included in the musculoskeletal examination are not covered in this chapter, although the practitioner should be skilled in their application. The practitioner should consult standard musculoskeletal or orthopedic examination textbooks for descriptions of these tests.

During the musculoskeletal examination, the patient is examined in several positions, including standing, seated, supine (i.e., lying on the back), prone (i.e., lying on the chest and abdomen), and occasionally, sidelying. If the treatment table or plinth has a hole in the center to accommodate the face, the patient may lie prone with the head straight in alignment with the spine; otherwise, the patient can turn his or her head to one side or the other.

When assessing symmetry or alignment of anatomic landmarks, the practitioner should use his or her dominant eye. The dominant eye is the one used for midline visualization while the other eye is used to visualize off midline for depth perception. Most people have one eye that is more dominant than the other. Anatomic landmarks should be observed with the dominant eye in the midline for accurate visual discrimination. The dominant eye can easily be determined by looking at a distant object, such as the corner of a room where the ceiling meets two walls, through the center of a hole made by the tips of forefingers and thumbs at the end of outstretched arms. By closing one eye at a time, the practitioner can notice that the dominant eye maintains visualization of the object in the center of the hole, but the other eye focuses off midline, and the object is viewed at an angle through that eye. The following method is one way to determine which eye is dominant:

1. Extend both hands and place the hands together making a small circle (as small as possible) with the thumbs and index fingers of each hand.
2. With both eyes open, look through the circle and sight an object at least 20 feet away.
3. Close the left eye. If the object can still be seen within the circle, this indicates right eye dominance. If the object does not remain in view within the circle, this indicates left eye dominance.
4. To validate this test, look through the circle at the object again with both eyes open.

5. Repeat the procedure, this time closing the right eye and observing the difference in the results.

There are several components to the structural examination. It entails visual and palpatory assessment of anatomic symmetry and active joint motion, followed by assessment of passive joint and soft tissue motion, tension and tenderness, and skin texture and turgor assessments. The examination may be thought of as being performed in three stages:

1. A *screening* or *general impression* examination entails assessment of symmetry of anatomic landmarks and active and passive regional motion tests. The practitioner takes a general view of the entire musculoskeletal system to answer this question: Is there a problem in the musculoskeletal system?

2. A *scanning* or *regional* examination entails palpating the soft tissues of the regions selected as having a problem based on the screening examination. It is a process of *localization* to answer this question: Where is the problem? The practitioner looks for evidence of abnormal structure; skin temperature, surface moisture, and colors (e.g., rubor); subcutaneous tension, texture, tenderness, and edema; and muscle tension or compliance.

3. A *segmental* examination entails defining and describing the specific joint, spinal segmental, or soft tissue dysfunctions localized in the scanning examination. Using standard terminology, the practitioner makes a specific diagnosis that enables a specific treatment with manual treatment. It answers this question: What is the problem?

Screening Examination

The practitioner notices the patient's appearance, nutritional status, gait, and any evidence of gross structural, joint motion, or soft tissue asymmetries or irregularities. Each body region is observed during active motion testing and palpated during passive motion testing. Joint motion testing assesses the range of motion and should detect any abnormalities in the quality of the motion. The practitioner should observe whether the motion being tested is smooth and equal in all possible directions or there is a feeling of excessive tension in the tissues even though the quantitative range of motion may be normal. The practitioner also notices the "end feel" of the passive motion; this is the quality of the motion as its end range is approached. Does the end feel seem smooth and supple, which is normal, or does it feel hard and abrupt, indicating soft or bony tissue restrictions that may result primarily or secondarily from underlying pathology?

The screening examination as outlined in this chapter may seem to have redundancies at first glance. There are static (i.e., patient does not move), active (i.e., patient moves), and passive (i.e., practitioner moves the patient) motion assessments of each body region. Some regions, however, have more than one of a particular type of assessment. For example, the lower extremities have two active motion assessments: one that is observational only (i.e., the squat test) and another that is palpatory and visual (i.e., the standing flexion test). There are two passive lower extremity motion tests: one that tests joint motions (i.e., sequential **f**lexion,

abduction, **e**xternal **r**otation, and **e**xtension [FABERE test]) and another that assesses hamstring muscle tension. Similarly, there are two active lumbar spine sidebending tests that are performed with the patient standing, one in conjunction with thoracic sidebending and the other in conjunction with active hip motion (i.e., the hip drop test). These tests enable assessment of the lumbar spine in relation to the regions above and below it. Focal regional thoracic and lumbar active and passive motion tests are then performed while the patient is seated, which stabilizes the pelvis. Although similar tests are performed, each is designed to provide specific and unique information that, when combined with the other tests, enable a fairly comprehensive screening evaluation of the musculoskeletal system for evidence of somatic dysfunction.

Abnormal findings on the general screening examination indicate regions of the musculoskeletal system that require further evaluation. The screening musculoskeletal examination can be organized by the position in which the patient is to be evaluated, because in clinical practice, it is most natural to have the patient move comfortably from standing to sitting and then to lying down. The tests can be grouped to conform to the patient's position:

Patient walking
   1. Active gait analysis
Patient standing
   2. Static postural anatomic landmark assessment, including head and facial symmetry and alignment
   3. Active scoliosis screening test
   4. Active iliosacral joint and lower extremity mobility test (i.e., standing flexion test)
   5. Passive hip shift test
   6. Active spine sidebending test
   7. Active hip drop test
   8. Active upper extremity mobility (i.e., quick test)
   9. Active lower extremity mobility (i.e., squat test)
Patient sitting
   10. Active and passive spine flexion, extension, sidebending, and rotation tests
   11. Active lumbar-sacroiliac joint mobility (i.e., seated flexion test)
Patient supine
   12. Static pelvic and lower extremity anatomic landmark symmetry assessments
   13. Active costal cage mobility with breathing assessment
   14. Passive hamstring muscle tension test (i.e., straight-leg raising test)
   15. Passive lower extremity mobility (i.e., FABERE test)
   16. Passive upper extremity mobility test
Patient prone
   17. Active 11th and 12th ribs mobility with breathing assessment
   18. Static assessment of leg-length symmetry

Patient Walking

• Gait analysis (Fig. 3.1) entails observing the patient walking to detect abnormalities in the motor system or musculoskeletal structures that are more pronounced during walking.

1. If possible, observe the patient's gait when he or she is not aware of being evaluated, such as when the patient is being escorted to the examination room.
2. Otherwise, observe the patient's gait by having him or her walk the length of the examination room several times.
3. Observe any abnormalities in the length of stride, arm swing, heel strike, and toe off; pelvic tilt; or any limping. Asking the following questions while observing may be helpful:

   Is the weight transferred in a smooth manner from heel strike to toe off?

   Do the toes point inward or outward?

   Is there excessive pronation or supination of the feet?

   Is there internal or external rotation of either leg?

- Abnormal gait may signify neurologic or musculoskeletal problems that require further regional and segmental evaluation.

Patient Standing
Postural Assessment

Postural assessment entails observation of static posture for alignment and visual and palpable assessment of paired anatomic landmarks for symmetry.

- The patient is instructed to stand still, with feet shoulder-width apart, face forward, and arms relaxed to the sides.
- The patient's posture should be evaluated from posterior, lateral, and anterior views.
- The practitioner should have his or her eyes at the level of the area being evaluated.
- The examiner should observe and palpate where appropriate in all views and levels.
  1. Posterior view (Fig. 3.2)
     Head carriage for sidebending or rotation off midline
     Mastoid processes level
     Shoulders level
     Inferior tips of the scapulae level

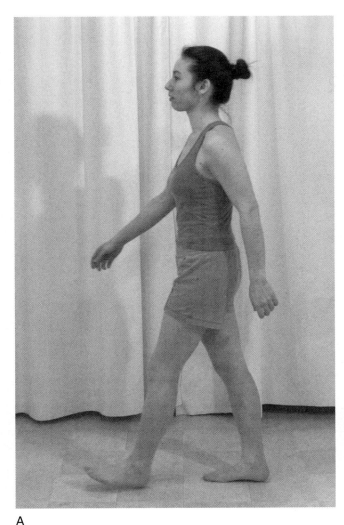

A

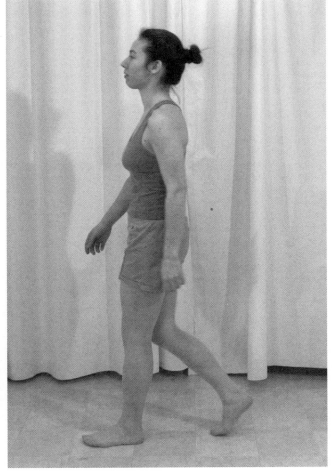

B

Figure 3.1   Gait cycle. **A,** heel strike. **B,** Midstance.

Continued

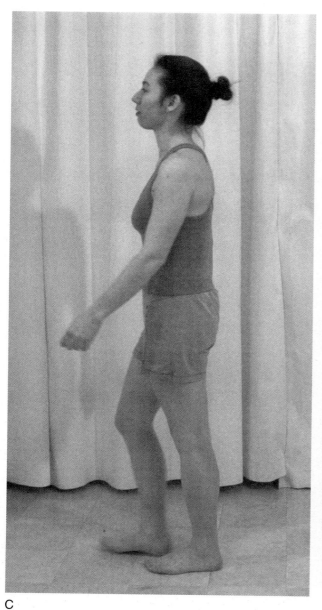

C

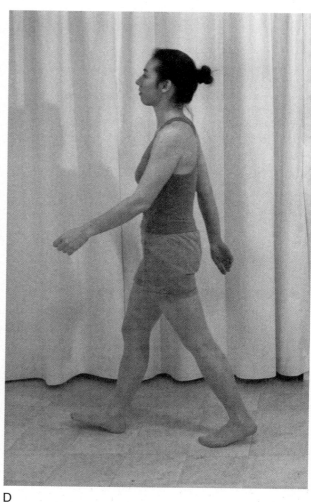

D

Figure 3.1, cont'd   **C,** Swing phase. **D,** Opposite heel strike.

Carrying angle of the elbows
Iliac crests level
Posterior superior iliac spine (PSIS) level
Greater trochanters level
Gluteal creases level
Fingertip lengths level
Popliteal lines level
Achilles tendons for lateral curvatures
Arches of the feet for flattening or high arches
Unilateral asymmetries in paired muscle groups, such as
    trapezius, erector spinae, gluteus maximus, hamstrings,
    or gastrocnemius

2. Lateral view (Fig. 3.3)
    Gravitational line
    Lateral symmetry of posture is evaluated by imagining a
        line drawn from the ceiling to the floor through the
        midline of the patient's body.
    Ideally, this line passes through the following points: the
        external auditory meatus, the acromioclavicular joint,
        the greater trochanter, and a point just anterior to the
        lateral malleolus.
    Anteroposterior cervical, thoracic, and lumbar spinal curves
    Anterior or posterior rotation of the pelvis
    Flexion or hyperextension of the knees

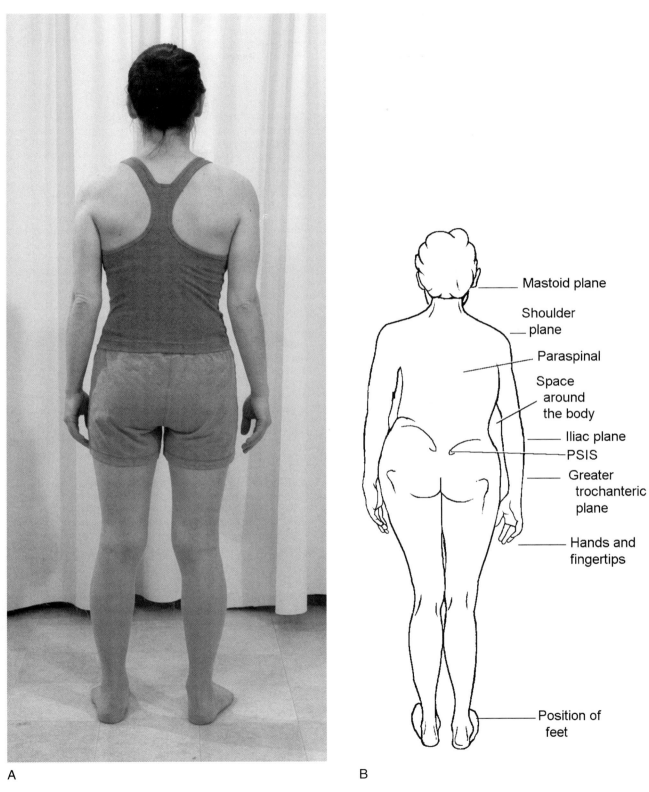

A   B

Figure 3.2   Postural assessment. **A,** Posterior view. **B,** Drawing of the posterior view of an asymmetric patient. PSIS, posterior superior iliac spine.

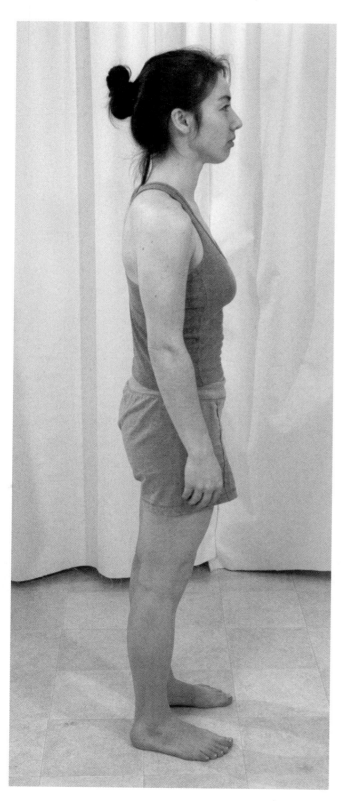

Figure 3.3 Postural assessment: lateral view.

3. Anterior view (Fig. 3.4)
   Head carriage
   Facial structural symmetry
   Jaw symmetry at rest and on opening
   Levelness of the shoulders
   Symmetry of the clavicles
   Rib cage and sternum configuration
   Carrying angle of the elbows
   Internal or external rotation of the upper extremities
   Iliac crest heights
   Anterior superior iliac spines
   Patella heights
   Valgus or varus deformities of the hips, knees, or ankles
   Pronation or supination of the feet

Observation of postural misalignment or asymmetries may indicate problems such as scoliosis, postural decompensation, anatomic short leg, previous trauma or surgery, or specific segmental somatic dysfunctions in the body regions where asymmetry is observed.

Scoliosis Screening Test

- The scoliosis screening test (Fig. 3.5) identifies lateral curvature of the spine due to congenital or acquired spinal abnormalities or muscle imbalances.
  1. The patient is standing comfortably with his or her back to the practitioner.
  2. The practitioner stands or sits behind the patient.
  3. The practitioner then asks the patient to bend forward and observes and palpates any asymmetries in the spinal column or rib cage contour. It is helpful if the practitioner visually observes at the horizontal level of the patient's flexed spine.
  4. If a lateral spinal curvature is identified, the practitioner then has the patient bend forward just to the level of the spinal region where the curve is located.
  5. The patient then swings his or her upper body to the left and then to the right.
  6. The practitioner observes any changes in the spinal curvature or rib cage contour as the patient performs this maneuver.
  7. Functional scoliotic curves can reduce or disappear with rotation, sidebending, or forward bending. Structural scoliotic curves do not change significantly with these motions.
- A positive scoliosis test result can signify vertebral anomalies, congenital defects, acquired deformities, compensation for a short leg, hip or lower extremity pathology that unlevels the sacral base, or muscle imbalance.

Standing Flexion Test

- The standing flexion test (Fig. 3.6) screens for iliosacral somatic dysfunction, defined functionally as somatic dysfunction of the innominate or lower extremity. It can be done while checking for thoracolumbar scoliosis.
  1. The patient stands with the feet comfortably apart, weight evenly distributed to the lower extremities, and his or her back to the practitioner.

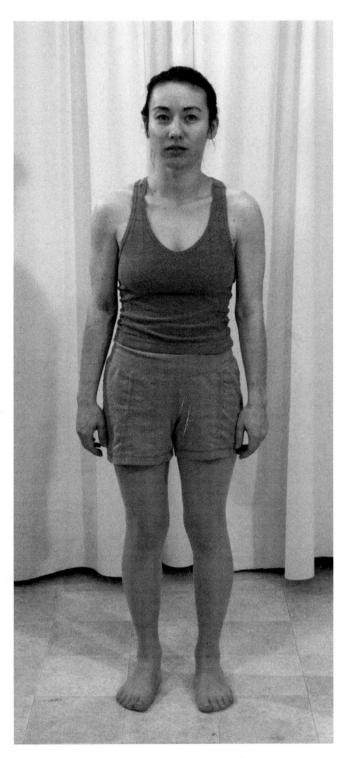

Figure 3.4 Postural assessment: anterior view.

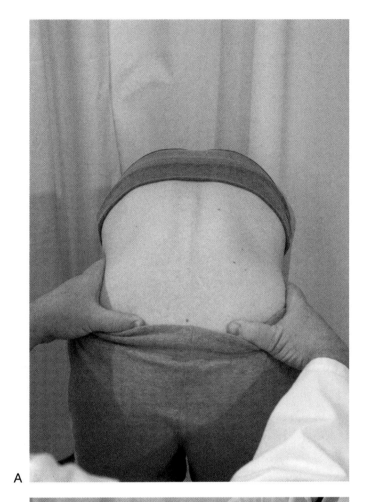

A

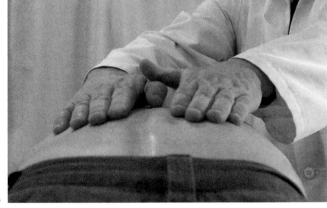

B

Figure 3.5 Scoliosis screen. **A,** Normal. **B,** Positive result. Notice the elevation of the right paraspinal region compared with the left (convexity of the lumbar curve is to the right).

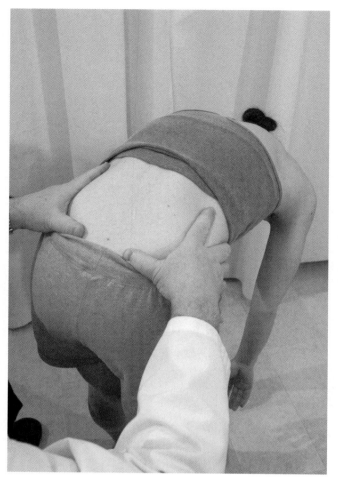

Figure 3.6   Standing flexion test.

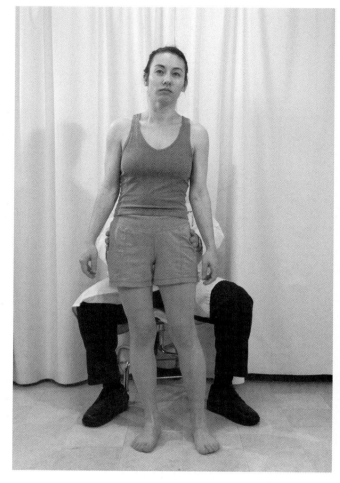

Figure 3.7   The hip shift test is measured by resistance to returning toward midline. The side with the most resistance is the side to which the hip is shifted.

2. The practitioner sits or kneels behind the patient and places his or her thumbs on the inferior slopes of the patient's PSISs.
3. The patient is then asked to bend forward from the waist with the arms hanging loosely and attempt to touch the floor.
4. The practitioner observes whether the PSISs move symmetrically (normal motion) or one PSIS is more superior or ventral than the other at the end of the forward bending motion (i.e., positive test result).
- A positive standing flexion test result indicates a somatic dysfunction in the innominate region or in the lower extremity on the side of the positive test result.

Hip Shift Test
- The hip shift test (Fig 3.7) identifies pelvic region somatic dysfunction typically in response to lumbar or lower extremity somatic dysfunction.[1,2]
  1. The patient stands with feet only slightly apart and with his or her back to the practitioner.
  2. The patient's arms hang loosely and are relaxed.
  3. The position of the feet is maintained steadfast while the hips are allowed to move freely.
  4. The practitioner stands or sits behind the patient.

5. The practitioner places his or her hands laterally on each of the patient's hips with finger pads in contact with the greater trochanters.
6. The practitioner gently introduces a translatory force from one side to the other, moving the patient's hips passively from side to side, first with one hand then the other.
7. In about one of every three patients, the practitioner encounters immediate resistance in attempting to move the hips back toward midline in one direction.
8. In the opposite direction, an easy range of freedom (i.e., compliance) is encountered.
- A positive hip shift test result indicates that the pelvis, lower extremities, and lumbar spine need further evaluation for evidence of somatic dysfunction.
  1. When there is asymmetry of palpatory findings (i.e., one direction resists more than the other) or bilateral resistance to this passive hip shift motion test, the hip shift test result is positive.
  2. In the case of asymmetry of motion, the direction of ease designates the side to which the hip is shifted. If a patient's hips translate easily to the right and resist movement

toward the left, the right hip shift test result is positive, meaning that the hip is shifted toward the right.

3. Typically, the patient bears weight on the ipsilateral leg of the shifted hip; in the example given with a right-shifted hip, the weight is mostly on the right leg.

Standing Spine Sidebending Test

- The standing spine sidebending test is helpful in identifying any regional sidebending restrictions in the thoracic or lumbar regions.
  1. The patient stands with his or her back to the practitioner.
  2. The practitioner sits or kneels behind the patient and places his or her hands on the superior borders of the patient's iliac crests.
  3. The patient is asked to place one hand on the lateral aspect of the thigh and then to sidebend to one side by slowly sliding the hand toward the floor.
  4. The patient sidebends without moving into flexion or extension and continues this motion until the practitioner can feel movement at the iliac crest on the side opposite the sidebending.
  5. The patient then repeats this procedure by sidebending to the opposite side.

6. The practitioner observes the following:
   The amount of sidebending achieved, which is normally about 40 degrees in each direction
   The induced lateral spinal curve; which should be a symmetric C-shape curve with paravertebral muscle fullness on the side of the convexity
   The shifting of the pelvis from side to side during sidebending
   Whether the weight bearing on the lower extremities appears symmetric
- Any straightening of the spinal segments within the induced lateral curve or paravertebral muscle fullness on the side of the concavity suggests somatic dysfunction of the vertebral segments at that spinal level. Pelvic side shift or asymmetric loading of the lower extremities may occur as compensatory movements resulting from somatic dysfunction in the lower thoracic or lumbar spinal regions.

Hip Drop Test

- The hip drop test (Fig. 3.8) identifies restriction of passive lumbar sidebending in response to active lowering of one hip by bending the ipsilateral knee.
  1. The patient is standing with his or her back to practitioner.
  2. The practitioner sits behind the patient.

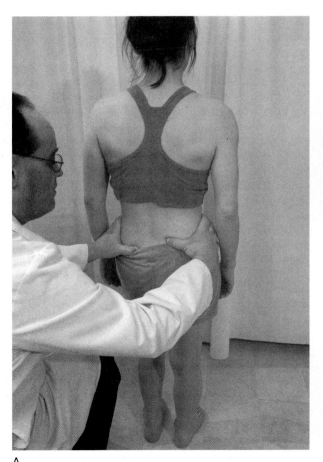
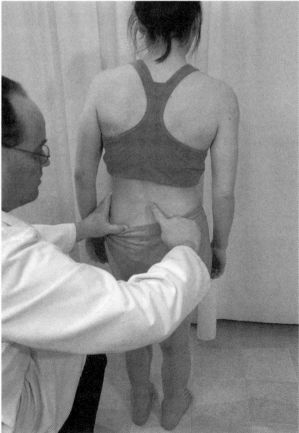

A   B

Figure 3.8   Hip drop test. **A,** When the left knee is flexed, the left hip drops. **B,** When the left hip drops, the lumbosacral spine should sidebend to the right in a smooth curve.

3. The practitioner evaluates the symmetry of patient's iliac crests in the standing position.
4. The patient then bends one knee with both heels flat on the ground. This movement tilts the pelvis to the side of the bent knee. The normal range of hip drop is 25 to 30 degrees.[3]
5. The practitioner observes how the lumbar spine bends to the side away from the dropped hip to accommodate the pelvic tilt.
6. The test is repeated on the opposite side, and the results of amount of hip drop and lumbar sidebending are compared.
7. The direction to which there is restricted lumbar sidebending is identified.

- A positive (asymmetric) hip drop test result indicates lumbar somatic dysfunction that may result primarily or secondarily from pelvic or lower extremity dysfunction. If primary lumbar somatic dysfunction is present, this test will display the level of lumbar spinal dysfunction by an angle or straightening of the normal C-curve induced by sidebending.

Upper Extremity Mobility Test

- The upper extremity mobility test (i.e., quick test) (Fig. 3.9) screens for soft tissue or joint motion restrictions in the upper extremity. Proper function of the upper extremities requires good mobility of the sternoclavicular, acromioclavicular, glenohumeral, and wrist and hand joints, as well as properly functioning soft tissues and supportive structures.
  1. The patient stands facing the practitioner. This test can also be done seated on the examination table or on a stool.
  2. The practitioner observes this motion from in front of the patient.
  3. The patient is instructed to raise (i.e., abduct) both arms in the coronal plane, as if reaching toward the ceiling, until the arms are fully overhead and then to bring the backs of the hands together (i.e., pronating the forearms).
  4. The patient's arms should be able to almost touch the ears (i.e., 180 degrees of abduction), and the backs of the hands should be able to completely come together.
- Asymmetry or decreased range or quality of motion of the upper extremities signifies dysfunction of one or more of these joints and warrants further evaluation by regional and segmental evaluations.

Lower Extremity Mobility Test

- The lower extremity mobility test (i.e., squat test) assesses active hip, knee, and ankle flexion and extension capabilities (Fig. 3.10). It is performed as follows:
  1. The patient is in the standing position.
  2. The practitioner views the patient from the side to observe the ability of the patient to keep the heels flat on the floor while performing the test.
  3. The patient is asked to squat down and then come back up to standing position while keeping the heels flat on the floor. The patient may extend his or her arms out in front to maintain balance.
  4. The practitioner observes the ability of the patient's hips, knees, and ankles to flex and extend.

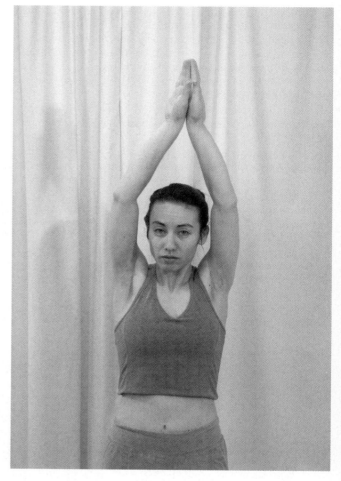

Figure 3.9   Upper extremity mobility assessment (quick test).

- Asymmetry, decreased range, or lack of ease of motion indicates a positive (abnormal) squat test result. If the patient's heels come off the floor or the patient is unable to flex the hips or knees to at least 90 degrees, further evaluation of the lower extremities for somatic dysfunction or other pathology is warranted.

Patient Seated
Seated Flexion Test

- The seated flexion test (Fig. 3.11) screens for sacroiliac somatic dysfunction, defined functionally as somatic dysfunction of the sacrum or lower lumbar spine.
  1. The patient sits with the feet flat on the floor and the knees comfortably apart.
  2. The practitioner sits or kneels behind the patient and places his or her thumbs on the inferior slopes of the patient's PSISs.

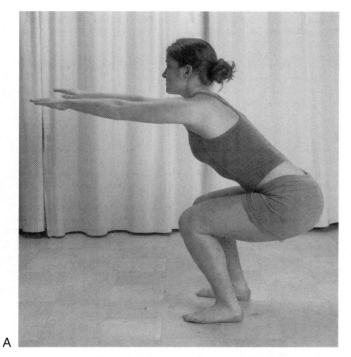

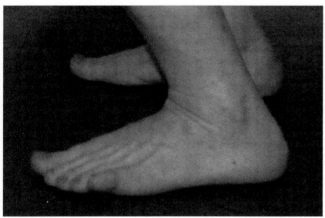

B

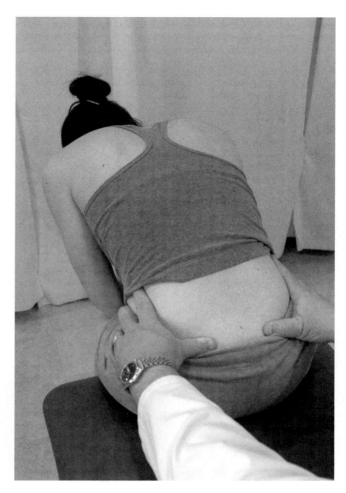

Figure 3.11   Seated flexion test.

Figure 3.10   Lower extremity mobility assessment (squat test). The practitioner observes, from the lateral view, the patient's ability to flex and extend the hips, knees, and ankles, making note of whether the heels remain flat on the floor during the maneuver, indicating good tone and compliance of the lower leg muscles, tendons, and ankle joints.

3. The patient is then asked to bend forward from the waist with the arms hanging loosely between the knees.

4. The practitioner observes whether the PSISs move symmetrically (i.e., normal motion is a negative test result) or one PSIS is more superior or anterior than the other at the end of the forward-bending motion (i.e., abnormal motion is a positive test result).

• A positive standing flexion test indicates somatic dysfunction in the lower lumbar vertebrae or the sacral region on the side of the positive test result.

Active and Passive Spine Mobility Tests

• The active and passive spine mobility tests are used to evaluate the mobility of the thoracic and lumbar regions. For both the active and passive motions, the following movements are tested: flexion, extension, left and right sidebending (i.e., lateral bending), and left and right rotation.

1. The patient is seated comfortably on the examination table or on a stool.

2. The practitioner stands or sits behind the patient.

3. For *flexion*, the patient is asked to bend forward slowly at the waist as far as comfortably possible. Normally, there are about 50 degrees of flexion in the thoracic spine and about 60 degrees of flexion in the lumbar spine.

4. The practitioner observes the degree of movement, the smoothness of the motion, and whether there is any deviation of the thoracic or lumbar spine to the left or right.

5. The patient then returns to the neutral position.
6. To observe *extension*, the patient is asked to lean backward by arching the lumbar spine and to look toward the ceiling. Normally, there are about 10 degrees of extension in the thoracic spine and about 25 degrees of extension in the lumbar spine.
7. The practitioner observes the amount of movement and the smoothness of the motion.
8. To observe *sidebending*, the patient is asked to sit erect with the arms at the sides and the fingertips pointing toward the floor.
9. The practitioner sits or kneels behind the patient and palpates the superior surfaces of the patient's iliac crests.
10. The patient is then instructed to sidebend to one side by slowly moving his or her hand toward the floor.
11. The patient sidebends without moving into flexion or extension and continues this motion until the physician can feel movement at the iliac crest on the side opposite the sidebending.

12. The degree of movement and the smoothness of the motion on each side can be compared.
13. The normal amount of combined sidebending motion in the thoracolumbar spine is about 30 degrees to each side.
14. *Rotation* is observed from behind the patient, who is asked to turn the shoulders toward one side, as if looking at his or her back.
15. This process is then repeated to the other side after the patient returns to a neutral midline position.
16. The practitioner observes for the amount and smoothness of the motion from side to side.
17. The normal amount of rotation in the thoracolumbar spine is about 45 degrees to each side.
18. These motions also should be assessed passively.
19. The practitioner can have the patient fold his or her arms and use the patient's shoulders as contact points to induce passive flexion, extension, and sidebending (Fig. 3.12A and B). The patient's shoulders or ipsilateral elbow can be the contact point for thoracolumbar spine rotation assessment (see Fig. 3.12C). The practitioner should observe smoothness and range of motion in each direction.

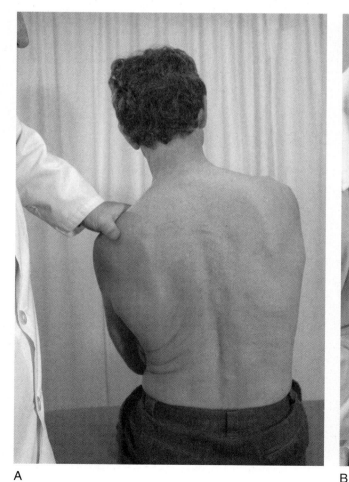
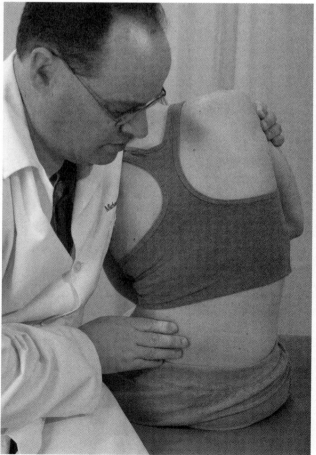

A   B

Figure 3.12   **A,** Passive assessment of thoracolumbar sidebending with the practitioner standing. **B,** Passive assessment of thoracolumbar sidebending with the practitioner seated.

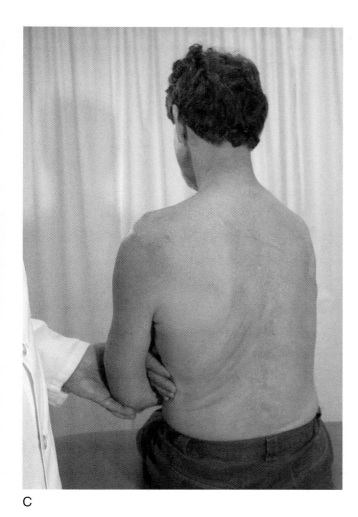

Figure 3.12, cont'd   C, Passive assessment of thoracolumbar rotation. The patient is seated with arms folded. The practitioner uses the patient's elbow to induce rotation by gently pulling posteriorly.

20. To avoid straining the low back during these maneuvers, the practitioner should maintain an erect posture when standing and use total body motion to passively move the patient, who needs to be instructed to relax and allow the motions to be tested without resistance. This is best performed by bending at the knees and maintaining normal lumbar lordosis throughout these maneuvers. It is also less strain on the low back to perform passive rotation and sidebending toward the side on which the practitioner stands.

- Asymmetry of any of these trunk motions indicates the need for further structural evaluation of the thoracic and lumbar vertebrae and the rib cage.

Cervical Spine Active and Passive Motion Assessments

- Cervical spine active and passive motion assessments (Fig. 3.13) screen for neck motion dysfunction. For both the active and passive motions, the following movements are tested: flexion,

extension, left and right sidebending (i.e., lateral bending), and left and right rotation.

1. The patient is seated comfortably on the examination table or on a stool.
2. The practitioner stands in front of or behind the patient.
3. For flexion, the patient is asked to move the chin toward the chest. The practitioner observes the degree of movement, the smoothness of the motion, and whether there is any deviation of the cervical spine to the left or right. Full flexion is accomplished when the chin, with the mouth closed, touches the patient's chest. Normally, there are about 60 degrees of flexion in the cervical spine (see Fig. 3.13A).
4. To observe extension, the patient is asked to raise the chin and look toward the ceiling. The practitioner observes the amount of movement and the smoothness of the motion. Normally, there are about 75 degrees of extension in the cervical spine (see Fig. 3.13B).
5. To observe sidebending, the patient is asked to try to touch one ear to the shoulder on the same side. This process is repeated on the opposite side. Make sure that the patient does not use a substitute movement by raising the shoulder to meet the ear. The degree of movement and the smoothness of the motion can be compared from side to side. The normal amount of sidebending in the cervical spine is about 45 degrees to each side.
6. Rotation is observed by asking the patient to turn the chin to one side so that the chin moves toward the shoulder. This process is then repeated to the other side. Do not allow the patient to use a substitute motion by rotating the trunk. Observe for the amount and smoothness of the motion from side to side. The normal amount of rotation in the cervical spine is about 80 degrees to each side (see Fig. 3.13C and D).
7. These motions also should be assessed passively.
8. The practitioner grasps the patient's head with one hand on the patient's forehead and the other on the patient's occiput.
9. The practitioner then moves the patient's head and neck into flexion and into extension and observes the motion of the cervical spine, evaluating the range of motion accomplished and the smoothness of the motion.
10. The practitioner then changes his or her hand position by placing one hand on each side of the patient's head.
11. The patient's head and neck are sidebent to the left and right and then rotated left and right.
12. The amount and smoothness of motion of the cervical spine is observed.
13. The normal range of degrees of motion for these passive movements is the same as those for active range of motion.

- Asymmetry in any of these ranges or quality of motion indicates the need for further regional and segmental evaluation of the cervical spine.

Patient Supine
Pelvic and Lower Extremity Symmetry Tests

- Tests of pelvic and lower extremity symmetry (Figs. 3.14 to 3.16) assess symmetry of anatomic landmarks (i.e., anterior superior iliac spine [ASIS], pubic symphysis, and medial malleoli) to

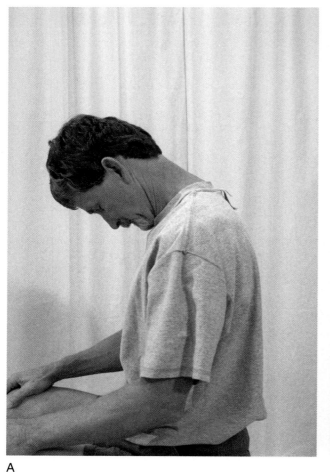
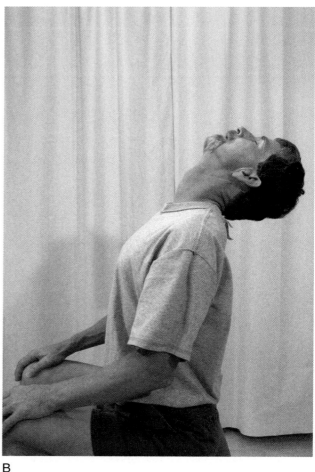

A   B

Figure 3.13   A, Assessment of active cervical spine flexion. **B,** Assessment of active cervical spine extension.

determine whether there are pelvic or lower extremity somatic dysfunctions or the possibility of an anatomic short leg.

1. The patient is supine.
2. The practitioner stands over the patient, making sure the patient's dominant eye is able to view the midline.
3. The patient's ASIS level is evaluated by placing each thumb horizontally under the inferior aspect of the patient's ASIS (see Fig. 3.14).
4. The patient's pubic symphysis level is assessed by placing each forefinger tip on the pubic tubercle and determining whether one is more superior than the other (see Fig. 3.15).
5. The practitioner evaluates the level of the patient's malleoli by having the patient first lift the pelvis off the table and set it down to ensure it is centered on the examination table. The practitioner then uses his or her index fingers as straight edges vertically along the inferior aspect of each medial malleoli (see Fig. 3.16).

- Asymmetric landmarks indicate pelvic or lower extremity somatic dysfunction or an anatomic short leg.

Rib Cage Motion Screening

- Assessment of motion restriction in the rib cage (Fig. 3.17) is performed using a combination of palpation by the practitioner and respiratory cooperation on the part of the patient. The rib cage is evaluated by observing motion in the upper rib cage (ribs 1 to 5), the lower rib cage (ribs 6 to 10), and then ribs 11 and 12 as a separate group (with the patient prone).

1. To evaluate the upper rib cage, the patient is supine on the examination table.
2. The practitioner stands at the side of the table that allows his or her dominant eye to be over the midline of the patient.
3. The practitioner places his or her hands over the anterior aspect of the upper rib cage, with the tips of the middle fingers in contact with the cartilage of the first ribs, just under the medial ends of the clavicles.
4. The patient is instructed to inhale deeply and then exhale fully.
5. The practitioner observes symmetry or asymmetry of the upper rib cage during both phases of respiration.
6. This portion of the evaluation assesses the pump-handle motion of the upper rib cage (ribs 1 to 5).
7. This process is repeated with the practitioner's hands placed over the anterolateral aspects of the patient's upper rib cage, allowing the practitioner to observe the bucket-handle motion of the upper rib cage.

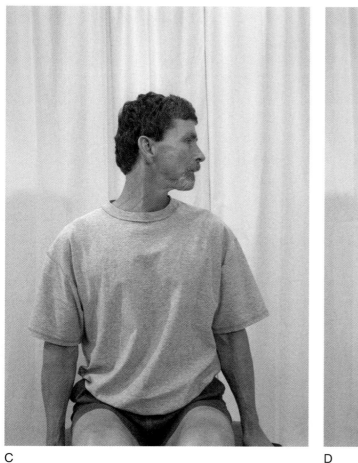

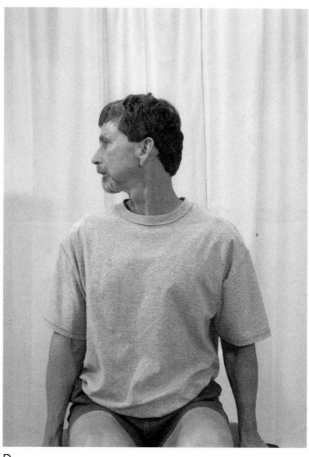

Figure 3.13, cont'd   **C,** Assessment of active cervical spine left rotation. **D,** Assessment of active cervical spine right rotation.

8. The practitioner next places his or her hands over the anterolateral aspects of the patient's lower rib cage bilaterally.
9. The patient is instructed to inhale deeply and then exhale fully.

10. The practitioner observes symmetry or asymmetry of the lower rib cage during both phases of respiration.
11. This portion of the evaluation assesses the predominantly bucket-handle motion of the lower rib cage (ribs 6 to 10).

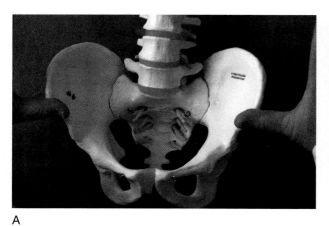

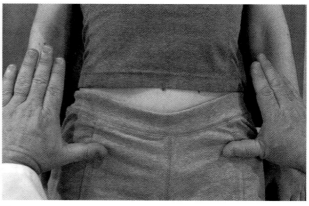

Figure 3.14   **A,** Pelvic and lower extremity symmetry assessment: location of the anterior superior iliac spines on a skeletal model.
B, Assessment of pelvic and lower extremity symmetry at the level of the anterior superior iliac spines.

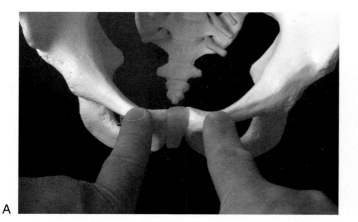

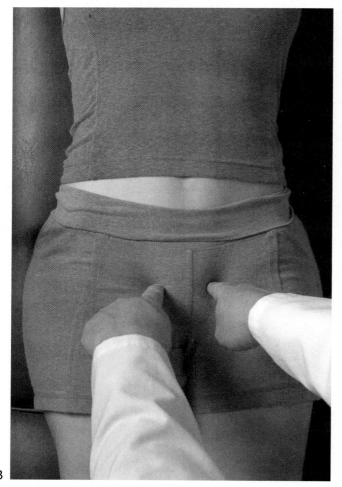

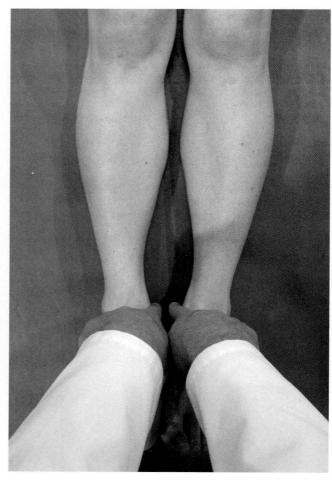

Figure 3.16   Assessment of pelvic and lower extremity symmetry at the level of the medial malleoli.

Figure 3.15   **A,** Pelvic and lower extremity symmetry assessment: location of the pubic tubercles on a skeleton model. **B,** Assessment of pelvic and lower extremity symmetry at the level of the pubic symphysis.

12. Ribs 11 and 12 are evaluated with the patient in the prone position (discussed later).
• Asymmetry of inhalation or exhalation movements of the rib cage requires further structural examination of the thoracic spine and rib cage for somatic dysfunction.

1. A group of ribs that have decreased excursion on one side more so than on the contralateral side is further evaluated segmentally to determine the most dysfunctional rib in the group.
2. Typically, if one rib does not move well due to a dysfunctional relationship with its associated vertebra or muscle attachments, the motion of the ribs above and below it is also affected.
3. For example, if a group of ribs moved easily and completely into its inhalation position but sluggishly moved into its exhalation position, it would be considered to be "held up" more in the inhalation position. This is usually caused by a rib in the group that is not moving well and that does not allow the rest of the ribs in the group to move inferiorly into their exhalation position.
4. The lower ribs in the group are evaluated one at a time to discern which one may be preventing the rest of the group from moving inferiorly as they should during exhalation.

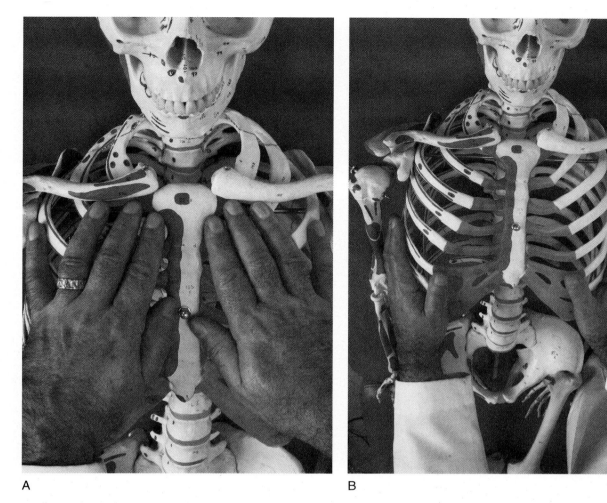

Figure 3.17 **A,** Hand positions on a skeletal model for assessment of the pump-handle motion of the upper ribs. **B,** Hand positions on a skeletal model for assessment of the bucket-bail motion of the lower ribs.

Hamstring Muscle Tension Test

- The hamstring muscle tension test (i.e., straight-leg raising test) (Fig. 3.18) is a passive test that assesses the tension in the posterior thigh or "hamstring" muscles that help to flex the knees and to stabilize the pelvis by their attachment to the innominates (i.e., hip bones). The hamstring muscle tension assessment is important for interpreting the findings from other tests that rely on hip bone mobility, such as the standing flexion test.

  1. The patient is supine on the examination table with his or her legs fully extended.
  2. The practitioner stands on either side of the table.
  3. The practitioner grasps one of the patient's ankles with one hand while placing the finger pads of the other hand on the opposite ASIS.
  4. The practitioner then lifts the extended leg until motion is first felt at the opposite ASIS, gaining an appreciation for the length of the hamstring muscle group on the side of the leg that is raised (see Fig. 3.18A).
  5. Another commonly used method is to hold the patient's distal femur just above the knee to maintain knee extension while lifting the leg from below the ankle with the other hand (see Fig. 3.18B).
  6. This maneuver is repeated on the opposite side.
  7. Asymmetry of motion indicates excessive tightness in the hamstring muscles on the side that demonstrates the lesser range of motion.
  8. The practitioner observes the degree of elevation before a restrictive motion barrier is perceived. The normal range is between 50 and 90 degrees of hip flexion.

- A tight hamstring muscle group may prevent the ipsilateral ilium from moving superiorly or anteriorly during the standing flexion test, potentially giving the practitioner signs of a false-positive test result on the contralateral (mobile) side. A tight hamstrings muscle group should be stretched, and then the standing flexion test should be repeated before interpreting its results. If pain is elicited that radiates posteriorly down the tested leg or even down the contralateral leg to the foot, a posterior lateral herniated lower lumbar disc impinging on the sciatic nerve root as it exits the intervertebral foramen should be suspected.

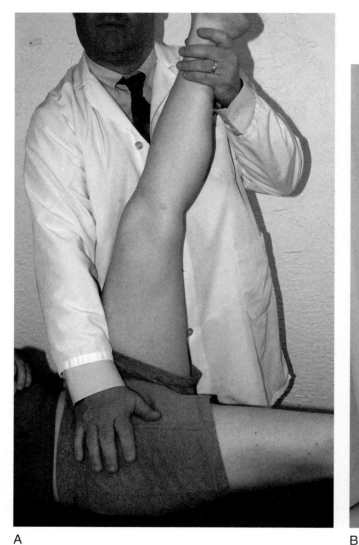

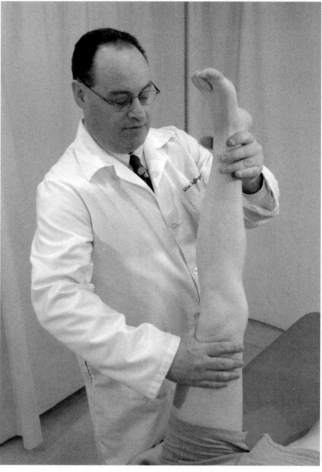

A   B

Figure 3.18 **A,** The hamstring muscle tension test with one hand raising the patient's left leg and the other monitoring motion of the patient's right hip, which begins to move after the hamstring muscle reaches its restrictive barrier. **B,** An alternative method for evaluating the hamstring muscle tension. Notice that the practitioner uses one hand to raise the patient's left leg while the other hand stabilizes the patient's left knee to keep it extended.

Hip and Lower Extremity Mobility Test

- The hip and lower extremity mobility test (i.e., FABERE test) assesses passive mobility of the hips, knees, and ankle joints (Fig. 3.19).
  1. The patient is supine on the examination table.
  2. The practitioner stands at one side of the table.
  3. The practitioner passively flexes the patient's knee and ankle and then passively flexes, abducts, externally rotates, and extends the patient's hip, knee, and ankle on that side. The mnemonic FABERE (i.e., Patrick's test) is derived from the initial letters of these motions.
  4. The practitioner then moves to the other side of the table and repeats this maneuver for the opposite hip joint.

- Any restricted motion noted suggests somatic dysfunction or possibly other pathology of the hip joint, knee, or ankle being examined.

Upper Extremity Mobility Test

- The upper extremity mobility test is a passive motion assessment of the shoulders, elbows, and wrist joints. It is performed as follows:
  1. The patient is supine on the treatment table.
  2. The practitioner stands on the side of the upper extremity to be assessed.
  3. The practitioner holds the patient's wrist with one hand and stabilizes the patient's elbow with the other hand.

4. The practitioner then passively flexes and extends the patient's shoulder, elbow, and wrist joints; circumducts, abducts, and adducts the shoulder and wrist joints; internally and externally rotates the shoulder; and supinates and pronates the forearm.

5. The practitioner repeats these procedures on the other upper extremity and compares the ranges and quality of motions of the two sides.

6. The practitioner observes any decreased range or abnormal quality of motion of the joints in the upper extremity.

- Asymmetric or decreased range or quality of motion indicates somatic dysfunction or other underlying pathology of one or more of the joints in the upper extremity and warrants further regional and segmental evaluation.

Patient Prone
Mobility Assessment of Ribs 11 and 12
- The 11th and 12th ribs are evaluated for caliper or pincer-type motion dysfunction as part of the rib cage screening examination (Fig. 3.20).

1. The patient is prone on the examination table.
2. The practitioner stands at the side of the table with his or her dominant eye over the patient's midline.
3. The practitioner then places his or her hands over the 11th and 12th ribs with the thumbs and thenar eminences over the medial aspects of the ribs and with the fingers of both hands pointing laterally and overlying the shafts of the ribs.
4. The patient is instructed to inhale deeply and then exhale fully. The practitioner observes symmetry or asymmetry of the 11th and 12th ribs during both phases of respiration.

- Asymmetry or decreased range or quality of motion indicates further regional and segmental evaluation of these ribs and their muscular attachments, especially the diaphragm and quadratus lumborum muscles.

Leg-Length Symmetry Assessment
- Assessment of the symmetry of leg lengths may be more reliable and accurate with the patient in the prone position. This test is used to determine whether there are sacral, pelvic, or

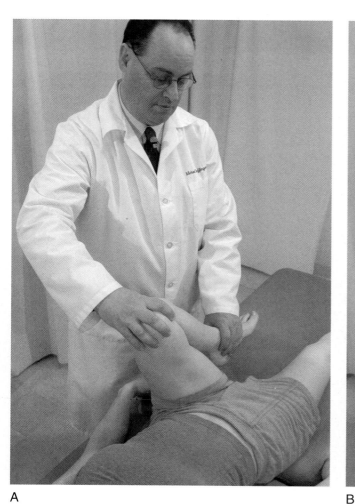
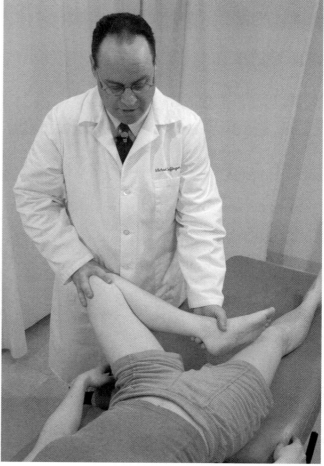

A   B

Figure 3.19 Hip and lower extremity mobility test (i.e., FABERE test). **A,** Hip flexion. **B,** Hip abduction, external rotation.

Continued

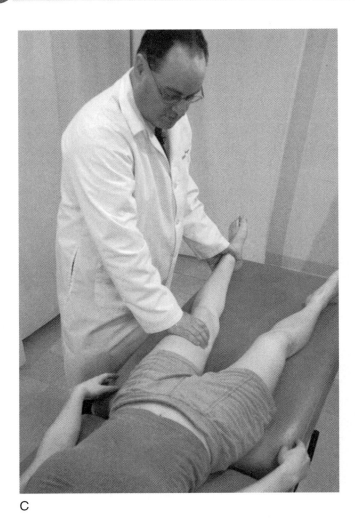

C

Figure 3.19, cont'd **C,** Hip extension.

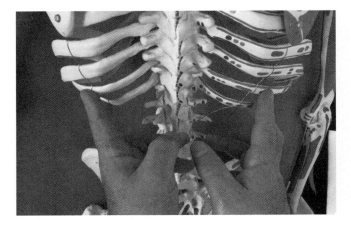

Figure 3.20 Hand positions on a skeletal model for assessment of pincer or caliper motion for ribs 11 and 12.

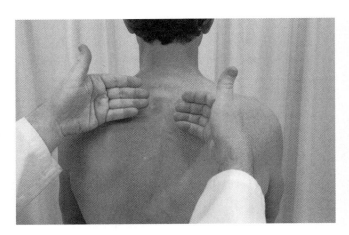

Figure 3.21 Regional assessment of radiant heat. In this example, the examiner assesses the thoracic paraspinal soft tissues.

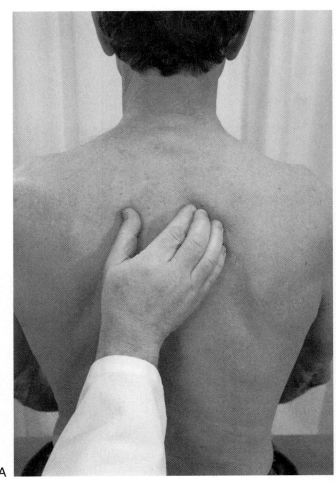

A

Figure 3.22 **A,** Soft tissue palpatory assessment. In this example, the examiner assesses the thoracic paraspinal soft tissues.

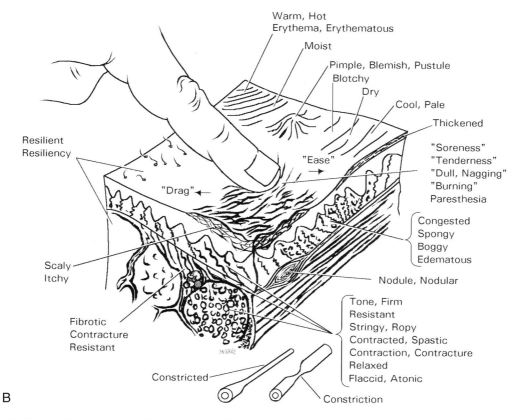

Warm, Hot
Erythema, Erythematous
Moist
Pimple, Blemish, Pustule
Blotchy
Dry
Cool, Pale
Thickened
"Soreness"
"Tenderness"
"Dull, Nagging"
"Burning"
Paresthesia
Congested
Spongy
Boggy
Edematous
Nodule, Nodular
Tone, Firm
Resistant
Stringy, Ropy
Contracted, Spastic
Contraction, Contracture
Relaxed
Flaccid, Atonic
Constriction
Constricted
Fibrotic
Contracture
Resistant
Scaly
Itchy
Resilient
Resiliency
"Ease"
"Drag"

B

Figure 3.22, cont'd   B, The drawing depicts a variety of palpatory findings and the underlying pathophysiology. From Kuchera WA, Kuchera ML, Osteopathic Principles in Practice, Second Edition Revised, Greydon Press, Columbus, OH, 1994:510. Used with permission.

lower extremity somatic dysfunctions and to evaluate the possibility of an anatomic short leg.

1. The patient is prone.
2. The practitioner stands over the patient, making sure his or her dominant eye is able to view the midline.
3. The practitioner evaluates the level of the patient's medial malleoli by using the index fingers as straight edges vertically along the inferior aspect of each medial malleoli.

- Asymmetric landmarks indicate sacral, pelvic, or lower extremity somatic dysfunction or an anatomic short leg.

Regional Examination Procedures

The scanning examination is performed using a combination of static and dynamic testing procedures. Static testing is done by feeling above the skin for radiant heat or areas of relative coolness using the posterior surfaces of the hands (Fig. 3.21), palpating the soft tissues (e.g., skin, subcutaneous tissues, muscles, ligaments, fascia) and looking for tissue texture abnormalities such as hypertonicity, ropiness, bogginess, or edema and increased or decreased skin moisture (Fig. 3.22). The tissues within the region may also be palpated for discrete trigger points or tender points (Fig. 3.23). Asymmetry of tissues or joint structures within a region may be observed and palpated.

The static and dynamic tests allow the practitioner to identify specific areas within body regions that may exhibit the presence

of somatic dysfunction. After these areas are identified, the practitioner proceeds to the segmental examination.

Segmental Examination

The final part of the structural evaluation is the segmental examination. In this part of the structural examination, a region

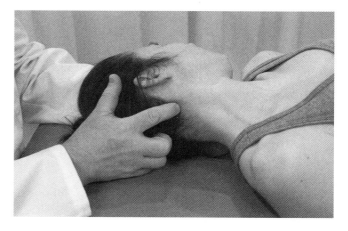

Figure 3.23   Assessment of tender points. In this example, the examiner assesses the right posterior C2 tender point.

identified by the screening and scanning examinations is further evaluated. Dysfunctional individual vertebral segments or peripheral joints are identified and given a specific somatic dysfunction diagnosis. The practitioner also identifies the specific motion restrictions that are present and the tissues that are most involved in the dysfunctional segment. The segmental examination is designed to answer the following questions:

- What specific segments are dysfunctional? In this context, a segment may be defined as a vertebra, rib, sacrum or one of the innominate bones, or a specific upper or lower extremity joint.
- What specific motion restrictions are present?
- What other tissues (e.g., muscle, ligaments, fascia) are involved?
- How are the somatic dysfunctions related to the patient's other health problems?

The diagnosis of somatic dysfunction depends on determining motion loss at a given segment and the associated tissue characteristics that accompany this motion loss. Having determined (during the regional examination) an area within a body region that may exhibit somatic dysfunction, the practitioner's goal is to determine the specific segment that is dysfunctional, the specific motions that are restricted, and the associated tissues that may be causing or contributing to the motion restriction. If there are several segments involved within a particular body region, the practitioner attempts to find the most restricted segment (i.e., the segment that exhibits the greatest amount of motion restriction and associated tissue texture changes).

- In the spinal regions, the practitioner may observe tissue texture changes in the form of increased paravertebral soft tissue fullness extending over the transverse process area of several vertebral segments on one side or the other of the spinal column.
- Part of this fullness can be attributed to rotation of one or more of these vertebral bodies toward the side of the fullness, with the result that the transverse processes of these vertebrae are posterior on the side of the fullness.
- If several segments are involved, the practitioner first determines (by palpation and observation) which segment demonstrates the most fullness (i.e., the most posterior transverse process). That vertebra is presumed to be rotated to the side of the posterior transverse process.

Diagnosing Somatic Dysfunction Summary

- Somatic dysfunction is defined as impaired or altered function of related components of the somatic (body framework) system: skeletal, arthrodial, and myofascial structures and related vascular, lymphatic, and neural elements.
- The distinguishing physical findings support a diagnosis of somatic dysfunction. Think of the ART of diagnosis (also designated as TART or other mnemonics):
  1. *A*symmetry of anatomic landmarks
  2. *R*ange or quality of motion abnormalities; usually *r*estriction of motion
  3. *T*issue texture abnormalities, including *t*enderness and palpable, localized *t*emperature changes indicative of hyperemia or ischemia

- *Screen* the body regions to get a general impression.
  1. Answer this question: Is there a problem in the musculoskeletal system?
  2. Perform gait and postural assessment, perform active and passive regional motion tests, and check the position of landmarks.
- *Scan* the region selected as having a musculoskeletal problem, based on asymmetry of range of motion or position of landmarks.
  1. Check the periarticular soft tissues for tension, tenderness, edema, and structural abnormalities.
  2. Answer this question: *Where* is the problem?
- *Define* the somatic dysfunction.
  1. Find the restrictive barrier in all planes of motion.
  2. Feel the local tissue response to passive or active regional or segmental motion tests.
  3. Perform digital pain provocation of muscles, tendons, ligaments, joint capsules, bursa, and surrounding connective tissues.
  4. Answer this question: *What* is the problem?
- Determine whether the problem is of musculoskeletal origin or is a systemic, organic disease (Table 3.1).
  1. Answer this question: Is there a more serious medical or surgical condition that needs attention beyond manipulation?
  2. If the answer is yes or the practitioner is unable to answer the question because of a lack of training, skill, experience, or scope of practice, an evaluation by a practitioner with the requisite training and experience is warranted before manipulation is provided.
  3. A radiograph is sometimes needed to rule out fracture in cases of acute traumatic injury, and ultrasound, other radiographic procedures, and blood, urine, or other diagnostic tests are indicated if the history and physical evaluations point to the possibility of systemic or organic conditions underlying the musculoskeletal dysfunction.
- After the diagnosis of somatic dysfunction is established, manipulative treatment is indicated.

VALIDITY AND RELIABILITY OF EXAMINATION PROCEDURES

- The ability to arrive at an accurate assessment of the musculoskeletal system depends on several factors, primarily the patient's medical history and history of the present illness, the examiner's experience and skills, and the validity and reliability of the examination procedures used.
- The validity and reliability of examination procedures has been a subject of controversy for hundreds of years. Because of the variety of procedures and professions using them and the lack of ability to validate many of them, it is difficult to establish gold standards for examination procedures.
- For internal organ disease diagnoses, the validity and reliability of palpatory diagnostic procedures are not as accurate or reliable as visual, auscultory, laboratory, or radiographic tests.[4] It is therefore understandable why palpatory diagnostic procedures as a primary method of gathering physical evidence

Table 3.1   Diagnosis and management of a patient with primary musculoskeletal pain versus one with secondary musculoskeletal pain

Findings and Treatment	Primary Musculoskeletal Pain	Secondary Musculoskeletal Pain Referred from Visceral Disease
History		
Pain is localized to a muscle or joint	Yes	No
Overuse, trauma or activity related at onset	Yes	Not usually, but possible (e.g., angina)
Pain relieved by rest	Yes	Not usually, except for angina or claudication
Pain worse at night	No	Yes
Unexplained weight loss	No	Yes
Physical Examination		
Passive joint motion restricted	Yes	No, although characteristic motion patterns and tissue changes occur
Muscle point tenderness on digital palpation	Yes	No
Pain reproduced by joint motion or muscle contraction	Yes	No
Management		
Amenable to manual treatment	Yes (as long as improvement is progressive as expected)	No (manual treatment is included secondarily for support of the patient's body systems)
Requires further workup, diagnosis, and treatment	No (unless patient does not steadily improve as expected)	Yes

to support a diagnostic impression for these diseases have fallen out of favor among physicians.

- Most of the examination procedures used by manual practitioners are palpatory in nature. Because each examiner is unique in skill level, experience, training, and education, there is a high degree of subjectivity involved in the interpretation of the findings.
- Although several palpatory diagnostic procedures have been shown to be valid and reliable, many are not. The practitioner of manual medicine should be aware that these procedures do have limitations.
- A systematic review of the literature on the reliability of spinal palpatory diagnostic tests revealed the following[5]:
  1. Landmark location, regional motion, and pain provocation tests have acceptable reliability (kappa values of 0.40 or greater).
  2. Pain provocation tests are the most reliable, and soft tissue paraspinal palpatory diagnostic tests are the least reliable.
  3. Regional ranges of motion tests are more reliable than segmental ranges of motion tests.
  4. Intraexaminer reliability is better than interexaminer reliability.
- The spinal palpatory examination may be more difficult to reliably perform because of small joints and limited mobility, but acceptable reliability has been demonstrated for the larger proximal joints of the extremities (e.g., shoulder, knee),[6,7] but not the smaller interphalangeal joints.[8]
- Some practitioners of manual medicine use instruments such as goniometers that measure range of joint motion to more accurately measure musculoskeletal dysfunction. Many, however, prefer to rely solely on their palpatory skills.

- Pain scales are one of only a few validated instruments with which to measure the accuracy of palpatory diagnostic procedures.[9] Practitioners are encouraged to use them with each patient complaining of pain, at each office visit, and before and after each intervention.
- When there is no gold standard test available, it is prudent to use more than one diagnostic test to support a diagnostic impression and management plan. For example, composites of pain provocation tests for the sacroiliac joints improve the accuracy of diagnosis more so than single tests for patients with low back pain.[10]
- Examiner bias and inconsistency create variability in procedures. This leads to unreliability of findings and inaccurate diagnoses. It is therefore imperative that each practitioner strives to limit personal bias and perform manual diagnostic procedures correctly and the same way every time in every patient.
- Professions that research and teach palpatory diagnostic and manual medicine procedures should work together to identify and develop the most valid and reliable tests.

DOCUMENTATION

- Findings should be documented using standard nomenclature for clarity. It is helpful to grade the severity of findings in each region to be able to more objectively evaluate improvement. A standardized form can be used to facilitate this process (see http://www.academyofosteopathy.org for examples of standard documentation forms).
  - 0: No ART changes
  - 1: Minimal and asymptomatic changes

Table 3.2   ICD-9 diagnostic codes for somatic dysfunction by body region

Body Region	ICD-9 Code
Head	739.0
Neck	739.1
Thoracic region	739.2
Lumbar region	739.3
Pelvis, sacrum	739.4
Pelvis, innominate	739.5
Lower extremity	739.6
Upper extremity	739.7
Costal cage	739.8
Abdomen	739.9
Unspecified area	739.9

2: Localized significant restriction and tissue changes; may be tender

3: Key restriction and tissue changes that create compensatory changes elsewhere; typically tender. Chronic dysfunction may be dull or numb to digital pressure.

- This diagnosis is coded in the ICD-9 system as 739.0-9, and each region is given a separate number (Table 3.2).

- No matter how many dysfunctions are found in one region, only one code is given for that region (see Chapter 12).

REFERENCES

1. Johnston WL: Hip shift: Testing a basic postural dysfunction. J Am Osteopath Assoc 63:923-930, 1964. (Reprinted in the American Academy of Osteopathy Yearbook. Indianapolis, IN, American Academy of Osteopathy, 1998, pp 47-55.)
2. Johnston WL: Hip shift. Part II. A continuing postural study. *In* Academy of Applied Osteopathy Yearbook. Indianapolis, IN, American Academy of Osteopathy, 1968. (Reprinted in the American Academy of Osteopathy Yearbook. Indianapolis, IN, American Academy of Osteopathy, 1998, pp 56-58.)
3. Kuchera WA, Kappler RE: Musculoskeletal examination for somatic dysfunction. *In* Ward RC (ed): Foundations for Osteopathic Medicine. Philadelphia, Lippincott Williams & Williams, 2003, pp 642.
4. McGee S: Evidence-Based Physical Diagnosis. Philadelphia, WB Saunders, 2001.
5. Seffinger MA, Najm WI, Mishra SI, et al: Reliability of spinal palpation for diagnosis of back and neck pain: A systematic review of the literature. Spine 29:413-425, 2004.
6. Chesworth B, MacDermid J, Roth J, et al: Movement diagram and "endfeel" reliability when measuring passive lateral rotation of the shoulder in patients with shoulder pathology. Phys Ther 78:593-601, 1998.
7. Malanga GA, Andrus S, Nadler SF, et al: Physical examination of the knee: A review of the original test description and scientific validity of common orthopedic tests. Arch Phys Med Rehabil 84:592-603, 2003.
8. Bellamy N, Klestov A, Muirden K, et al: College of Rheumatology classification criteria for hand, knee and hip osteoarthritis (OA): Observations based on an Australian Twin Registry study of OA. J Rheumatol 26:2654-2658, 1999.
9. Najm WI, Seffinger MA, Mishra SI, et al: Content validity of manual spinal palpatory exams: A systematic review. BMC Complement Altern Med 3:1, 2003.
10. Laslett M, Aprill CN, McDonald B, et al: Diagnosis of sacroiliac joint pain: Validity of individual provocation tests and composites of tests. Man Ther 10:207-218, 2005.

CHAPTER 4

Treatment Procedures Overview

Although manual treatment has been applied to most maladies that afflict humans for several millennia, this textbook focuses on manual treatments for the following common clinical conditions:

- Low back pain
- Neck and upper back pain
- Cervicogenic headache
- TMJ dysfunction
- Shoulder pain
- Carpal tunnel syndrome
- Ankle sprain

Myriad manual techniques have been created, developed, and passed down through the ages in several cultures across the globe to treat these common conditions. The techniques included in this textbook were chosen on the basis of their safety profile, applicability to patients of all ages, ease and wide range of use across professions worldwide, and clinical efficacy. They represent the main techniques taught in osteopathic medical schools in the United States. The high-velocity, low-amplitude (HVLA) and osteopathy in the cranial field (OCF) manual techniques are omitted because of the higher level of skill required and difficulty in application. Although HVLA has an excellent safety profile in the hands of trained professionals, greater force is generated by these maneuvers to correct articular dysfunctions, and the chance for side effects and the potential for harm are also increased when used incorrectly or inappropriately. OCF manual techniques are also safe and efficacious in the hands of trained professionals, but they require a higher level of palpatory sensitivity, and if forces are applied inaccurately to the cranium, untoward side effects will likely result.

Each technique is introduced in a standard format:

- Classification
- Definition
- Mechanism
- Applications
- Procedure
- Improving efficacy

CLASSIFICATION OF MANIPULATIVE PROCEDURES

Manipulative techniques can be classified as one of three methods:
1. Direct: toward the restrictive barrier and increased tissue tension and restriction

2. Indirect: away from the restrictive barrier and toward a sense of ease and increasing tissue compliance
3. Combined: a combination of direct and indirect methods applied concomitantly or sequentially

Direct Techniques

- The practitioner passively moves or holds tense tissues toward their restrictive barrier, engages the barrier, employs an activating and corrective force, and then moves through the restrictive barrier as permitted by the response of the tissues to the procedure.
- Advantages: The technique is expedient and addresses restricted joints and hypertonic muscle groups.
- Disadvantage: The technique has a limited range of applicability in patients with comorbidities and low levels of vitality.
- Table 4.1 compares direct procedures.

Indirect Techniques

- The practitioner guides, moves, or holds the patient's body into positions that enable the soft tissues around a restricted joint to relax or become less tender to palpation. This is accomplished by moving away from the restrictive barrier in directions toward increasing ease of motion and tissue compliance.
- Advantage: The technique has a wide range of applicability in patients of all ages and levels of health.
- Disadvantage: It may take 5 seconds to 2 minutes before release of tension or a significant decrease in tenderness occurs.
- Table 4.2 compares indirect procedures.

Combined Techniques

- The practitioner uses direct and indirect approaches in tandem or simultaneously.
- The patient may be instructed to actively assist by using, for example, respiration or eye movements.
- Advantage: The technique enables real-time adjustments to tissue responses.

Table 4.1   Comparison of direct action procedures

Technique	Characteristics	Advantages	Disadvantages
Soft tissue	Axial or lateral stretch of muscles and connective tissues uses repetitive or sustained force until tension yields.	Increases blood flow to the region; relaxes hypertonic muscles	Does not necessarily mobilize restricted joints
Myofascial release (direct)	Maintain sustained tension at the restrictive barrier until tension yields by using direct contact on myofascial tissues or through contact with bony structures to which the myofascial tissues are attached.	Addresses regional fascial tension patterns, large muscles, and muscle groups	Does not necessarily mobilize restricted joints
Articulatory	Practitioner stabilizes one bone of the restricted joint while passively and repetitively, without thrust, moves the other through the restrictive barrier until normal physiologic range of motion is obtained.	Mobilizes restricted joints	Requires repetitive motions to obtain lasting results
Muscle energy	Practitioner-controlled resistance to patient's gentle counterforce	Joint and muscle group specific	Requires patient effort and cooperation

• Disadvantages: It requires skill and experience in using direct and indirect methods.

CONTRAINDICATIONS AND PRECAUTIONS

General Principles

It is inappropriate to apply these procedures to an alert, oriented, and coherent adult patient who refuses to be touched or treated with manual techniques. It is also inappropriate to manipulate a somatic dysfunction when there is a more urgent or life-threatening problem, such as hemorrhage, vascular occlusion, or other emergency, which should be attended to first. Although written consent has not become the standard of care for the techniques in this textbook, it is prudent to obtain verbal consent after informing the patient of the diagnosis and proposed treatment plan. Any potential side effects also should be mentioned.

Complications from manual medicine procedures are rare events. Those that have been reported in the literature are mostly from HVLA thrust procedures used on the upper cervical spine and occasionally on the lumbar spine. Complications from the clinical application of the procedures included in this textbook have not been identified by literature search. Although there may be underreporting of complications to these procedures, we have used and taught them for decades without experiencing or hearing of any complications.

Table 4.2   Comparison of indirect procedures

Technique	Characteristics	Advantages	Disadvantages
Functional	Practitioner passively moves adjacent body regions or limbs in directions that elicit increasing compliance of the monitored soft tissues around a restricted joint.	Identifies spinal reflex relationships between the movements of different body regions; no side effects	Requires considerable skill and training to master
Strain-counterstrain	Practitioner employs positional release of tender points located on bones, within muscles, or on ligaments.	Easy to learn and perform	Can take 90 to 120 seconds to achieve at least 50% reduction in tenderness per tender point
Myofascial release	Using direct contact on the tissues or through contact with bony structures to which the myofascial tissues are attached, practitioner maintains myofascial soft tissues away from the restrictive barrier towards increasing compliance.	Addresses regional fascial tension patterns, large muscles, and muscle groups	Does not necessarily mobilize specific joints

Direct Techniques

Precautions and Contraindications to Direct Manipulation Techniques for Joint Mobilization

These contraindications do not apply to soft tissue or myofascial techniques, which are discussed later. Contraindications to direct techniques include applications to specific joints that have any of the following:

- Acute trauma (e.g., fracture, dislocation, open wound, sprains [unstable joints])
- Congenital or acquired malformations (e.g., fused hemivertebra, spinal laminectomy, spinal rods, joint replacement [immobile or altered joint anatomy])
- Friable, acutely inflamed, or infected bony or soft tissues (i.e., unstable tissues)
- Hemarthrosis (e.g., ruptured tissues, hemorrhage)
- Hypermobility (i.e., instability such as ligamentous laxity or rupture)
- Nearby venous thrombosis, arterial aneurysm or dissection (i.e., vascular instability)
- Primary joint, metabolic, or cancerous bone disease (i.e., bony instability)

Some conditions indicate treatment with caution in applying direct techniques to joints:

- Anatomic deformities (i.e., abnormal joints)
- Brain injury or trauma or hemiplegia (i.e., abnormal reflexes and muscle activity)
- Connective tissue or rheumatic diseases (i.e., inflamed joints and soft tissues)
- Disc herniation resulting in radiculopathy (i.e., may worsen condition)
- Hemophilia (i.e., may have increased risk of bleeding)
- Metastatic bone cancer (i.e., anatomic and physiologic derangement of joints)
- Anticoagulation therapy (i.e., may have increased risk of bleeding)
- Spinal cord injury (i.e., muscles and joints do not respond normally)

Precautions and Contraindications to Direct-Action Soft Tissue and Direct Myofascial Release Techniques

Contraindications to soft tissue and myofascial release (MFR) techniques include the following:

- Congenital connective tissue diseases or abnormalities (e.g., Ehlers-Danlos syndrome, a condition of hyperelasticity of connective tissue [abnormal soft tissue response])
- Friable or ruptured skin or subcutaneous soft tissues; acutely inflamed or infected soft tissues (i.e., unstable soft tissues)
- Hypersensitivity to touch (i.e., complex regional pain syndromes [patient intolerability])
- Muscle splinting or guarding due to underlying disease, fracture, or inflammation (i.e., abnormal response of soft tissues)

Precautions to direct-action soft tissue and MFR techniques include the following:

- Patients with a history of "easy bruising" (i.e., may cause bruising)
- Recent surgical incisions (i.e., can disrupt scar healing)

Indirect Techniques

Contraindications and Precautions

Indirect techniques have few contraindications and precautions.

- Immediately after acute trauma (e.g., fracture, dislocation, open wound [unstable tissues])
- Friable, acutely inflamed, or infected bony or soft tissues (i.e., unstable tissues)

SIDE EFFECTS

Side effects of the techniques, when done correctly as described in this textbook, are minimal and self-limiting and last between 24 and 48 hours. Side effects include the following:

- Myalgias or arthralgias, aches, and fatigue
- Soft tissue redness from increased circulation
- Occasionally, headache or dizziness from upper cervical manipulation techniques
- Bruising or subcutaneous hemorrhage with soft tissue or myofascial-type direct techniques (can occur in patients with easy-bruising or friable skin)

Side effects often can be minimized by applying ice to the affected or to sore areas for 20 minutes after the procedure.

DESIGNING A MANAGEMENT PLAN FOR SOMATIC DYSFUNCTION

The management plan for somatic dysfunction entails making a manipulative prescription, developing a maintenance and prevention plan, and selecting the manual methods or techniques to be used. As with any therapeutic procedure, the practitioner should explain the choice of manual treatment procedure selected, its goals, and its potential side effects and should obtain the patient's permission before applying it.

The Manipulative Prescription

Like a medicine prescription, a manual treatment prescription entails the following components:
1. Goals
2. Dose
3. Frequency
4. Duration

Goals of Manual Treatment

Manual treatments alleviate somatic dysfunction, improve joint motion, mobilize body fluids, and decrease pain. The International

Federation of Manual Medicine (FIMM) developed a consensus definition of the goal of manipulation in 1983: "The goal of manipulation is to restore maximal, pain-free movement of the musculoskeletal system in postural balance."[1] American trained osteopathic physicians define their manipulation treatment goals as follows: "Osteopathic manipulative treatment (OMT) is described as the therapeutic application of manually guided forces by an osteopathic physician to improve physiologic function and support homeostasis, which is accomplished via a variety of techniques."[2]

Ideally, manual treatments can treat the cause of any dysfunction, but they sometimes may be used to alleviate symptoms related to a disease process to help the patient feel better. When combined with medical treatment, manual treatments reduce the requirements for medications that often cause unwanted side effects.[3-5]

In summary, the goals of manual treatment include the following:

- To improve posture and motion
- To restore joint range of motion and flexibility
- To improve circulation and venous and lymphatic drainage (i.e., fluid flow)
- To alleviate myofascial tender points
- To integrate central and peripheral motor control mechanisms
- To improve the patient's responsiveness to stress and medications
- To maximize the patient's health potential

Dosage Guidelines
The dose of treatment entails the amount of time spent with the patient and the amount of energy expended by the patient during the procedure. Patients with acute illnesses require smaller, more frequent doses at first. Chronic conditions may require larger doses, meaning more time spent using a variety of techniques, including direct and combined techniques, which may entail patient participation as part of the treatment.

Frequency of Treatment
Frequency varies for the ambulatory patient with a primary musculoskeletal problem.

- For an acute condition, treatment is usually once or twice weekly.
- For a chronic condition, treatment is usually once or twice monthly.
- Re-evaluate before and after each treatment to determine the treatment response, the need for follow-up, and the next treatment interval.
- If no improvement occurs from treatment to treatment despite adjusting the frequency interval between treatments, re-evaluate the diagnosis and management plan.
- As the patient improves, decrease the frequency of treatments.

Duration of Treatment
The duration of treatment refers to how long (e.g., days, weeks, months, years) a patient should be treated with manual methods for any given problem. The following are general guidelines:

- For acute conditions, treatment should continue until normal function is restored or the condition is returned to baseline or a plateau.

- If unable to effect continued improvement, the practitioner should reassess and adjust the management plan.
- For chronic conditions, the duration of treatment is determined by the nature of the condition and the patient's response and needs.

Maintenance and Prevention

To maintain the goals obtained by manual treatments and prevent recurrence of somatic dysfunctions, the following guidelines are offered:

- Encourage exercises to strengthen and stretch core postural muscles and maximize cardiovascular capacity.
- Educate patients regarding proper postural biomechanics.
- Re-evaluate the musculoskeletal system for evidence of somatic dysfunction at each office visit.
- Incorporate the structural examination into initial office visits, especially as part of a complete history and physical examination.

Methods of Treatment

Although there are many methods of manual treatment, this textbook covers these six basic methods:

1. Soft tissue techniques
2. Articulatory techniques
3. Myofascial release techniques
4. Muscle energy techniques
5. Functional technique techniques
6. Counterstrain techniques

Soft Tissue Techniques
Classification
- Soft tissue techniques are direct action techniques.

Definition
- Soft tissue techniques are applied to hypertonic muscles and involve lateral stretching, linear stretching, deep pressure, traction, and separation of muscle origin and insertion while monitoring tissue responses and motion changes by palpation.[2]
- Soft tissue techniques are procedures directed against tissues other than skeletal or arthrodial elements.
- Soft tissue techniques are passive techniques that are performed by the practitioner while the patient is relaxed.

Mechanisms
Soft tissue techniques relax hypertonic muscles by several mechanisms.
- Sustained pressure and stretch fatigue hypertonic muscles.
- Alteration of afferent information from stretch receptors in the tendons and muscle spindles attenuates the efferent limb of the myotatic reflex (i.e., the alpha motor neurons and gamma efferents).
- Increased blood flow helps to remove toxic metabolic waste products that build up from sustained muscle contraction.

Increased warmth is felt in the soft tissues after application of soft tissue procedures due to increased blood flow.

- Connective tissue is separated, and crosslinks are broken by the forces used, the stimulation of glycosaminoglycans (GAGs), and the increase in water content in the connective tissue matrix; these effects increase compliance and pliability of the soft tissues.[6]

Applications

- Soft tissue techniques are used to lengthen or relax hypertonic muscles and connective tissue.
- These techniques are often used to loosen the periarticular soft tissues in preparation for more definitive and localized joint-specific techniques.

Procedure

- The procedure entails the following steps:
  1. The patient should be as relaxed as possible. Most of the muscles can be treated with the patient supine or prone. The positioning must not cause the patient pain or any uncomfortable feeling.
  2. The practitioner applies the soft tissue manipulation while monitoring (i.e., palpatory feedback) the tissue response and motion changes.
  3. Manual traction (i.e., tension) is applied in one of the following directions:

     Longitudinal traction (i.e., in the direction of the muscle fibers) or pull at one or both ends of the muscle, separating origin and insertion (i.e., directly stretching the muscle)

     A push or pull on the muscle perpendicular to the long axis of the muscle (i.e., stretching the muscle as if pulling or pushing a bow string)
  4. The force should have the following characteristics:

     It should be slowly applied. Suddenly applied tension may result in increased resistance.

     It should have low intensity.

     It should be of sufficient duration to give the desired tissue response, which often involves fatigue of the muscle.

     Slow, long-duration stretching may be more effective when treating more fibrous connective tissue such as fascia or ligaments.

     Changes in soft tissue structure (i.e., GAGs and crosslinks in the connective tissue) usually require a minimal stretch of 20 to 30 seconds.

     It should be released slowly.
  5. The tension or pull is applied gradually and then slowly released, as stretch (i.e., relaxation) is sensed. Pressure or tension is reapplied rhythmically at the same or another point or area.
  6. A counterpressure may be used to increase effectiveness.
  7. The tissues are usually not pressed directly against bone.
  8. The practitioner should not allow the hand or fingers to slide or rub over the skin.
  9. Operator fatigue can be avoided by using proper postural mechanics, leverage, and body weight rather than muscle force.
  10. The fingertip pads, palms, and thenar or hypothenar eminences are most commonly used to contact the soft tissues, although an elbow occasionally is used for deep pressure, as in the cases of large spastic muscles such as the gluteus medius or resistant trigger points.
  11. Deeper pressure is used when treating the more deeply located tissues.

Improving Efficacy

- Move slowly into the restrictive barrier and wait for the tissues to begin to relax before proceeding with increasing force. Some practitioners refer to this as *tissue speed*, meaning the speed at which the tissues respond best or at which they can relax and comply with the forces provided by the practitioner.
- Instead of working on one specific area over and over, move up and down through a region with each application of force to avert having too much blood flow build up in one area.
- When working on the paraspinal muscles with the patient in the prone position, the table height should be below waist level to gain the mechanical advantage of trunk movement to apply the forces necessary to get the tissues to relax. Do not use arm muscle forces, because this approach expends too much energy and leads to fatigue; keep the elbows extended and locked during application of forces against the soft tissues.

Articulatory Techniques
Classification

- Articulatory procedures are direct techniques.

Definition

- Articulatory techniques, also known as springing techniques, are low-velocity, moderate- to high-amplitude direct techniques in which a joint is passively carried toward its physiologic range of motion with the therapeutic goal of moving through any restrictive barriers and improving the range and quality of motion. The activating force is extrinsic and is carried out as a repetitive springing motion or repetitive concentric movement of the joint through a restrictive barrier.[2]

Mechanisms of Articulatory Techniques

- Articulatory techniques mobilize joints, including facets (i.e., zygapophyseal intervertebral joints) within their physiologic ranges of motion. Mobility of restricted joints is improved by stretching tight muscles and myofascial connective tissue.
- Articulatory techniques enhance connective tissue lubrication, produce GAGs, and decrease joint adhesions.
- These methods elicit pain-relieving effects by joint mechanoreceptor activity that stimulate faster-conducting (e.g., group IA) myelinated afferents that "close the gate" on (i.e., inhibit the transmission of) afferent information from slower-conducting afferents (e.g., group C fibers that transmit nociceptive information). Joint manipulation stimulates inhibitory monoamine interneurons within the spinal cord and prevents the transmission of nociception by second-order neurons to the thalamus and somatosensory cortex.[7]

Applications

- Articulatory techniques are used in patients with somatic dysfunction to stretch restricted muscles, ligaments and joint capsules and to decrease myofascial tissue tension, enhance lymphatic flow, and stimulate increased joint circulation.
- Articulatory techniques are particularly valuable as a preparation for an HVLA or thrust technique, but they can be combined with all other manual treatment procedures.
- Very young or very old patients respond very well to articulatory techniques because of the ease of localizing direction and amount of force, as well as the duration of treatment. They are also less likely to experience post-treatment stiffness and discomfort compared with patients treated with HVLA.
- Because the treatment movements are slow, deliberate, and controlled, practitioners can carefully monitor the patient with visual and palpatory feedback to adjust the appropriate conditions.
- For hospitalized patients or patients with respiratory conditions such as infections or obstructive diseases, articulatory techniques may be specifically used to improve thoracic respiratory mechanics through methods such as rib mobilization with the patient in the seated or supine position.
- Articulatory techniques are especially useful in treating transitional zones (e.g., cervicothoracic, thoracolumbar, lumbosacral) that are common areas for somatic dysfunction.

Procedure

- The procedure entails the following steps:
  1. The patient is relaxed and in a position that enables localization of movements at the restricted joint. This can be in any position, but there usually are optimal positions for each joint. The cervical spine is best articulated with the patient supine to prevent a sense of disequilibrium: the thoracic spine with the patient seated, the lumbar spine with the patient seated or sidelying, the ankle joint with the patient supine or seated, the wrist joint and ribs with the patient seated, and the shoulder with the patient sidelying.
  2. The practitioner stands or sits in such a way as to be mechanically efficient and balanced in posture. The practitioner sits at the head of the table for cervical articulatory procedures, sits or stands alongside of the seated patient for thoracic procedures; stands or sits alongside the seated patient and stands to the side of the table for the lateral recumbent patient for lumbar procedures, stands in front of the patient who is seated for wrist or rib articulatory procedures, stands or sits at the end of table for ankle procedures for the supine patient and in front of the seated patient, and stands to the side of the table for shoulder articulatory procedures with the patient sidelying.
  3. The practitioner isolates and stabilizes one bone of the restricted joint and locates the restrictive barrier in one plane at a time.
  4. The other bone of the restricted joint is moved slowly toward its restrictive barrier, moving steadily and smoothly but with not enough force to cause discomfort in the patient. The smooth motion is continued slightly through the restrictive barrier.
  5. The practitioner returns the joint to the middle of its range and then repeats step 4.
  6. Steps 4 and 5 are repeated, extending slightly past the restrictive barrier each time until the physiologic barrier is restored.
  7. The practitioner retests the range of the joint after each set of 10 articulations.
  8. Steps 3 through 6 are repeated for each direction of motion: flexion, extension, sidebending, and rotation to each side and, for the extremities, internal and external rotation, abduction, and adduction.

Improving Efficacy

- Movement must be slow and steady through the restrictive barrier and performed at the speed at which the soft tissues around the joint will comply.
- Improving motion in the primary direction for a particular joint will increase the range in other directions. For example, the occipitoatlantal joint and the L5-S1 joint are primarily flexion-extension joints, and improving flexion-extension ranges will likely increase the sidebending and rotation ranges, which are secondary motions for the joints.
- The patient must be totally relaxed to be able to move the joint through the restrictive barrier without resistance from voluntary muscle contraction.

Myofascial Release
Classification

- MFR procedures can be direct, indirect, or combined.

Definition

- The term *myofascial tissues* refers essentially to all connective tissues of the body, which includes fascia surrounding muscles, muscle tendons, ligaments, capsules and their membranes, and the linings of body cavities.
- MFR procedures are manual medicine treatments in which the practitioner identifies resistant or tight myofascial tissues in a particular body region or related to a localized muscle spasm and uses direct or indirect engagement of the restrictive barrier sense to obtain a release of myofascial tension.
- Direct MFR involves engaging a myofascial restrictive barrier, loading the tissue with a constant force until tissue (tension) release occurs.[2]
- Indirect MFR involves guiding the dysfunctional tissues along the path of least resistance until free movement is achieved.[2]
- The practitioner controls the dose, which is measured in terms of the amount of force and duration of time applied.

Mechanisms

- There are mechanical soft tissue biomechanical principles as well as neuroreflexive principles used to explain the mechanism of effectiveness in MFR procedures.
- Direct MFR techniques cause continued deformation (creep) in the myofascial tissues by using a combination of traction, compression, and twist maneuvers. These procedures may also increase GAGs and the fluid content in the myofascial tissues, which separate the connective tissues and decrease

connective tissue crosslinks, increasing compliance and pliability of the myofascial tissues.[6]

- MFR techniques alter afferent information from proprioceptors in the myofascial tissues that attenuates the efferent limb of the myotatic reflex (i.e., alpha motor neurons and gamma efferents) to effect a change in muscle or myofascial tension.

Applications

- As tolerated by the patient, MFR may be used to address all soft tissue or joint restrictions in patients of all ages.
- MFR procedures can be used in conjunction with other manual medicine procedures.

Procedure

- The procedure entails the following steps:
  1. The practitioner selects a direct, indirect, or combined approach based on the patient's clinical presentation and response of the tissues to the procedure.
  2. The patient can be in any position (i.e., seated, supine, prone, or lateral recumbent) that facilitates the effectiveness of the technique.
  3. The restrictive barrier sense is engaged (i.e., direct action), or the myofascial tissues are moved away from the restrictive barrier (i.e., indirect action).
  4. As the patient's soft tissues respond to the sustained load of the extrinsic force, the practitioner follows the loosening of the patient's myofascial tissues in the direction toward increasing compliance until no further relaxation is felt.
  5. The patient can be asked to assist by tightening opposing muscle groups, holding the breath, or holding body positions that enhance increase tension or release of the myofascial tissues being treated.
  6. A reassessment on provocative mechanical challenge by the practitioner usually shows improved passive motion of the region's myofascial tissues. Typically, affiliated joint range of motion also improves.

Improving Efficacy

- Maintain the tension on the myofascial tissues at the restrictive barrier long enough to allow them to begin to release. Attached tight muscles need to relax, and connective tissue needs to undergo deformation or adaptation to the load applied.
- Follow the response of the tissues to the new restrictive barrier when using direct-action MFR or, in the case of indirect action MFR, away from the restrictive barrier.

Muscle Energy Techniques
Classification

- Muscle energy techniques are classified as direct-action or active techniques in which the patient contributes to the corrective force.

Definition

- Muscle energy treatment entails the patient voluntarily moving the body as specifically directed by the practitioner from a precisely controlled position against a defined resistance by the practitioner.[2]

- There are several types of muscle energy techniques, but those presented in this textbook include the following:
  1. Isometric (most commonly used)
  2. Isotonic
  3. Eccentric or isolytic
  4. Reciprocal (antagonistic) inhibition

- *Isometric* muscle energy technique is a manual medicine treatment procedure that involves the voluntary contraction of patient's muscle or group of muscles in a precisely controlled direction at various levels of intensity against a distinctly executed counterforce applied by the practitioner. The contracted muscle maintains the same length throughout the duration of the contraction. It employs a post-isometric relaxation stretch procedure to lengthen a shortened, contracted, or spastic muscle or to move a bone into its proper position.
- The patient can control the dose, but the practitioner determines how much counterforce the patient should push against.
- Dose is measured in terms of the number of times the procedure is repeated and how much counterforce is used by the practitioner against which the patient is instructed to push during one treatment session, such as 2 pounds of force or two or three fingers of counterforce.
- *Isotonic* muscle energy technique entails voluntary muscle contraction by the patient against a steady but yielding counterforce of the practitioner, allowing the contracted muscle to maintain its tone throughout a range of motion.
- *Eccentric or isolytic* muscle energy technique entails voluntary contraction of patient muscle against a stronger counterforce by the practitioner. As the muscle contracts, it is forced to elongate.
- Antagonistic inhibition muscle energy techniques use isometric forces to reciprocally inhibit antagonistic muscles that are hypertonic. These techniques are useful when isometric technique applied to the hypertonic muscle is ineffectual.

Mechanisms

- Isometric muscle energy techniques reset the intrafusal and extrafusal muscle fiber lengths during the postcontraction relaxation phase; about 2 to 3 seconds after a muscle contracts, there is a refractory period during which the muscle can be passively stretched without the muscle being able to contract or resist this stretch. These techniques decrease alpha motor neuron efferent activity when the muscle is at rest. The stretch reflex is reset to a decreased resting muscle tone and increased resting length of the muscle's fibers.
- Isotonic muscle energy techniques essentially exercise a muscle against resistance to strengthen the fibers (i.e., increase their girth and force of contraction).
- Eccentric or isolytic muscle energy techniques are designed to break collagen crosslinks and fibrous adhesions to improve motion of the affected joints.
- Antagonistic inhibition muscle energy techniques use the agonist-antagonist spinal cord reflex of a hypertonic muscle to reciprocally inhibit the hypertonic muscle tone.
- The patient's muscle effort requires energy, and the process of muscle contraction results in carbon dioxide, lactic acid, and other metabolic waste products that must be transported

and metabolized. The patient frequently experiences some increase in muscle soreness within the first 12 to 36 hours after a muscle energy technique treatment. Muscle energy procedures provide safety for the patient because the activating force is intrinsic and the patient can easily control the dosage (i.e., amount of force applied against the practitioner's counterforce).

Applications
- Muscle energy procedures are used to restore normal motion to joints that are restricted due to somatic dysfunction.
- They can be used alone or in a complementary manner with other manual medicine procedures.
- The most common type used is the isometric muscle energy technique, which can be used to lengthen a shortened, contracted, or spastic muscle or to move a bone into its proper position by holding the bone into which the muscle inserts steady while letting its origin pull the attached bone toward the insertion.
- Isotonic muscle energy techniques are used to strengthen hypotonic muscles.
- Isolytic muscle energy techniques are used to stretch fibrous muscle tissue or lyse adhesions.
- Reciprocal inhibition muscle energy procedures decrease the tone of hypertonic antagonist muscles.
- Muscle energy procedures can influence the function of any articulation in the body that can be moved directly or indirectly by voluntary muscle action.

Procedures
- Each *isometric muscle energy* treatment entails the following steps:
  1. The patient's position is selected in consideration of the patient's comfort, the mechanical advantage needed to treat the somatic dysfunction, and the effectiveness of the technique in a particular position.
  2. The practitioner's position is selected to maximize the efficiency of the applied forces with the least amount of practitioner strain or effort.
  3. The practitioner's handhold and contact points on the patient vary according to the dysfunctional joint that needs to be treated.
  4. The practitioner passively motion tests (e.g., flexion or extension, rotation, side bending to both sides) and locates the restrictive barriers in three planes.
  5. The practitioner then supports the patient's relaxed body in the position that brings the restricted joint up to its restrictive barrier.
  6. The practitioner instructs the patient to apply an intrinsic, or active, isometric muscle contraction force against the practitioner's equal counterforce using the tight restrictive muscles. This is in the direction of the midline resting position, which is also toward the direction of ease of motion or diagnostic position of the dysfunctional joint. However, no motion occurs because the practitioner is holding the patient's body position steady with equal counterforce.

7. This isometric contraction is held for 5 to 6 seconds.
8. The patient is then directed to fully relax this effort.
9. The practitioner then engages the new restrictive motion barrier in all three planes at the dysfunctional joint. This resets the resting length of the shortened, tight muscles.
10. Steps 5 through 8 are repeated three to five times with a final stretch of the dysfunctional joint into the restrictive barriers (e.g., flexion or extension, rotation, sidebending) after the final repetition.
11. The patient is retested.
- The amount of patient effort may vary from a minimal muscle twitch to a maximum muscle contraction.
- The duration of the effort is usually 3 to 5 seconds.
- Typically, the procedure is repeated three to five times during one treatment session before rechecking the joint motion.
- Each *isotonic muscle energy* treatment entails the following steps:
  1. The patient is resting in a stable position.
  2. The practitioner isolates the muscle to be strengthened.
  3. The patient contracts the muscle, moving the affected joint through its range of motion.
  4. The practitioner maintains a sustained and steady counterforce that is weaker than the patient's force, allowing a full range of joint motion against resistance. Because the amount of resistance is constant, the patient's force of contraction also remains constant.
  5. Steps 3 and 4 are repeated several times until the desired strengthening effect is achieved.
  6. The practitioner can increase the resistive counterforce to the level of the patient's tolerance and responsiveness.
  7. Strength of the muscle is retested after three to five isotonic contractions.
- The *isolytic or eccentric contraction muscle energy* procedure entails the following steps:
  1. The patient is resting in a stable position.
  2. The practitioner isolates the muscle to be stretched.
  3. The patient contracts the muscle, moving the affected joint through its range of motion.
  4. The practitioner overcomes the patient's contraction and takes the joint into the opposite direction, lengthening the muscle (eccentric) while the patient is contracting it. The practitioner's counterforce is stronger than the patient's force.
  5. Steps 3 and 4 are repeated several times until the desired lengthening effect is achieved.
  6. The practitioner can retest the length and compliance of the muscle after three to five eccentric contractions.
- The *reciprocal inhibition muscle energy* procedure entails the following steps:
  1. The patient is resting in a stable position.
  2. The practitioner isolates the antagonist muscle group to the ones that are hypertonic. For example, if the right rotators of a joint are hypertonic, the left rotators are isolated to set up the antagonistic contraction. If the flexors are hypertonic, the extensors are used.
  3. The patient is instructed to contract the antagonist muscle with about 3 pounds of force and hold for 3 to 7 seconds against an unyielding practitioner counterforce.

4. The practitioner maintains a sustained and steady counter-force that is equal to the patient's force, creating a sustained isometric contraction and inhibition of the hypertonic antagonist muscle.
5. Steps 3 and 4 are repeated several times until the desired relaxation of the hypertonic muscle is achieved.
6. The practitioner can retest the relaxation and compliance of the muscle and its affected joints after three to five isometric contractions.

Improving Efficacy
- Monitor motion with palpation to ensure the forces are localized to the dysfunctional joint being treated.
- Have the patient use the least amount of force necessary to obtain the desired goal of treatment.
- Use the least amount of counterforce necessary to assist the patient in also using less force, reducing the potential for muscle soreness. Consider using only a fingertip or two for the patient to push against initially.
- Retest all planes of motion after treatment, even though only one or two main motions were treated.
- For isometric muscle energy treatment
  1. Ensure the muscle contraction is held for at least 3 seconds, although up to 7 seconds sometimes may be necessary to get the proper recruitment of muscle fibers to achieve the desired result.
  2. It may not be necessary to localize the restrictive barrier in all three planes[8]; consider the main motion of a particular joint, and use the restrictive barrier in that direction. For example, the C1-2 (atlantoaxial) cervical joint primarily rotates, and it can be treated solely in rotation.
  3. Allow the patient to totally relax before repositioning to the new restrictive barrier.
  4. Wait for 2 seconds after the patient completely relaxes the muscle before applying the stretch to take full advantage of the refractory muscle spindle activity.

Functional Technique
Classification
- Functional techniques are classified as indirect action procedures in which both the practitioner and patient contribute to the activating force.

Definition
- Functional methods involve finding the dynamic position of balance (of tension of periarticular tissues) of a dysfunctional joint and applying a passive guiding force to relieve the dysfunction.
- The dysfunctional area is palpated during the procedure to obtain a continuous feedback of the physiologic response to the passively induced motion. The practitioner guides the dysfunctional part to create a decreasing sense of tissue resistance (i.e., increased compliance).[2]
- Functional technique is a manual medicine treatment procedure in which the practitioner monitors the tissue tension around a restricted joint while attempting to decrease this tension by passively moving adjacent body regions or limbs and has the patient use respiratory cooperation to further enhance compliance and ease of the monitored soft tissues around the joint.
- The practitioner controls the dose, which is measured in terms of number of times the procedure is repeated.
- Duration of the procedure is 3 to 15 seconds.

Mechanisms
- Functional technique is an afferent reduction technique; the stimulation of joint and soft tissue afferents from mechanoreceptors, proprioceptors, and nociceptors is diminished as much as possible by finding positions of ease and relaxation of soft tissues around a restricted joint.
- The lack of afferent information going into the spinal cord extinguishes the reflexive efferent discharge (i.e., alpha motor neurons), and the myofascial tissues innervated at that spinal cord level become compliant, relaxed, and desensitized.
- The facilitated, or sensitized, spinal cord becomes quiescent and normalized.

Applications
- Functional technique is used in all patient populations, including post-trauma patients, children, women during pregnancy, and elderly, ill, or frail patients.
- It is used to calm facilitated or sensitized spinal cord segments that are involved in somatic or visceral reflexes.
- It can be used in conjunction with other manual medicine procedures.

Procedure
- Diagnose a dysfunctional segment or joint by palpation and passive motion tests.
  1. Identify areas of somatic dysfunction (i.e., facilitated or sensitized segment) by shearing and motion testing.
  2. The dysfunctional segment has a distinct palpatory and response to motion characteristics. Passive motion in one direction induces reflex tightening in the dysfunctional segment, but passive motion in the opposite direction induces reflex loosing, or increased compliance.
  3. Adjacent body regions or limbs are often employed to elicit a tissue tension or relaxation response, also called *bind-ease*, at the dysfunctional segment.
- Functional technique is performed according to the following guidelines[9]:
  1. While carefully focusing attention on the tissue tension in the monitored tissue, the practitioner passively induces six motions (around three axes and in three planes), one direction at a time.
  2. The three axial (i.e., rotating around an axis) motions are
     Flexion and extension
     Sidebending left or right
     Rotation left or right
  3. The three translatory motions are
     Lateral translation to the left or right
     Anteroposterior translation
     Inferosuperior translation
  4. Motion directions are selected such that there is an immediately decreasing sense of resistance to pressure at the

finger pads monitoring the response at the tense dysfunctional segment.

5. Motions are away from the direction in which increasing resistance is encountered.

6. The introduction of motion in any one direction is minimal (i.e., not full range), with minimal forces applied; just enough motion is introduced to elicit a palpable response in the tissues being monitored.

7. Single elements of axial and translatory directions that elicit the most relaxation of the monitored tissues are combined ("stacked"), creating an eventual smooth arc of passive body movement.

8. The order of introduction of these elements is not important.

9. The final step of the indirect procedure involves request for a specific direction or phase of active respiration (inhalation or exhalation), which contributes further to the increasing ease.

10. For inhalation, the request is for the patient to take a deep breath slowly and hold it briefly while the practitioner fine-tunes the movements that allow for the maximum compliance in the tense tissues being monitored.

11. If unsuccessful at relieving the somatic dysfunction, the practitioner can repeat the procedure and again introduce the six motions into increasing compliance during the phase of respiration that produces maximum compliance.

12. The practitioner then retests.

Improving Efficacy

- Take the time to ensure that the correct direction of each of the six motions and the correct phase of respiration are identified and used to get maximal afferent reduction.
- Refine the six directions of motion while the patient is breathing in the phase of respiration that increases compliance of the monitored tissues.
- Continuously induce passive motion into the directions that enhance increasing compliance of the tense tissues being monitored while the patient is breathing as directed (in contrast to holding a position as is done with counterstrain, for example).

Counterstrain
Classification

- Counterstrain techniques are classified as indirect action in which the passive positioning itself contributes the corrective force.

Definition

- Counterstrain is a manual treatment procedure that applies a position of mild strain in the direction exactly opposite to that of the inappropriate strain reflex that created the somatic dysfunction and related tender points to inhibit it and resolve the dysfunction. This is accomplished by specific directed positioning around the point of tenderness to achieve the desired therapeutic response.[2]
- Counterstrain involves passive positioning of the patient such that the tenderness at a tender point is diminished by at least two thirds of its original level.[10]

- The practitioner controls the dose, which is measured in terms of the number of times the procedure is repeated and how many tender points are treated in a region during one session. No more than three points per region per session is recommended for the highest efficacy and least side effects.

Mechanisms

- Shorten and relax strained muscles and connective tissue.
- Interrupt inappropriate nociceptive and proprioceptive activity.
- Reduce afferent neuronal activity that facilitated central and peripheral sensitization.

Applications

- These procedures are safely used on almost all patients, even those who have severe osteoporosis, metastatic bone cancer, or acute injuries, unless gently moving the patient into the specific treatment position is contraindicated or not tolerated (e.g., if a patient gets dizzy or lightheaded with neck extension and rotation, placing the patient in this position for 90 seconds to resolve a tender point or cervical somatic dysfunction would not be appropriate).
- Counterstrain can be used in conjunction with other manual medicine procedures.

Procedure

- Counterstrain is performed as follows:

  1. Locate tender points in a region related to somatic dysfunction by using slight digital pressure (one-fourth blanching of the thumb fingernail or less); Table 4.3 and the text describe locations of these points.

  2. A strain is produced in a muscle during an injury, which contracts and prevents movement away from the position of injury. The practitioner must passively place the patient in the position that allows that muscle to release its hypertonic contracted state, which is usually the position in which the muscle or joint was in during the strain injury.

  3. Surrounding muscles also relax as a result of returning the primary muscle strain to its normal resting state.

  4. When the strained muscle is relaxed, the associated tender point decreases in its intensity after about 90 to 120 seconds, which is the time it takes for the spinal cord to abolish the abnormal reflexes maintaining the tender point.

  5. A posterior muscle strain usually has a tender point associated with it on the contralateral anterior side in the same region.

  6. A lateral muscle strain or ligamentous sprain usually has a tender point associated with it on the contralateral side.

  7. Ensure the patient rates the level of tenderness before and after positioning and after treatment to be able to assess improvement (Table 4.4).

  8. Flexing or "folding" the body region involved over the tender point often reduces tenderness. Table 4.5 provides more keys to successful treatment.

Improving Efficacy

- Have the patient rate the pain before positioning.[11]
- Reassess the patient's pain after positioning.

Table 4.3   Determining locations of tender points

Activity	Method
Use somatic dysfunction as a clue.	Perform screening musculoskeletal structural examination.
	Find regions of asymmetric structure, motion, or tissue tension.
	Locate segmental somatic dysfunction in the affected regions.
	Palpate for the tender points within the affected region.
Evaluate and palpate for variations from ideal posture. Patients tend to unconsciously bend their bodies around tender points to shorten and relieve tense myofascial (strained) tissues.	Look at the apex or focal point of the concavity of the patient's position.
	Locate the flattened thoracic kyphotic curve, and look for posterior thoracic tender points.
	Locate the excessive kyphotic curve, and look for anterior thoracic tender points.
Scan for regional tender points. This is based on clinical history and presenting complaints.	Reproduce the initial position of injury.
	Look for tender points around areas of pain.
Use firm but gentle palpation, and apply pressure gradually.	Use a few milligrams of pressure up to 4 kg of force.
	The better conditioned the patient is, the more pressure may need to be applied to elicit tenderness.
Determine if a tender point is clinically significant.	Check the same spot on the opposite side.
	Check for other tender points in the general area.
Check for any other pathology that may induce the tenderness. These areas are not related to neuromusculoskeletal tender points.	Examine for local areas of irritation, infection, inflammation, and underlying visceral disease.

Table 4.4   Quantifying the level of tenderness

Activity	Procedure
Patient directly assesses the pain.	While applying firm pressure on the tender point, the practitioner asks the patient to express his or her level of tenderness.
	The pressure is then released, and the practitioner uses only light contact to maintain location of the point while passively adjusting the patient's position to further decrease the tenderness.
	On obtaining a new position, the practitioner again gradually applies firm pressure to the tender point and asks the patient to rate the level of tenderness.
	Positioning and questioning continues until the tenderness is reduced by at least 70% or is gone.
Patient uses a pain scale.	Different scales may be used:
	Scale of 0 to 10, with 10 being equal to the initial tenderness and 0 representing no pain. This may be expressed verbally or drawn on a prepared line scale.
	Scale of 0 to 100
	Whole numbers and even percentages or fractions can be used by the patient to indicate the amount of tenderness remaining, as the practitioner continues to reposition the patient around the tender point.
	These are examples of how to instruct the patient:
	"If you had one dollar's worth of pain when we started, how much money do you have left?"
	"Tell me if the pain is better, worse, or the same."

Table 4.5   Keys to treating a tender point with counterstrain

1. The closer the tender point is to the midline, the more flexion or extension is required for treatment.
2. The more distant the tender point is from the midline, the more sidebending and rotation is required for treatment.
3. Treatment of the most intensely painful tender point in a region often alleviates less intense tender points within that region.
4. Reduce tenderness by placing the patient in a position of maximal comfort.
5. The patient must be able and willing to relax his or her muscles.
6. Fine tune the position until the tenderness has been reduced by at least 70% (preferably by 100%).
7. Hold the position for 90 seconds (120 seconds for rib tender points).
8. Maintain continuous light contact with the tender point during treatment so that the retest occurs in exactly the same spot. Firm pressure is not required for treatment; firm pressure is applied only when trying to elicit tenderness.
9. Slowly return the patient to a neutral position without the patient's muscular assistance.
10. Retest the tender point.

- Reassess the patient's pain after treatment.
- Reduce the tenderness to 30% or less than its original level.
- Return the patient to the resting position passively and slowly to prevent stimulation of nociceptors or proprioceptors.

CHOICE OF PROCEDURE

Numerous factors influence the practitioner's decision to use one type of manual technique over another. Some of the main factors include the following:

- Previous or present therapies and their effects
- Acuteness or chronicity of the problem
- Age or tolerance of the patient to active versus passive techniques
- Effectiveness of a particular technique for a specific dysfunction
- General physical condition of the patient
- Preferences of the patient or practitioner
- The practitioner's size and ability
- The response of the tissues to a type of manipulative procedure

The techniques can be used sequentially or combined, depending on the tissue response as perceived by the practitioner.

- Muscle strains that result in muscle spasm can be treated effectively with any of the techniques taught in this textbook. It is often prudent to start with soft tissue and then use MFR to get a sense of the degree of irritability of the tissues and calm down hyperirritability. Isometric muscle energy treatment can then be used if a direct-action approach is deemed appropriate for the clinical situation. If the practitioner and patient prefer indirect approaches, indirect MFR, functional, and counterstrain techniques can be employed.
- For functional technique to be effective, there must be a softening or increased compliance of the soft tissues around the dysfunctional joint when the body is moved in one direction and tightening or increased resistance palpated in the tissues when it is moved in the opposite direction.
- For counterstrain to be effective, there must be point tenderness elicited on digital provocation that is relieved by at least 70% with passive body positioning.
- When the muscle is inflamed or the spasm is not responsive to isometric muscle energy procedures, antagonistic inhibition muscle energy or deep inhibitory pressure of the muscle motor end plate in the belly of the muscle is usually effective.
- When there is myofascial hypertonicity throughout an entire body region, starting with MFR and soft tissue techniques is often most productive.
- Somatic dysfunction is often associated with tenderness on digital provocation of the bony and soft tissues in its proximity. This tenderness may not go away after treatment of the dysfunction with soft tissue, articulatory, MFR, muscle energy, or functional techniques. However, persistent tender points can be treated with counterstrain procedures if the degree of tenderness significantly changes (decreases to less than 30% of the initial pain evaluation) with passive positional changes.

- In some patients, especially those who are ill and weak, the practitioner may select to use functional or counterstrain and other indirect techniques first because they do not require the patient to expend energy.
- Paraspinal myofascial tensions surrounding dysfunctional segments can be assessed and treated with myofascial or soft tissue procedures.
- If the soft tissue surrounding a segmental dysfunction or group of dysfunctions tightens, or binds, in response to passive movement of the head or extremities, functional treatments are indicated.

CLINICAL PEARLS

- *Control* body position and forces (intrinsic, or patient generated, and extrinsic, or practitioner generated).
- *Balance* posture for relaxation of the patient and practitioner.
- *Localize* forces for accuracy.

Spinal somatic dysfunction can be challenging to treat. It is common to have a single segment dysfunction (i.e., type II mechanics) within or at the inferior or superior end of a group (i.e., type I mechanics) spinal somatic dysfunction. Usually, type II dysfunctions are more acute and symptomatic, and type I dysfunctions are compensatory and chronic. However, because it is sometimes difficult to discern which one is primary and which is compensatory, the practitioner should treat one type of dysfunction, reassess the findings, and treat the other dysfunction if it is still present.

REFERENCES

1. Greenman PE: Principles of Manual Medicine, 3rd ed. Philadelphia, Lippincott Williams & Wilkins, 2003.
2. Educational Council on Osteopathic Principles: Glossary of osteopathic terminology. In Ward RC (ed): Foundations for Osteopathic Medicine, 2nd ed. Philadelphia, Lippincott Williams & Wilkins, 2003.
3. Andersson GB, Lucente T, Davis AM, et al: A comparison of osteopathic spinal manipulation with standard care for patients with low back pain [published correction appears in N Engl J Med 342:817, 2000]. N Engl J Med 341:1426-1431, 1999.
4. Noll DR, Shores JH, Gamber RG, et al: Benefits of osteopathic manipulative treatment for hospitalized elderly patients with pneumonia. J Am Osteopath Assoc 100:776-782, 2000.
5. Goldstein FJ, Jeck S, Nicholas AS, et al: Preoperative intravenous morphine sulfate with postoperative osteopathic manipulative treatment reduces patient analgesic use after total abdominal hysterectomy. J Am Osteopath Assoc 105:273-279, 2005.
6. Jones HJ: Somatic dysfunction. In Ward RC (ed): Foundations for Osteopathic Medicine, 2nd ed. Philadelphia, Lippincott Williams & Wilkins, 2003, pp 1153-1161.
7. Skyba DA, Radhakrishnan R, Rohlwing JJ, et al: Joint manipulation reduces hyperalgesia by activation of monoamine receptors but not opioid or GABA receptors in the spinal cord. Pain 106:159-168, 2003.
8. Mitchell FL Jr, Mitchell PKG: The Muscle Energy Manual, vol 3. East Lansing, MI, MET Press, 1999.
9. Johnston WL, Friedman HD, Eland D: Functional Methods, 2nd ed. Indianapolis, IN, American Academy of Osteopathy, 2005.
10. Jones LH: Strain-Counterstrain. Indianapolis, IN, American Academy of Osteopathy, 1995.
11. Glover JC, Rennie PR: Strain and counterstrain techniques. In Ward RC (ed): Foundations for Osteopathic Medicine, 2nd ed. Philadelphia, Lippincott Williams & Wilkins, 2003, pp 1002-1016.

CHAPTER 5

Mechanical Low Back Pain

DEFINITION

- Pain in the posterior lumbar spine, sacral spine, or paraspinal soft tissues is of musculoskeletal origin.
- It is characterized by the presence of muscle spasm, decreased range of motion, and pain that is worse with movement and better with rest.
- It can be associated with tendonitis, trigger points, or joint inflammation.
- There is a lack of systemic pathology to account for the pain.

EPIDEMIOLOGY

Age

- Simple mechanical LBP occurs in people 10 to 64 years old; the highest clinical prevalence is observed in those between 55 and 64 years old.
- Disabling LBP occurs most often in people between 35 and 54 years old.
- Between 30% and 50% of teenagers 13 to 18 years old have LBP.[1,2]

Gender

- Low back pain (LBP) affects males and females equally.

Prevalence

- Approximately 80% of adults have LBP sometime in their lifetime. Lifetime prevalence estimates are 50% to 85%.[2]
- Up to 50% of the population experiences LBP each year. The 1-year prevalence rates are 10% to 50%.[2,3] Using data from the National Health Interview Survey, the annual prevalence of back pain in America (work related and non–work related), was estimated at 17.6%, and the prevalence of lost-workday back pain was approximately 4.6%.[3,4]
- About one fourth of American adults have LBP at any given time. The international point prevalence rates are 6% to 35%.[2]

- LBP is the most common reason for patients to see a doctor or health care practitioner for a musculoskeletal dysfunction. LBP is the third most commonly reported symptom. It is second most common pain complaint; headache is the first.

Natural Clinical Course

- In 90% of cases, an acute episode of LBP resolves within 6 weeks, and another 5% resolve by the end of 12 weeks.
- When LBP is accompanied by sciatica neuralgia (i.e., radiating pain down the posterior leg into the heel or lateral and plantar foot), 50% recover within 1 month.[5]
- Researchers and clinicians categorize LBP as acute if symptoms last for less than 6 weeks, subacute if between 6 and 12 weeks, and chronic if longer than 3 months.
- One third of patients with acute LBP will have a recurrent, intermittent, and episodic problem.[2]

Effect on Society

- LBP causes more disability among working-age adults than any other disability.
- LBP is the second most frequent cause of worker absenteeism[4] and the most costly ailment of working-age adults in the United States.[2]
- The average cost of a single work-related back injury is $8000,[6] and with 1 million cases nationally per year, the minimal direct cost is approximately $8 billion.[3] The combined direct and indirect costs of LBP disability in the United States is estimated at $50 billion.[3]
- Costs of care for patients with LBP are higher for older patients and patients with higher pain at baseline, and costs are lower for patients with lower education levels and those with higher physical and emotional functioning.[7]

Risk Factors

- The most common causes of mechanical LBP are bending, twisting, and lifting movements with inefficient biomechanical postures, trauma, and prolonged repetitive activities, including prolonged standing.[2]

- The strongest known predictor of a future episode of LBP is the history of previous episodes.[2]

FUNCTIONAL ANATOMY

Lumbar Region

- There are five lumbar vertebrae (Fig. 5.1). The contiguous superior and inferior surfaces of the vertebral bodies are held together by intervertebral discs. The lumbar vertebrae increase progressively in height and in circumference from L1 to L5, with L5 being the largest of the lumbar vertebrae (Fig. 5.2).
- Each vertebra consists of two components: the body and the vertebral arch (Fig. 5.3). The vertebral arch is the portion that extends posteriorly from the vertebral body and that helps to formulate the vertebral foramen. The vertebral arch protects the spinal cord and the meninges, which are enclosed within the vertebral canal. The arch consists of two pedicles that extend posteriorly from the vertebral body and continue posteriorly to form the two laminae. The laminae then join at the midline. Several processes are part of the vertebral arch. On each side, at the junction of the pedicle and the lamina, there extends a transverse process, as well as a superior process and an inferior articular process. The superior and inferior articular processes have facets that formulate articulations with neighboring vertebrae. The transverse processes allow for attachment of muscles and ligaments. The spinous process extends posteriorly from the junction of the two laminae at the midline (see Fig. 5.3).
- The vertebrae are able to articulate with each other by two types of joints. Fibrocartilaginous joints lie between the vertebral bodies, and synovial joints exist between the vertebral arches. There are ligaments associated with each of these types

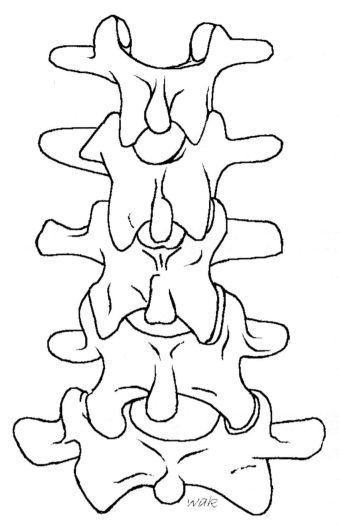

Figure 5.2 Posterior view of the lumbar vertebrae.

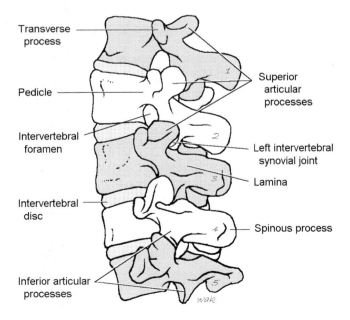

Figure 5.1 Lateral view of the lumbar vertebrae.

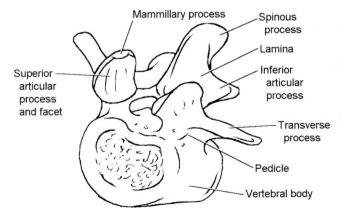

Figure 5.3 Superolateral view of a typical lumbar vertebra.

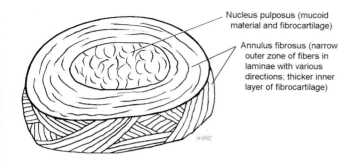

Figure 5.4 Lumbar intervertebral disc.

of joints. The fibrocartilaginous joint between vertebral bodies is essentially the inner vertebral disc (Fig. 5.4). The disc resists displacement of vertebrae on one another while at the same time allowing for some movement between vertebrae. The disc dissipates forces that are transmitted along the vertebral column. The disc consists of a fibrocartilaginous ring, called the annulus fibrosis, and an inner more gelatinous type of mass, called the nucleus pulposus.

- Several ligaments are associated with the lumbar vertebral bodies and intervertebral joints. The anterior and posterior longitudinal ligaments run in an uninterrupted fashion on the respective surfaces of the vertebral bodies. These ligaments resist anterior and posterior displacement of the vertebrae on one another. The laminae and the spinous and transverse processes of the vertebrae also have ligaments that run between them. The ligamentum flavum connects the laminae of adjacent vertebrae. A thin intraspinous ligament attaches along the superior and inferior portions of spinous processes. The supraspinous ligament is a stronger ligament that connects the tips of the spinous processes. Intertransverse ligaments connect the transverse processes of adjacent vertebrae.

- The musculature associated with the lumbar spine can be divided into posterior and anterior groups. The posterior muscles include the superficial, intermediate, and deep muscle layers (Figs. 5.5 to 5.7). The roof of the superficial layer consists of the lumbodorsal fascia, which stabilizes the thoracolumbar and pelvic regions and enables a firm attachment for the latissimus dorsi muscles that insert onto the humerus (see Fig. 5.5). The intermediate layer includes the erector spinae muscle group, which is made up of the iliocostalis, longissimus, and the spinalis muscles (see Fig. 5.7). These muscles can function bilaterally to produce extension of the lumbar spine and can function in a unilateral fashion to provide ipsilateral sidebending or lateral flexion. The deep layer contains the quadratus lumborum muscle, which functions in a bilateral fashion to produce lumbar extension and unilaterally to produce lateral flexion. This layer also contains the multifidi, rotatores, and intertransversarii muscles that help to control the movements of the individual vertebrae relative to one another. They also may function bilaterally to produce extension of the vertebrae and can function unilaterally to produce ipsilateral lateral flexion with contralateral rotation.

- The piriformis muscle functions primarily as an external rotator of the femur and aids in abduction of femur. Hypertonicity of

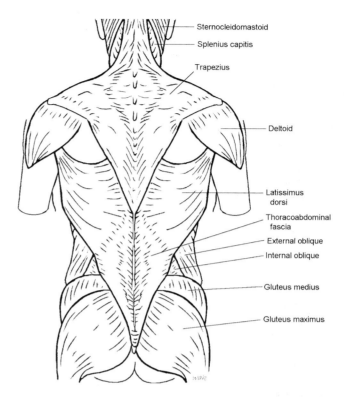

Figure 5.5 The superficial back muscles. With permission from Gray's Anatomy 35th British Edition, Saunders Co., Philadelphia, 1973:533

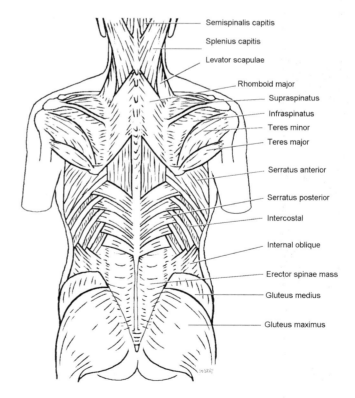

Figure 5.6 The intermediate back muscles. With permission from Gray's Anatomy 35th British Edition, Saunders Co., Philadelphia, 1973:533

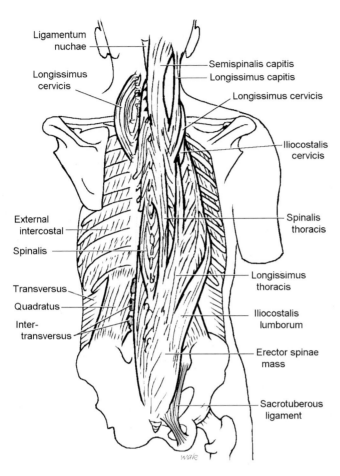

Figure 5.7   The intermediate (right side) and deep (left side) back muscles.

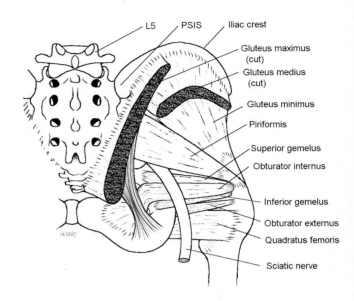

Figure 5.8   The piriformis muscle and its relation to the sciatic nerve. PSIS, posterior superior iliac spine. With permission from Travell JG and Simons DG. Myofascial Pain and Dysfunction. The Trigger Point Manual. Volume II. The Lower Extremities. Baltimore: Williams and Wilkins 1992:91.

this muscle may produce irritation of the sciatic nerve, resulting in low back and gluteal pain syndromes (Fig. 5.8).

- Anteriorly, the abdominal muscles generally act together to produce flexion of the lumbar spine (Fig. 5.9). The external oblique muscle (see Fig. 5.9B) functions unilaterally to produce rotation of the vertebral bodies to the contralateral side while the internal oblique muscle functions unilaterally to produce rotation of the vertebral bodies to the ipsilateral side (see Fig 5.6). The psoas muscle functions as a hip flexor, but when the hips are fixed in position, the psoas can act as a lumbar flexor muscle (Fig. 5.10).
- The lumbar nerve roots form the lumbar plexus. This plexus is positioned anterior to the transverse processes of the lumbar vertebrae and posterior to the psoas major muscle. The plexus is made up of the ventral rami of L1 through L4, with the first lumbar nerve also receiving a branch from the T12 spinal nerve.

Pelvic Region

- The two innominate bones and the sacrum form the bony pelvis. The components of the pelvis are described in this section.

Innominates

- Each innominate bone is formed by the conjoining of three parts: the ilium, the ischium, and the pubis (Fig. 5.11). The ilium has a wing-shaped appearance. The upper margin of the ilium is called the iliac crest. The anterior and posterior terminations of the ilium are the anterior superior iliac spine (ASIS) and the posterior superior iliac spine (PSIS), respectively. Generally, the ASIS is palpable and visible as a prominence. The PSIS is also palpable and is usually marked by the presence of a dimple in the skin. The PSISs are level with the plane of S2 and can be used to locate the position of the sacroiliac joints. The superior-most portion of the iliac crests is level with the spinous process of L4.
- The ischium forms the most posteroinferior portion of the innominate bone. Its major landmark, the ischial tuberosity, can be palpated through the soft tissues of the buttock. The sacrotuberous ligament runs from this tuberosity to the sacrum. The ramus projects forward from the body of the ischium, and the ischial spine projects backward and somewhat medially. The sacrospinous ligament extends from this spine to the sacrum.
- The pubis forms the anterior portion of the pelvis. The bodies of the two pubic bones articulate anteriorly to form the pubic symphysis. From each pubic bone there extends a superior ramus that joins the ilium and ischium near the acetabulum and an inferior ramus that joins with the ramus of the ischium. The pubic rami, along with the ischium and its ramus, form the boundaries of the obturator foramen. The superior surface of the body of the pubis is known as the pubic crest. This crest terminates just lateral to the midline at the pubic tubercle. The inguinal ligament runs from the ASIS to the pubic tubercle.

Sacrum

- The sacrum is a large, triangular bone formed by the fusion of five sacral vertebrae (Fig. 5.12). It is located at the posterosuperior

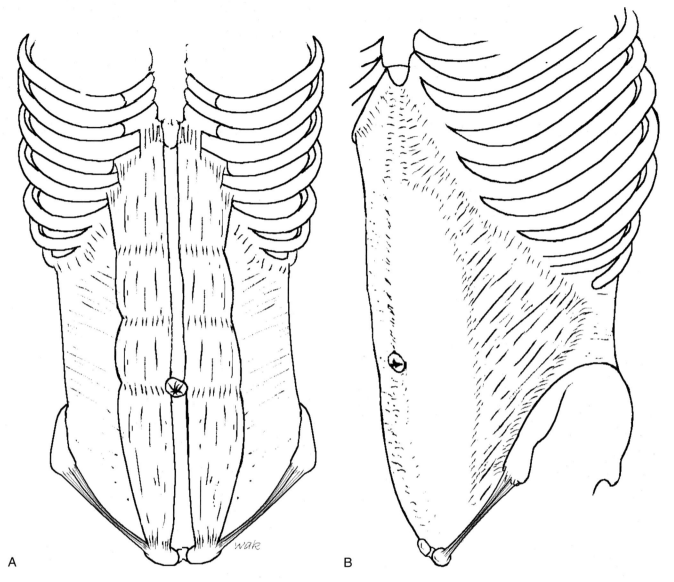

Figure 5.9 **A**, The rectus abdominis muscle. **B**, The external oblique abdominal muscles. With permission from Simons DG, Travell JG, Simons LS: Myofascial Pain and Dysfunction, Vol. I: Upper Half of the Body, Second Edition, Baltimore, Williams and Wilkins, 1999:948-949.

part of the pelvis and is situated like a wedge between the two innominate bones of the pelvis. The inferior portion of the sacrum is narrow and blunted to form an apex, which articulates with the coccyx. The superior portion consists of a wide base with articulatory processes for the fifth lumbar vertebra. The sacrum is curved longitudinally so that it forms a convex posterior surface and a concave anterior surface.

- The dorsal surface of the sacrum displays a midline raised area, known as the median sacral crest, which also bears with it four spinous tubercles. Below the fourth tubercle is a gap in the posterior wall of the sacral canal known as the sacral hiatus (see Fig. 5.12).
- Four pairs of sacral foramina transmit the ventral rami of the upper four sacral spinal nerves (Fig. 5.13).

- The lower portion of the sacrum curves medially, and the point at which this change of direction occurs is known as the inferior lateral angle (ILA). Each lateral surface of the sacrum reveals an articular surface shaped somewhat like an inverted L. This surface joins in articulation with the ilium. When articulated with the ilia, a depression known as the sacral sulcus can be palpated along each sacroiliac joint just medial to the PSIS of each ilium (Fig. 5.14).
- A number of important ligaments are associated with the sacrum (Fig. 5.15). The interosseous sacroiliac ligament is the chief ligament joining the sacrum to the ilium. It is a large ligament, consisting of superficial and deep layers. The dorsal sacroiliac ligament overlies the interosseous ligament and extends from the lateral margins of the sacrum obliquely to

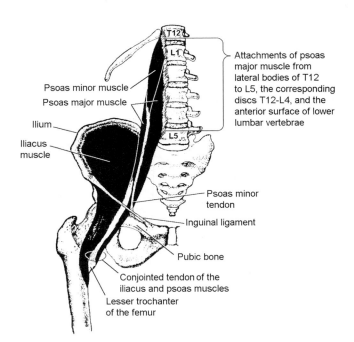

Figure 5.10 The iliopsoas muscle. With permission from Travell JG and Simons DG. Myofascial Pain and Dysfunction. The Trigger Point Manual. Volume II. The Lower Extremities. Baltimore: Williams and Wilkins 1992:91.

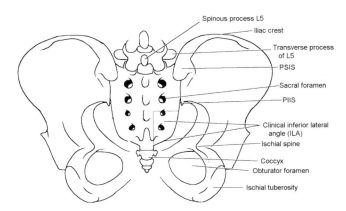

Figure 5.12 Posterior view of the bony pelvis. PIIS, posterior inferior iliac spine; PSIS, posterior superior iliac spine.

the PSIS and the inner edge of the posterior aspect of the ilium. The ventral sacroiliac ligament performs a similar function, extending from the ventrolateral surface of the sacrum to the mediolateral surface of the ilium.

- The sacrotuberous ligament is attached to the PSISs, the lower transverse tubercles of the sacrum, and the lateral margins of

the lower sacrum and coccyx. It extends inferolaterally and forms a thick band that attaches to the medial aspect of the ischial tuberosity (see Fig. 5.15B).

- The sacrospinous ligament is a smaller, triangular ligament that extends from the spine of the ilium medially to the lateral margins of the sacrum and coccyx. Its fibers are mingled with those of the sacrotuberous ligament.

Variations in Sacral Anatomy

- There are variations in sacral articulations with L5. Both L5 and sacral facets can be asymmetric, with one side facing posteriorly and the other medially. There are crescentic facets and flat facets.
- There is also significant variation in the lateral articular surfaces of the sacrum. The average articular surface is somewhat flat and roughened in appearance. In one variation, this surface is convex anteroposteriorly, whereas in another variation, this surface is concave. A given sacrum can have one type of lateral articular surface on one side and another type on the opposite side. The lateral articular surfaces of the sacrum complement the corresponding surfaces on the innominates. Structural asymmetry can increase the incidence of LBP.

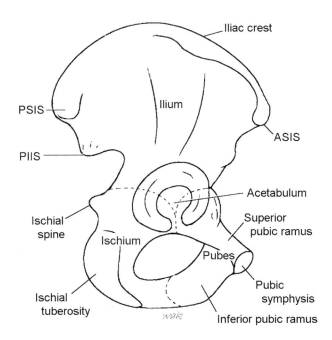

Figure 5.11 Lateral view of the bony pelvis. ASIS, anterior superior iliac spine; PSIS, posterior superior iliac spine.

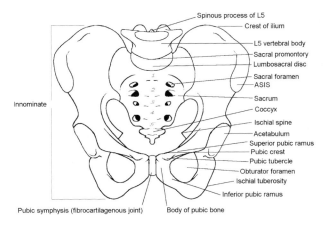

Figure 5.13 Anterior view of the bony pelvis. ASIS, anterior superior iliac spine.

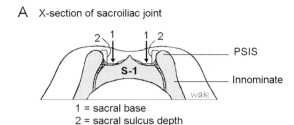

A   X-section of sacroiliac joint

PSIS

Innominate

1 = sacral base
2 = sacral sulcus depth

B   View from the head

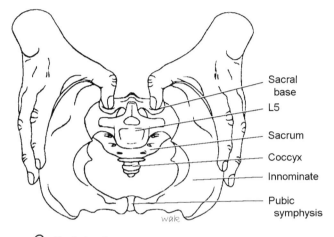

Sacral
base
L5
Sacrum
Coccyx
Innominate
Pubic
symphysis

C   Posterior view

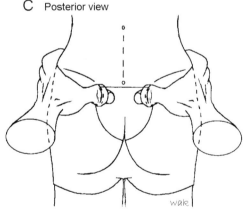

Figure 5.14   Location of the sacral sulcus. **A**, Cross section of the sacroiliac joint. **B**, Superior view of the cross section of the sacral sulcus palpated with practitioner's thumbs. **C**, Palpation of the sacral sulcus medial to the posterior superior iliac spine (PSIS) with the practitioner's thumbs' distal interphalangeal joints flexed.

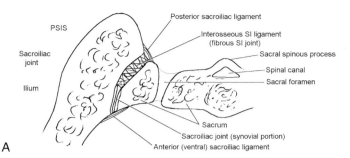

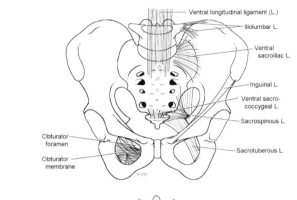

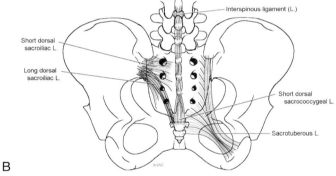

B

Figure 5.15   **A**, Horizontal section showing the sacroiliac ligaments. **B**, Anterior and posterior views of the sacroiliac ligaments. PSIS, posterior superior iliac spine.

PATHOPHYSIOLOGY

- Ninety-seven percent of LBP or leg pain is mechanical (i.e., nonorganic musculoskeletal dysfunction) in origin.[8]
- Degenerative processes of the vertebra and discs, herniated lumbar intervertebral discs, spinal stenosis, osteoporotic compression fractures, and spondylolisthesis are considered etiologically collectively in about 23% of LBP or leg pain patients.[8]

- In less than one third of patients, the cause of acute LBP is pathologic (Table 5.1).
- In 2% of patients, LBP is referred pain of visceral origin.[8]
- Although there often is overlap of etiologic conditions, at least 70% of LBP is caused by somatic dysfunction.[8]
- Somatic dysfunction is characterized by segmental *a*symmetry of structural position, altered *r*ange of motion (typically segmental restriction), and palpable *t*issue texture abnormalities or *t*enderness (ART or TART).
- Five anatomic sites of somatic dysfunction that cause or exacerbate LBP are amenable to manipulation (Table 5.2).
  1. Lumbar intervertebral joints
  2. Myofascial paraspinal soft tissues
  3. Lumbosacral-pelvic (sacroiliac) joints
  4. Lumbosacral and lumbopelvic ligaments
  5. Ilium-pelvic (iliosacral) joints

Table 5.1   Pathologic causes of low back pain*

Type of Pathophysiology	Examples
Mechanical	Spinal arthritis
	Degenerative or ruptured disc disease
	Facet arthritis
	Fracture
	Spondylolysis
	Spondylolisthesis
	Congenital disorders
	Genetic malformations
	Achondroplasia
Nonmechanical	Viscerogenic
	Renal colic
	Inflammatory bowel disease
	Endometriosis
	Vasculogenic
	Aortic aneurysm
	Ischemic claudication
	Epidural venous anomaly
Neoplastic	Primary tumor
	Myeloma
	Sarcoma
	Neural cancer
	Secondary (metastasis)
	Prostate cancer
	Lung cancer
	Breast cancer
	Kidney cancer
Rheumatologic	Rheumatoid arthritis
	Seronegative spondyloarthropathies
	Ankylosing spondylitis
	Psoriatic arthritis
	Reiter's syndrome
	Behçet's syndrome
	Fibromyalgia
	Polymyalgia rheumatica
Infection	Discitis
	Herpes zoster
	Osteomyelitis
Metabolic	Osteoporosis
	Paget's disease
Psychosocial	Compensable injury
	Seeking disability
	Seeking drugs
Psychiatric	Somatoform disorder
	Delusional disorder
	Depression

*In 30% or less of patients, the cause of acute low back pain is pathologic.

- Somatic dysfunction can be primary[9-11] or result from other comorbid conditions. For example, it can be reactive to underlying anatomic deformations or peripheral or central nervous system aberrations (see Chapter 2).
- The recurrent nature of LBP due to herniated intervertebral disc disease likely results from the body's attempt to compensate for the anatomic defect, which may include hypersensitivity of the neural structures and persistence of inflammatory tissues within the disc tissue, as well as engorgement of venous and lymphatic drainage from the area. The relatively ischemic nature of the fibrotic tissue further compromises the healing process.
  1. Gross changes can be visualized on plain radiographs, computed tomography (CT), and magnetic resonance imaging (MRI).
  2. Microscopic analysis of the intervertebral herniated disc tissues in patients with chronic LBP that required surgical treatment revealed higher incidence of dense granulation tissue and neovascularization into the ruptured areas of the disc, causing chronic inflammation.
  3. The inflammatory granulation tissue likely produces some proinflammatory cytokines and mediators, such as prostaglandin E_2, interleukin-6 (IL-6), and IL-8, that can sensitize the nociceptors within the painful discs.
  4. LBP from herniated discs is thought to occur when the intradiskal pressure increases with trunk motions such as flexion or extension, which stimulates these sensitized nociceptors.[12,13]
- Underlying anatomic short leg, previous traumas, and prior operations complicate the clinical presentation and should be considered in determining the cause of the LBP.

DIFFERENTIAL DIAGNOSIS

- Ninety percent of low back complaints are caused by mechanical factors that can be diagnosed by a thorough history and physical examination, including a palpatory assessment of the musculoskeletal system.
- A comprehensive history, thorough physical examination, and appropriate radiographic and laboratory tests can also identify the organic or systemic causes of LBP that require immediate further evaluation and treatment.
- A patient presenting with LBP usually falls into one of five categories (Table 5.3). The history, physical examination, laboratory tests, radiographs, and clinical course help to differentiate among them and to identify the organic or systemic causes of LBP that require immediate further evaluation and treatment.
- Differential diagnosis and management, including manual treatments, may be carried out using a cost-conservative, algorithmic approach.[14]

HISTORY

- Answers to questions about the patient's history and a review of systems help to discern the underlying pathophysiology.
- Key factors include the patient's age; presence or absence of constitutional symptoms (e.g., fever, weight loss); onset, character, location, duration, aggravating and alleviating factors, and temporal aspects of the pain; patient's medical history, operations, and trauma; family medical history; psychosocial stressors; physical activities at work and home; medications;

Table 5.2   Five types of somatic dysfunction associated with low back pain*

Lumbar Vertebral Joint Somatic Dysfunctions	Myofascial Somatic Dysfunctions	Lumbosacral-Pelvic (Sacroiliac) Dysfunctions	Ligament Sprain	Ilium-Pelvic (Iliosacral and Pubic) Dysfunctions
Flexed rotated sidebent right (FR_RS_R)	Erector spinae	Left sacral torsion on left axis (L/L)	Iliolumbar ligaments	Superior ilial shear
Flexed rotated sidebent left (FR_LS_L)	Gluteal muscles	Left sacral torsion on right axis (L/R)	Sacroiliac ligaments	Inferior ilial shear
Extended rotated sidebent right (ER_RS_R)	"Hamstrings"	Right sacral torsion on left axis (R/L)	Sacrotuberous ligaments	Anterior rotated ilium
Extended rotated sidebent left (ER_LS_L)	Multifidi rotatores	Right sacral torsion on right axis (R/R)		Posterior rotated ilium
Neutral sidebent left rotated right (NS_LR_R)	Pelvic diaphragm	Unilateral sacral flexion		Ilium inflare
Neutral sidebent right rotated left (NS_RR_L)	Piriformis	Unilateral sacral extension		Ilium outflare
	Psoas-iliacus	Bilateral sacral flexion		Superior pubic symphysis shear
	Quadratus lumborum	Bilateral sacral extension		Inferior pubic symphysis shear
	Lumbodorsal fascia	Lumbosacral joint compression		

*In 70% of patients, the cause of acute low back pain is neuromusculoskeletal (somatic) dysfunction characterized by segmental asymmetry of structural position, altered range of motion, and tissue texture abnormalities or tenderness (ART).

Table 5.3   Differential diagnosis of low back pain using Waddell's classification

	Spinal Pathology	Simple LBP	Work-Related LBP	LBP Radiating Below Knee	Inflammatory Disorder
Red Flags					
History	Age of presentation before 20 years or onset after 55 years Violent trauma, such as a fall from a height, MVA Constant, progressive, nonmechanical pain Thoracic pain History of carcinoma Systemic corticosteroids Drug abuse HIV Difficulty with micturition Fecal incontinence	Ages 20-55 years Pain may be in lumbar and sacral spine, buttocks and thighs, but does not radiate below knee Mechanical in nature Pain varies with physical activity and time	Heavy manual work Lifting and twisting Postural stress Whole-body vibration Monotonous work Lack of personal control Low job satisfaction Smoking	Unilateral leg pain more than back pain Pain generally radiating to foot or toes Numbness and paresthesias in the same dermatome distribution	Gradual onset Marked morning stiffness Family history
Physical examination	Systemically unwell Weight loss Persisting severe restriction of lumbar flexion Structural deformity Loss of anal sphincter tone Saddle anesthesia around the anus, perineum or genital Widespread (more than one nerve root) or progressive motor weakness in the legs or gait disturbance	Patient well Lumbosacral spine or pelvic somatic dysfunction present	Low-level physical fitness Inadequate trunk strength	Nerve root irritation signs Reduced SLR, which reproduces leg pain Motor, sensory or reflex change is limited to one nerve root	Iritis, rashes (e.g., psoriasis), colitis, urethral discharge Persistent limitation of spinal movements in all directions Peripheral joint involvement
Laboratory tests and radiography	Radiograph: look for vertebral collapse or bone destruction CT or MRI: look for cauda equina compression	Nondiagnostic	Nondiagnostic	Nondiagnostic or MRI: look for disc herniation with compression of peripheral nerve root	Nondiagnostic or blood tests: look for Rh factor or seronegative arthropathy; ESR > 25 Radiographs shows evidence of arthritis

Continued

Table 5.3   Differential diagnosis of low back pain using Waddell's classification—cont'd

Red Flags	Spinal Pathology	Simple LBP	Work-Related LBP	LBP Radiating Below Knee	Inflammatory Disorder
Course	If pain not resolved in 6 weeks, ESR and radiographs should be considered.	Prognosis is good; 90% recover from acute attack in 6 weeks, but most have recurrences throughout life. Manipulation and exercise provide pain relief and improved mobility and may shorten course.	Usually resolves within 6 weeks Responsive to manipulation and exercise and to use of proper posture and ergonomics Prolonged recovery is possible if secondary gain is involved.	Prognosis is reasonable; 50% recover from acute attack within 6 weeks.	Usually resolves with anti-inflammatory medication Episodic course

CT, computed tomography; ESR, erythrocyte sedimentation rate; HIV, human immunodeficiency virus infection; LBP, low back pain; MRI, magnetic resonance imaging; MVA, motor vehicle accident; SLR, straight-leg raising.

Adapted from Waddell G: The Back Pain Revolution. New York, Churchill Livingstone, 2004.

drug and alcohol abuse; and previous therapies and their effectiveness or failures.
- Obtaining a pain diagram at each visit along with a pain scale determination is helpful in monitoring progress and helping the patient to quantify her or his experience (see Table 5.3).

PHYSICAL FINDINGS

- The physical examination may entail the following:
  1. A thorough neurologic examination, which includes evaluation of lower extremity motor, sensory, deep tendon, and pathologic reflexes
  2. Assessment of peripheral pulses
  3. Straight-leg raising tests
  4. Hip flexion, abduction, external rotation, and extension (FABERE) tests
  5. Peripheral joint visual and palpatory evaluations
  6. Abdominal, pelvic and rectal examinations
  7. Gait, posture, and stance evaluations
  8. A series of visual and palpatory regional and segmental joint motion tests of the lumbosacral spine, paraspinal soft tissues, and bony pelvis
- The findings from these tests should be within normal limits in cases of simple LBP.
- In simple LBP, there are findings of *t*issue texture abnormalities, *a*symmetry of structural landmarks, *r*ange of motion abnormalities, and *t*enderness (TART), indicative of the presence of somatic dysfunction (see Tables 5.2 and 5.3).
- Asymmetry[15] and pain provocation are easier to measure reliably than tissue texture changes and motion tests.[16]

LABORATORY AND RADIOGRAPHIC FINDINGS

- Radiographs and laboratory evaluations are useful if the injury is unresolved after 6 weeks or when "red flags" are present in the history or physical examination (see Table 5.3).

- In simple LBP, there are nonspecific or normal radiographic findings.

MANUAL MEDICINE

Manual treatments for patients with LBP are provided by licensed and regulated health care professionals, such as doctors of chiropractic (DC), doctors of osteopathic medicine (DO), doctors of medicine (MD), diplomats of osteopathy (DO), physical therapists (PT), naturopathic doctors (ND), oriental medical doctors (OMD), massage therapists (MT), and by unlicensed professionals and the lay public. It is estimated that more than 100 million patients with mechanical LBP receive spinal manipulation each year.

Best Evidence

In 1975, the National Institutes of Health (NIH) sponsored the first of a series of interdisciplinary conferences inquiring into the research status of spinal manipulative treatment in the United States.[17] After that conference, the NIH established funding resources to investigate spinal manipulation. Numerous studies have evaluated this method's effectiveness and efficacy. The preponderance of the studies has been on the topic of LBP.
- The results of clinical trials examining the efficacy of spinal manipulative treatment for patients with mechanical LBP that ensued over the next 15 years demonstrated the medical and economical value of manual treatment approaches in that patient population.
- Many of the review articles of these scientific endeavors are included in the reference section.[6,18-28]
- This led to the inclusion of spinal manipulation treatment in the Agency for Health Care Policy and Research (now the Agency for Healthcare Research and Quality [AHRQ]) guidelines for the management of acute low back pain, which was published in 1994.[18,29]

- Six other countries recommend spinal manipulation for patients with LBP in their national guidelines[30]: United Kingdom, Switzerland, Sweden, New Zealand, Germany, and Denmark.
- Tables 5.4 and 5.5 provide practice recommendations based on the Cochrane Review, Institute for Clinical Systems Improvement, and other systematic reviews of the literature.
  1. Manual treatment for patients with acute or chronic mechanical LBP is as effective as standard treatments.[31,32]
  2. Manual treatment is recommended for adult patients with mechanical LBP.[33]
  3. Manual therapy provides more effective short-term pain relief for patients with acute or subacute LBP and better than a placebo treatment for patients with chronic LBP.[19,27]
  4. There is moderate, although conflicting, evidence to recommend spinal manipulation for chronic nonspecific or mechanical back pain sufferers[27,28] for short-term relief of symptoms, which may enable increased activity levels and less reliance on medications.
- Meta-analysis of the few osteopathic clinical trials shows benefits of osteopathic manipulative treatment, demonstrating decreased pain and decreased use of physical therapy and medications compared with standard medical care.[34,35] Numerous randomized clinical trials (RCTs) in the chiropractic and some in the medical and physical therapy literature demonstrate greater effectiveness of manual treatment compared with standard medical care. However, many of the studies are lacking in quality and power.[22,27,28]
- In reviewing the RCTs, the following results were found:
  1. There is strong evidence that manual therapy provides more effective short-term pain relief for patients with acute or subacute LBP.
  2. Manual therapy provides better than a placebo treatment for patients with chronic LBP (grade A evidence).[27]
- However, a systematic review[36] of sham-controlled, double-blind, randomized clinical trials of spinal manipulation (i.e., high-velocity, low-amplitude [HVLA] procedures) challenges this conclusion because it demonstrated no clinically significant specific therapeutic effects.
- There is moderate evidence (i.e., grade B) that manual therapy is more effective than usual care by the general practitioner, bed rest, analgesics, and massage for short-term pain relief of patients with acute and chronic LBP.[37]
- Taking into account effect sizes, a meta-analysis of RCTs of spinal manipulation for patients with LBP with less than 3 months' duration demonstrated effectiveness over placebo, no treatment, massage, and short-wave diathermy. There was no difference in outcomes within the first 4 weeks of therapy compared with exercise, physiotherapy, and standard medical care (i.e., grade A evidence).[38]
- Although most workers disabled with LBP return to work within 2 months, those with chronic LBP disabled for more than 3 months have not responded well to any therapeutic intervention, including medication, surgery, manual medicine physical modalities, exercise, and education.
  1. A 2-year study of workers in six nations with chronic LBP (defined as sick-listed for 90 days) showed no therapeutic interventions by any health care practitioner effective for improving work resumption, decreasing pain intensity, or increasing back function.

Table 5.4 Department of Defense and Veterans Administration practice guidelines for primary care: management of low back pain, May 1999

Evaluate for serious health problems.	A. Look for red flags during history taking, neurologic assessment, and physical examination: Major trauma Major muscle weakness Age > 50 years Bladder or bowel dysfunction Persistent fever Saddle anesthesia History of cancer Decreased sphincter tone Metabolic disorder Unrelenting night pain B. Refer patient with bowel or bladder symptoms immediately to orthopedic surgery or neurosurgery. C. For non-emergent red flag cases, assess with diagnostic tests for consultation or referral.
Provide conservative treatment for patients with acute LBP (<6 weeks' duration).	A. NSAIDs and acetaminophen are the drugs of choice; opiates and muscle relaxants give no additional proven benefit. B. Modified light activity improves outcome. C. Instruct patient in self-care. Note: 70% of patients improve by 2 weeks; 90% improve by 4+ weeks.
Evaluate patients who get worse.	Re-evaluate worsening patients quickly.
Evaluate patients who do not improve or call if pain gets worse.	A. Radiographs and MRI scans have proven benefit only in specific situations. B. Bed rest of more than 48 hours has no additional proven benefit. C. Manipulation may be helpful if the patient does not have sciatica. D. Re-evaluate after 4 to 6 weeks. E. Take a history and perform a physical examination to rule out other serious problems. F. Use self-report questionnaires for psychological distress or risk factors.
Manage chronic (>6 weeks' duration) lower back pain or sciatica (i.e., radiating pain below the knee).	A. Do appropriate diagnostic tests for consultation or referral. B. For active-duty soldiers with either condition (not improving in more than 6 weeks), assess for disposition.

LBP, low back pain; MRI, magnetic resonance imaging; NSAIDs, nonsteroidal anti-inflammatory drugs.

From Guideline Working Group, Veterans Health Administration, Department of Veterans Affairs, and Health Affairs, Department of Defense: Low Back Pain or Sciatica in the Primary Care Setting. Evidence-Based Clinical Practice. Office of Quality and Performance publication 10Q-CPG/LBP-99. Washington, DC, Veterans Health Administration and Department of Defense, November 1999.

Table 5.5   Highest level of evidence-based practice recommendations

Evidence Level*	Recommendation	Studies and Sources
A	Manual treatment for patients with acute or chronic mechanical low back pain is as effective as standard treatments.	Assendelft et al, 2003[31] Assendelft et al, 2004[32] http://www.cochrane.org/ chochrane/revabstr/ AB000447/htm
A	Manual treatment is recommended for adult patients with mechanical low back pain.	Institute for Clinical Systems Improvement (ICSI), 2004[33] (grade I; classes A, M, R) http://www.icsi.org/ knowledge/detail.asp? catID=29&itemID=149
A	Manual therapy provides more effective short-term pain relief for patients with acute or subacute low back pain and is better than placebo treatment for patients with chronic low back pain.	van Tulder et al, 2000[27] Bronfort et al, 2004[19]
A	Spinal manipulation is more effective for patients with low back pain of less than 3 months' duration.	Ferreira et al, 2003[38]

*Evidence levels: A, randomized, controlled trials, meta-analyses, and systematic reviews; B, case-control or cohort studies, retrospective studies, and certain uncontrolled studies; C, consensus statements, expert guidelines, usual practice, and opinion.

2. Surgery for herniated discs was helpful in some countries but not in others.
3. Work resumption in the first year depended on lower age, male gender, lower psychological and physical demands at work, better work control, not having received earlier treatment for the current LBP episode, and back surgery in Sweden only.[39]
4. The goal of treatment of an acute LBP episode is to prevent it from lingering and developing into a chronic LBP episode, especially one that lasts longer than 3 months.
- There is limited and conflicting evidence of any long-term effects of manual therapy for patients with LBP (grade C).
  1. Results from RCTs comparing treatments for patients with LBP have demonstrated that equivocal functional outcomes are observed at 6 and 12 months after initiation of treatment regardless of therapy or comparative intervention, such as manipulation, physical therapy, education, and medication.
  2. However, an RCT by physical therapists demonstrated that manual therapy for patients with LBP between 2 and 8 months improved significantly, more so than if treated only with exercise therapy.[40]
  3. Childs and colleagues[41,42] developed a clinical prediction model to identify patients between 18 and 60 years old with LBP most likely to benefit from a standard spinal manipulation procedure performed by physical therapists. Symptom duration of less than 16 days and no symptoms

extending distal to the knee were associated with a good outcome with spinal manipulation or mobilization plus exercises.[43]

4. In England, an unprecedented RCT with chiropractors, nonphysician osteopaths, and physical therapists performing an agreed on standard set of manual procedures was able to demonstrate, relative to "best care" in general practice, that manipulation followed by exercise achieved a moderate benefit at 3 months and a small benefit at 12 months; spinal manipulation achieved a small to moderate benefit at 3 months and a small benefit at 12 months; and exercise achieved a small benefit at 3 months but not at 12 months. Manipulation alone was more cost-effective than manipulation plus exercise.[44-46]

- It seems reasonable to use a combination of manual treatment along with exercise and medication as the best practice based on the evidence.
- There are a limited number of RCTs that evaluate all three types of care for patients with LBP provided by the primary treating physician. The doctor providing the manipulation approach would also choose the medication regimen for the patient at each visit and the exercise regimen.
  1. This shifts the paradigm such that manipulation is not looked on as a separate variable but interlaced with the decision-making process of the treating physician.
  2. This makes it difficult to separate the effectiveness of the manual approach from that of the medicine approach. However, this type of paradigm is necessary to examine the effectiveness of a physician who uses the two approaches in an integrated manner, as do many American osteopathic physicians.
- A U.S. trial of osteopathic manipulation used an integrated approach, including medications with manipulation at the discretion of the treating physician.[47]
  1. The results of this clinical trial were published in the November 4, 1999, issue of the *New England Journal of Medicine*. It was a prospective, randomized, ambulatory clinical trial of the efficacy of comprehensive osteopathic care (i.e., medical plus manipulative treatment) versus standard medical care in patients presenting with subacute LBP of 3 weeks to 6 months' duration.[47]
  2. The patients were equally satisfied with their care, irrespective to which group they were assigned, and outcomes were equivocal, but the osteopathic physician used less medication and physical therapy referrals.
  3. The study was not able to determine cost-effectiveness.
- Although there is conflicting evidence for any long-term effects treatment of patients with LBP regardless of therapy or intervention, giving patients with mechanical LBP a short trial of one or two nonforceful manipulative treatments to correct the somatic dysfunction diagnosed, along with teaching proper biomechanics and giving low back exercises, has proved to provide at least short-term benefit with minimal risk to the patient.
  1. Reassessment in 3 to 7 days is sufficient, with repeat treatment of the somatic dysfunction if still present.
  2. Manipulative treatment should be continued only if there is continued demonstration of improvement and no further progression of neurologic findings.
  3. This protocol is reasonable, quite effective, and cuts down significantly on medication and physical therapy use.

4. Strickland[48] is a family physician who, on review of the literature, recommends manipulative treatment by the primary care physician or referral to other health professional skilled and trained in spinal manual care for patients with mechanical LBP.

- It is difficult to readily apply the data gathered in clinical trials on spinal manipulation to clinical practice. Some of the characteristics of clinical trials on spinal manipulation make it difficult for various practitioners to apply the data to clinical practice:
  1. Unknown training of the manipulator (most are chiropractors)
  2. Unknown diagnosis (i.e., LBP)
  3. Unspecified treatment (most are single treatment, such as HVLA)
  4. Artificial scenario
  5. Difficult to control variables
  6. Difficult to prevent dropouts
  7. No perfect sham treatment
  8. Patients who self-treat
  9. Physicians (DO and MD) likely to combine all interventions available
  10. Multidisciplinary care becoming a more common practice
  11. Psychosocial and behavioral issues to be factored in to the outcome equation
- Many practitioners lack education and training in manual diagnostic and treatment methods.
  1. Although 200 to 400 hours of education and training in manual medicine theory and methods are generally considered minimal requirements for proficiency, an interesting study reported on the effect on patient care of an 18-hour, limited (low back) manual therapy training course for family physicians.[49]
  2. One outcome was that patients with acute LBP who received intensive manual therapy at each visit (within the first month) had a quicker return to functional recovery than others receiving limited manual therapy or the control group.
  3. Two years after the study, a survey of the 31 family practitioners (MDs) who participated revealed that 50% still used manual therapy, mostly muscle energy techniques, two to three times weekly.
  4. The physicians had changed their management of patients presenting with acute LBP by performing more complete examinations and by touching their patients more. Their practices also had less use of narcotics, reduced referrals to specialists, and increased referrals to chiropractors.
  5. They believed they were improving patient outcomes.
- A rational approach is to combine the best-evidence practices with clinical experience and judgment, follow the patient's response, respect his or her values, and adjust the management plan accordingly.

Risks

- Reviews of the literature on complications from spinal manipulation procedures have shown it to have relatively high benefit and low risk, being one of the safest methods of treatment for a wide variety of illnesses and injuries.[23,50,51]

- The risk for complications from HVLA rotatory manipulation of the lumbar spine is estimated at 1 in 100 million.[24] There have been fewer than 310 reported cases of complications from manual medicine since 1925.[23] There have only been a few cases of disc herniation (<10) and cauda equina syndrome (<20).[23] No complications have ever been reported during an RCT of spinal manipulation.[52]
- Two of the practitioner-dependent reasons for complications proposed by retrospective researchers are inadequate manipulative skill of the practitioner and incorrect or incomplete diagnosis. Side effects from spinal manipulation for patients with LBP are typically muscle soreness or pain that resolves within 24 to 48 hours.[53]
- There have been no reports of complications from any of the indirect or nonforceful (i.e., non-HVLA) procedures. They are among the safest procedures ever designed for manipulation of the spinal joints and surrounding paraspinal soft tissues.
- As long as the practitioner has arrived at a correct diagnosis of mechanical LBP, with findings of TART consistent with somatic dysfunction, has ruled out all other causes by complete history and physical examination, and is aware of precautions, it is highly unlikely there will be any complications.

Benefits

- Manual diagnosis and treatment to correct somatic dysfunction of the bony and soft tissue structures of the spine and pelvis can enable a quicker return to normal functional status with less dependency on medication and physical therapy.
- Common outcome findings from RCTs (i.e., grade A evidence)[19,27,31,36,40,47] on spinal manipulation include the following:
  1. Pain reduction
  2. Earlier return to work
  3. Shortened disability and impairment
  4. Reduced medication use
  5. Reduced physical therapy visits
  6. Increased patient satisfaction

Practice Recommendations

- The U.S. Department of Defense has developed clinical guidelines for the management of LBP in military personnel that includes the option for spinal manipulation (see Table 5.4).
- Chiropractic care is available to all military personnel, and military personnel can obtain manual treatment for LBP from MD, DO, DC, or PT practitioners.
- Most organized medical societies around the world have recognized the utility of and have supported the use of manipulation for mechanical LBP.
- Practitioners of musculoskeletal manipulation include physicians and surgeons (DO and MD), chiropractors, naturopaths, physical therapists, massage therapists, nurses, nurse practitioners, physician assistants, and the lay public.
- Further education and training for practitioners in the use of manual procedures for patients with LBP are available through various postgraduate institutions and medical societies devoted to educating health care practitioners in manual medicine.

1. Since 1992, the American Academy of Family Physicians has invited its members to become familiar with osteopathic manipulative medicine procedures by offering introductory courses during their annual scientific assemblies.
2. The American Back Society has some seminars at its annual meetings.
3. The American College of Rehabilitation Medicine sponsors seminars at selected continuing medical education (CME) programs.
4. The American Academy of Osteopathy offers a wide array of osteopathic manipulative treatment procedure courses.
5. Michigan State University offers a wide array of manual medicine courses.
6. The American Osteopathic Association requires demonstration of competency in osteopathic palpatory diagnosis and manipulative treatment in its postgraduate residency programs.
7. The International Federation of Manual Medicine (FIMM) is composed of unlimited licensed physicians devoted to the scientific investigation and development of the field of manual medicine, including the development of international guidelines. They hold international conferences every 3 years to update the knowledge accumulated during that time and to share information.
8. There are educational programs, evidence-based literature reviews, practice guidelines, books, web sites, and manipulation courses for practitioners through specialty colleges of practitioners that primarily treat problems of the musculoskeletal system (e.g., orthopedic surgeons, physical medicine and rehabilitation specialists, rheumatologists, osteopaths, chiropractors, physical therapists, naturopaths, massage therapists).

MANUAL DIAGNOSTIC PROCEDURES

- The ICD-9 diagnostic code for lumbar somatic dysfunction is 739.3.
- The ICD-9 diagnostic code for pelvic (sacrum or sacroiliac) somatic dysfunction is 739.4.
- The ICD-9 diagnostic code for pelvic (innominate or iliosacral) somatic dysfunction is 739.5.
- Patients complaining of LBP should be evaluated standing, seated, prone, and supine. The musculoskeletal screening and scanning (lumbar regional) examination (see Chapter 3) should be performed. Lumbar and pelvic regions will likely show asymmetric landmarks and restriction of motion. Positive findings on the lumbar and pelvic regional examinations lead the practitioner to investigate for the presence of a segmental somatic dysfunction. Examination of the patient in the standing and seated positions is performed as part of the 12-step structural examination described in Chapter 3. Key positive findings in that examination that lead to the segmental examinations described in this chapter include the following:
1. Decreased lumbar lordosis (lateral postural examination)
2. Lumbar scoliosis (scoliosis screening test) (Fig. 5.16)
3. Decreased lumbar sidebending (hip-drop test)

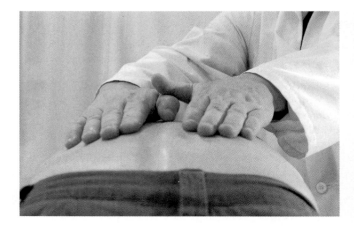

Figure 5.16   Lumbar scoliosis. Standing flexion assessment demonstrates a functional group curve, or scoliosis, with a convexity to the right (i.e., rotated right, sidebent left).

4. Decreased lumbar flexion, extension, sidebending or rotation (active and passive motion tests)
5. Asymmetric iliac crest heights
6. Unlevel PSIS landmarks (i.e., posterior postural screen)
7. Positive standing and seated flexion test results
8. Positive hip-shift test result

Lumbar Spine Anatomic Landmarks

- In general, the superior or inferior length of each lumbar spinous process is equivalent to the height of its associated lumbar vertebra. The superior margins of the spinous processes lie approximately in the same horizontal plane as the corresponding transverse processes. The length of the transverse processes varies with each lumbar vertebra. The transverse processes increase in length from L1 to L3 and then decrease in length from L3 to L5. L3 has the longest transverse processes of all the lumbar vertebrae, extending approximately 2 inches laterally from the spinous process.
- To locate L1, palpate the 12th rib and trace the rib to its attachment to T12. L1 is the first vertebra immediately below T12 (Fig. 5.17).
- To locate L2, palpate the tip of the 11th rib. A horizontal line drawn from this point to the midline locates the spinous process of L2 (see Fig. 5.17).
- To locate L3, palpate the tip of the 12th rib. A horizontal line drawn from this point to the midline locates the spinous process of L3 (Figs. 5.17 and 5.18).
- To locate L4, palpate the apex of the iliac crest. A line drawn horizontally from this point to the midline locates the vertebral body of L4 (see Fig. 5.17).
- To locate L5, palpate the PSIS (Fig. 5.19A). From this point, a line drawn medially and superiorly toward the midline at a 30-degree angle locates the spinous process of L5 (see Fig. 5.19B). The transverse processes can be located by first placing the thumbs or fingertips on each PSIS and then moving them

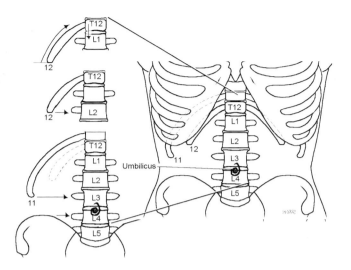

Figure 5.17 Locations of the lumbar vertebral landmarks.

medially and superiorly, just lateral to the spinous process of L5 (see Fig. 5.19C).

Anatomic Variations

- Anatomic variants occur in the lumbosacral area. Lumbarization of sacral segments and sacralization of lumbar segments are seen occasionally. It may be necessary to verify the exact number of lumbar vertebrae present in a given patient. One method of checking this is as follows:
  1. Locate L4 as described previously, and palpating superiorly, count the spinous processes until L1 is located (verifying the location of T12 as described previously can also accomplish this).
  2. Locate L1, and palpating inferiorly, count the spinous processes until the sacrum is located.
  3. Any discrepancy in correlating these counts may indicate the presence of an anatomic variant resulting in an abnormal number of lumbar vertebrae.

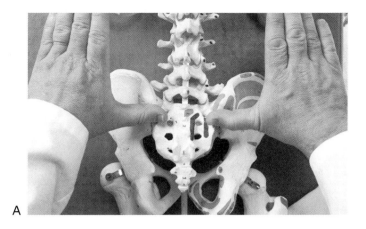

A

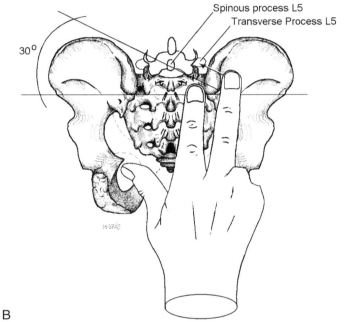

B

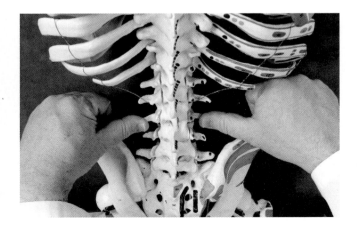

Figure 5.18 Locating the level of the L3 vertebra.

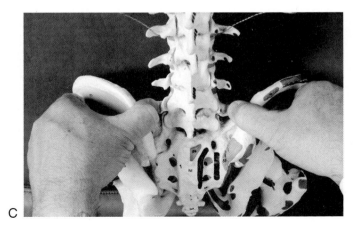

C

Figure 5.19 **A**, Location of both posterior superior iliac spine (PSIS) landmarks. **B**, Relationships between the right PSIS, sacral sulcus, L5 spinous process, and the right L5 transverse process. **C**, Locating the L5 vertebra transverse processes with the thumbs.

Lumbar Somatic Dysfunction Diagnosis

- For most of these diagnostic procedures, the practitioner usually stands behind the patient, and the patient can be seated in one of the following positions:
  1. At the end of the treatment table, with legs straddling the table, facing toward the length of the table
  2. Sitting on the table with feet on a chair for stability
  3. On a stool with feet flat on the floor
- Assessment of temperature variation
  1. Using the dorsal aspect of the hands positioned approximately 1 inch away from the patient's skin, the practitioner palpates for heat radiation, noticing changes from segment to segment or between groups of segments.
  2. Such variations indicate an alteration of blood flow due to inflammation or ischemia (Fig. 5.20).
- Assessment of tissue texture changes
  1. The practitioner feels the paraspinal soft tissues one segment at a time assessing for tissue texture abnormalities, such as

dry or moist skin, numbness or tenderness, and swelling or ropy and firm (Fig. 5.21).
  2. Some practitioners find it helpful to run two fingers down the spine along either side of the spinous processes, eliciting a "red reflex" or cutaneous vasodilatory response. This response may be altered at dysfunctional spinal segments and provide an indication for where to look for spinal somatic dysfunction (Fig. 5.22).

  An area that has persistent red streak marks for 3 minutes, which is about how long it takes for normal skin to return to normal color after the provocative test, is considered to have an abnormal autonomic and local vasodilator response due to spinal sensitization or facilitation.

  The examiner observes any deviation of the spinous processes from the midline while eliciting the red reflex.
- Segmental motion examination
  1. The practitioner finds an area along the spine that demonstrates structural asymmetry or tissue texture abnormalities and tests for motion asymmetry one segment at a time in that area (Fig. 5.23).

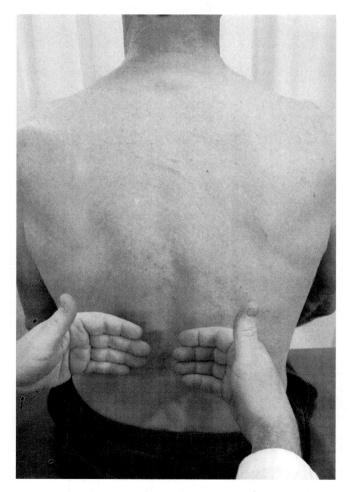

Figure 5.20 The practitioner assesses temperature variations overlying the lumbar paraspinal soft tissues, looks for asymmetries, and compares side to side and each successive vertebral level.

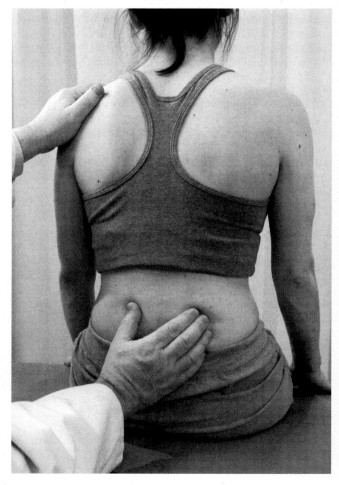

Figure 5.21 Assessing tissue texture in lumbar paraspinal soft tissues.

the transverse processes if necessary (i.e., if unable to feel the transverse processes through the erector spinae muscle mass).

5. The practitioner instructs the patient to flex or bend forward until the lumbar vertebra being palpated is in the flexed position (Fig. 5.24A).

6. The practitioner checks the transverse processes with thumb tip digital pressure at that level.

7. The practitioner assesses for asymmetry around the vertical axis in the coronal plane (i.e., whether a transverse process is more posterior on one side or the other in the horizontal plane).

8. The practitioner instructs the patient to extend the lumbar spine to the level of the dysfunctional segment being evaluated by the practitioner (see Fig. 5.24B).

9. The practitioner again checks for asymmetry of the transverse processes, observing whether any transverse process is more posterior than its counterpart on the opposite side at the same level.

10. If one segment has a posterior transverse process compared with the contralateral side at the same level, the practitioner should also check the segment above and the one below to compare symmetry.

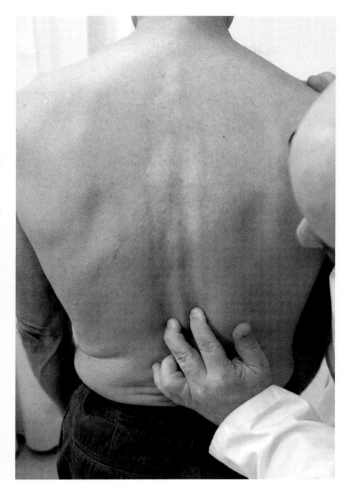

Figure 5.22   The practitioner assesses red reflex responses in lumbar paraspinal soft tissues and observes any deviation of the spinous processes from the midline.

2. The segmental examination can be performed actively or passively with the patient in the seated position or prone.

Active Segmental Motion Examination

- Examination of active segmental motion can be performed with patient in the seated position as follows:

  1. The practitioner palpates the paraspinal soft tissue tension at each lumbar spinal level and selects the level that has the greatest amount of tension, as determined by resistance to compressive thumb tip digital pressure.

  2. The practitioner places his or her thumbs on the transverse processes at the vertebral level where the most paraspinal muscle tension was found and observes whether there is a more posterior transverse process on one side compared with the contralateral side.

  3. The practitioner presses posterior to anterior with his or her thumbs overlying the transverse processes.

  4. The practitioner presses lateral to medial with his or her thumb tips contact on the lateral tips of the transverse processes, lateral to the erector spinae mass, to help locate

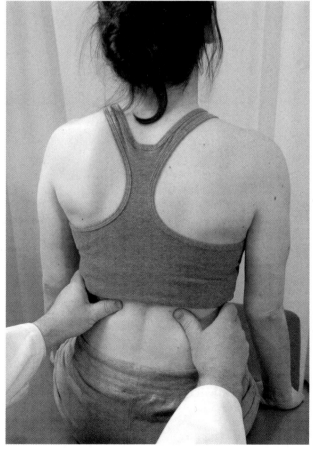

A

Figure 5.23   A, Palpating the L1 transverse processes with the patient seated.

Continued

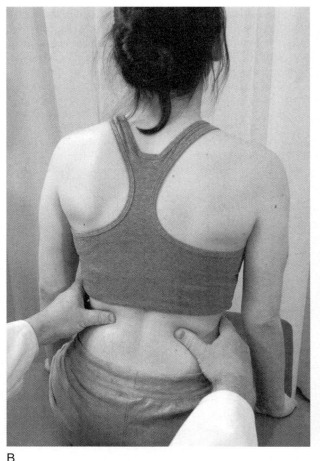

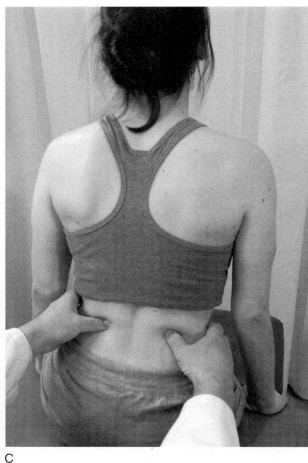

B

C

Figure 5.23, cont'd B, Palpating the L2 transverse processes with the patient seated. C, Palpating the L3 transverse processes with the patient seated.

Passive Segmental Motion Examination

- Lumbar segmental diagnosis can also be done by passively flexing and extending the seated patient while monitoring the transverse processes of the suspected dysfunctional segment as identified by posterior fullness of the paraspinal tissues at that segment (Fig. 5.25). This can be done as follows:
  1. The patient is seated.
  2. The practitioner stands behind the patient or sits facing in the opposite direction of the patient on the examination table.
  3. The practitioner locates the segment to be examined by noticing which segment in the area of the posterior soft tissue fullness has the most posterior transverse process (discussed earlier).
  4. The practitioner places the pads of the thumb and index finger (or the index and middle fingers) of one hand over the posterior aspects of the transverse processes of the vertebra being examined.
  5. The practitioner places his or her other arm across the patient's upper chest, with the practitioner's axilla resting on one of the patient's shoulders and the hand resting on the patient's opposite shoulder.

6. The practitioner moves the patient's lumbar spine passively into flexion until motion is felt at the segment being palpated. The practitioner then observes whether the posterior transverse process has become more or less symmetric in the horizontal plane.
7. Step 6 is repeated with the practitioner moving the patient's lumbar spine passively into extension until motion is felt at the segment being palpated. The practitioner again notices whether the posterior transverse process has become more or less symmetric in the horizontal plane.

Prone Segmental Motion Examination

- Lumbar segmental diagnosis can be performed with the patient prone. The examination can be done as follows:
  1. The patient is prone on the examination table.
  2. The practitioner stands to the side of the patient with his or her dominant eye over the midline of the lumbar spine.
  3. Practitioner evaluates symmetry of the lumbar spine vertebrae in neutral and in extension by pressing anteriorly over the transverse processes at each level (Fig. 5.26).

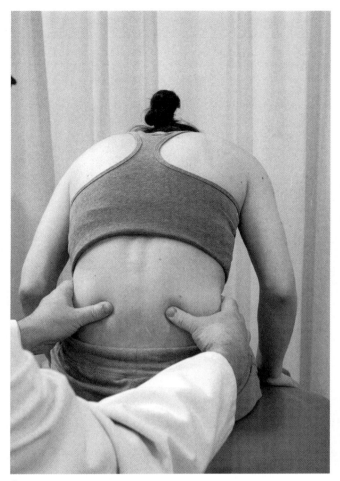

A

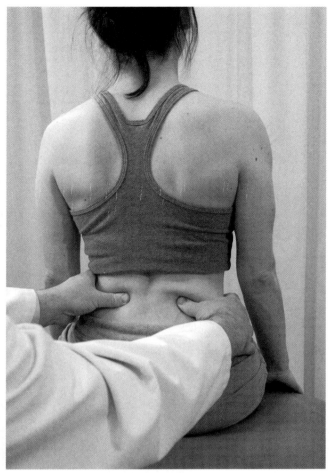

B

Figure 5.24 **A**, Lumbar segmental evaluation using active motion: flexion. **B**, Lumbar segmental evaluation using active motion: extension.

Interpretation of Segmental Examination Findings

- If one transverse process is felt sooner than its counterpart with the same amount and depth of digital pressure, the practitioner can deduce that that transverse process is more posterior and that the vertebra is slightly rotated to that side.
- If there is a posterior transverse process only in the flexed position and the transverse processes become symmetric in extension, an extended segmental somatic dysfunction is present.
  1. If this is a single-segment somatic dysfunction (i.e., a type II dysfunction), sidebending occurs to the same side as the rotation.
  2. If the segment is rotated right, most notably in flexion, and the transverse processes are symmetric when extended, the segment is determined to be extended, rotated right, and sidebent right (ER_RS_R). This is the position of ease of motion.
  3. The segment resists flexion, rotation left, and sidebending left (FR_LS_L).
  4. This can be documented as a position of ease (ER_RS_R) or as motion restriction restricted in flexion, left rotation, and left sidebending.
- If there is a posterior transverse process only in the extended position and the transverse processes become symmetric in

flexion, a flexed segmental somatic dysfunction is present. The segment is relatively more flexed and resists extension. This is the position of ease of motion.
  1. If this is a single-segment somatic dysfunction (i.e., type II dysfunction), sidebending occurs to the same side as the rotation.
  2. If the segment is rotated right, most notably in extension, and the transverse processes are symmetric when flexed, the segment is determined to be flexed, rotated right, and sidebent right (FR_RS_R). This is the position of ease of motion.
  3. The segment resists extension, rotation left, and sidebending left.
  4. This can be documented as position of ease (FR_RS_R) or as motion restriction: restricted in extension, left rotation, and left sidebending.
- If a vertebra has a posterior transverse process in neutral, flexed, and extended positions, it is likely part of a group of vertebrae that is dysfunctional.
  1. The practitioner should continue checking superiorly and inferiorly from the asymmetric segment until a symmetric segment is identified to make an accurate interpretation of the findings.

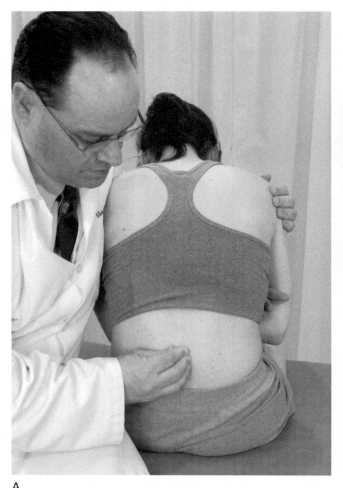 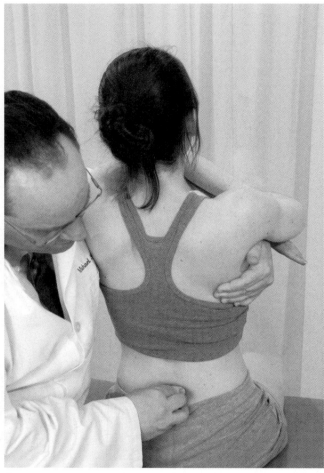

A

B

Figure 5.25   **A,** Lumbar segmental evaluation using passive motion: flexion. **B,** Lumbar segmental evaluation using passive motion: extension.

2. If there is a group (i.e., three or more) of successive vertebrae with transverse processes all found posterior on one side, they are likely rotated in neutral and therefore constitute a type I somatic dysfunction (i.e., in a scoliotic-type curve). Rotation and sidebending occur in opposite directions for type I somatic dysfunctions.

3. The transverse processes of neutral or type I group somatic dysfunctions cannot obtain symmetry in any position. They remain rotated, even if not as much, to the same side as in the neutral position.

4. The group of segments is determined to be neutral, rotated right, and sidebent left. This is the position of ease of motion.

5. The segment resists flexion, extension, rotation left, and sidebending right.

6. This can be documented as a position of ease (NR_RS_L) or as motion restriction: restricted in neutral, left rotation, and right sidebending.

- Consider the following clinical scenario. The practitioner notices paravertebral fullness from L1 to L4 on the right side of the patient, with the most fullness (i.e., the most posterior transverse process) at L3.

  1. Example: The transverse processes become more symmetric when the patient's lumbar spine is in the flexion position. The L3 structural diagnosis is L3 FR_RS_R.

  2. Example: The transverse processes become more symmetric when the patient's lumbar spine is in the extension position. The L3 structural diagnosis is L3 ER_RS_R.

  3. Example: The transverse processes are most symmetric when the patient's lumbar spine is in the neutral position. The structural diagnosis is L1 through L4 NR_RS_L.

- Assessment of tender points

  1. Posterior and anterior tender points of the lumbar and pelvic regions can be associated with segmental somatic dysfunctions.

  2. Tender points can persist after the joint dysfunction seemingly has been resolved by other manual procedures.

- Assessing for posterior lumbar and pelvic tender points can be done as follows:

  1. The patient is prone on the examination table.

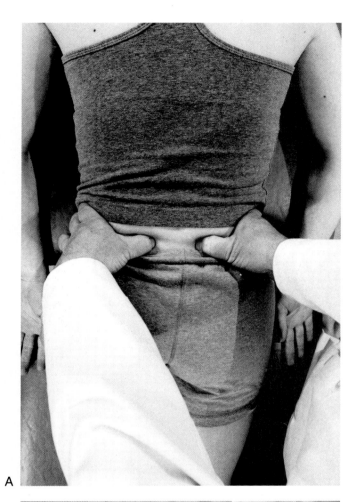

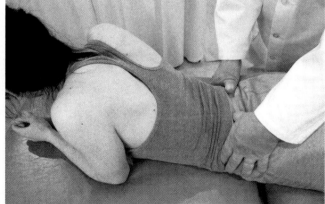

Figure 5.26   **A,** Assessing symmetry of the lumbar transverse processes with the patient prone (i.e., at rest or in a neutral position). **B,** Assessing symmetry of the lumbar transverse processes: extension. The patient extends (i.e., sphinx position) while the practitioner evaluates the symmetry of the lumbar transverse processes.

2. The practitioner stands to the side of the table with his or her dominant eye over the midline of the lumbar spine and pelvis.
3. The practitioner assesses some of the most common posterior lumbar and sacral tender points for tenderness (Fig. 5.27 and 5.28):

   Along the lateral aspects of each of the lumbar spinous processes

   Just above and below the PSIS bilaterally

   Overlying the belly of the piriformis muscle, over the sciatic notch, bilaterally
4. The practitioner then selects the three most tender points in the region to later treat with strain and counterstrain manual procedures (discussed later).

• Assessment for anterior lumbar tender points can be done as follows:
1. Patient is supine on the examination table.
2. Practitioner is standing alongside and facing patient.
3. Practitioner assesses the common anterior lumbar tender points for tenderness on each side (Fig. 5.29):

   Assess medial to the ASIS.

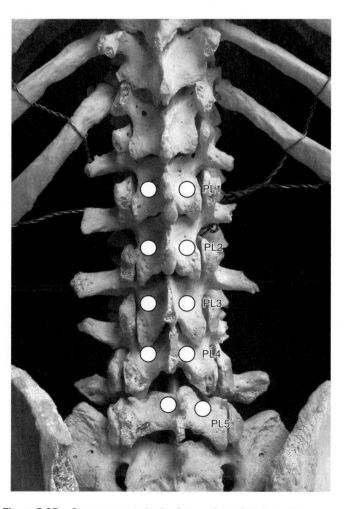

Figure 5.27   Common posterior lumbar tender points posterior lumbar 1 (PL1) through posterior lumbar 5 (PL5).

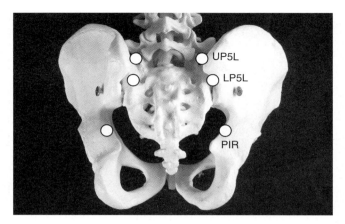

Figure 5.28 Common posterior pelvis tender points upper pole lumbar 5 (UPL5), lower pole lumbar 5 (LPL5), and piriformis (PIR).

Assess medial, lateral, and inferior to the anterior inferior iliac spine (AIIS).

Assess along the inguinal ligament and pubic ramus.

4. The practitioner selects the three most tender points for treatment using strain and counterstrain procedures (discussed later).

- For assessment of associated muscle tension, the practitioner should also palpate all muscles in the lumbar region for orientation and evaluation of any abnormalities. The tension of the psoas muscles, which play a role in the creation and maintenance of lumbar segmental somatic dysfunctions, can be assessed as follows (Fig. 5.30):
  1. The patient is prone on the examination table.
  2. The practitioner stands at either side of the table.
  3. The practitioner flexes the patient's knee to 90 degrees and grasps the patient's thigh just above the knee with one hand.
  4. The practitioner extends the patient's hip until the ASIS on that side rises off the table.
  5. This procedure is repeated with the patient's opposite leg.

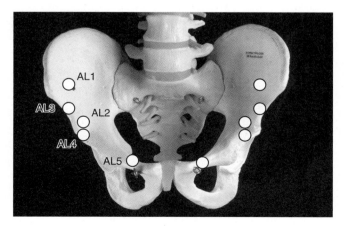

Figure 5.29 Common anterior lumbar tender points anterior lumbar 1 (AL1) through anterior lumbar 5 (AL5).

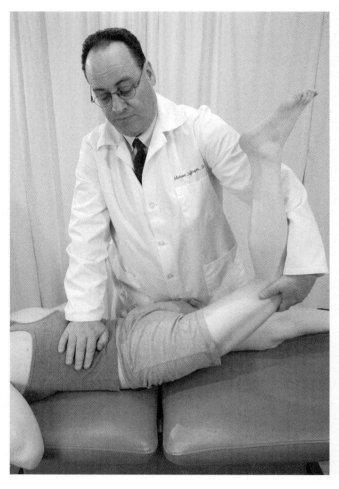

Figure 5.30 The psoas tension test.

6. The practitioner observes the range and quality of the hip extension motion on each side.

- Restriction in the range or quality of motion on either side indicates tightness of the iliopsoas muscle on that side.

Pelvic Anatomic Landmarks

Pubic Symphysis

- The pubic symphysis is examined as follows:
  1. The patient is supine on the examination table.
  2. The practitioner stands at the side of the table with his or her dominant eye over the midline.
  3. The practitioner places the palm of one hand on the lower abdomen and moves it inferiorly until the heel of the hand meets the superior aspect of the pubic symphysis (Fig. 5.31A).
  4. The practitioner then places the pads of his or her index fingers on the superior aspect of the pubic symphysis in the midline.
  5. The index fingers are moved laterally until they palpate the superior aspects of the pubic tubercles (see Fig. 5.31B and C).

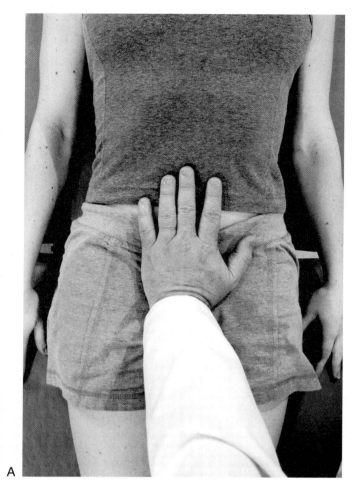

A

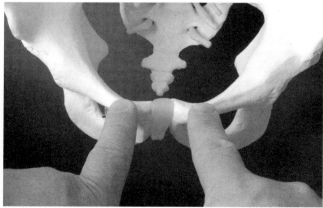

B

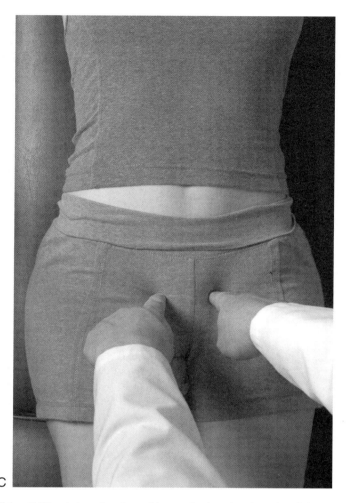

C

Figure 5.31 **A**, Locating the pubic symphysis using the palm of the hand. **B**, Locating the superior aspects of the pubic tubercles with the tips of the index fingers. **C**, Palpating the superior aspects of the pubic tubercles with the index fingertips.

6. The practitioner establishes the level of the two pubic tubercles to determine whether one is more superior or inferior than the other.

Anterior Superior Iliac Spines
- The ASISs are examined as follows:
  1. The patient is supine on the examination table.
  2. The practitioner stands at the side of the table with his or her dominant eye over the midline.

3. The practitioner places his or her thumbs on the most prominent aspects of the ASISs. The practitioner then slides his or her thumbs below the ASISs and then slides the thumbs superiorly to contact the inferior slopes of the ASISs (Fig. 5.32). For patients who are particularly ticklish or sensitive around the ASIS, the practitioner should use the palms to identify the ASIS on each side and then slide the thumbs underneath the ASIS to contact the inferior slopes.

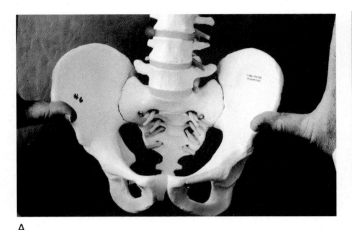
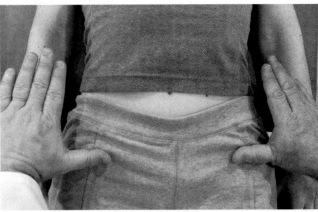

A   B

Figure 5.32 **A,** Locating the anterior superior iliac spine (ASIS) bilaterally. **B,** Palpating the ASIS bilaterally.

4. The practitioner determines the level of the two ASISs to determine whether one innominate is more superior or inferior than the other.
5. The practitioner (using his or her hand or a measuring device such as a tape measure) also establishes the distance of each ASIS from some midline point, such as the umbilicus or the tip of the xiphoid process, to determine whether one innominate is more medial or lateral than the other.

Posterior Superior Iliac Spines

• The PSISs are examined as follows:
1. The patient is prone on the examining table.
2. The practitioner stands at the side of the table with his or her dominant eye over the midline.
3. The practitioner places his or her thumbs on the most prominent aspects of the PSISs.
4. The practitioner then slides his or her thumbs below the PSISs and then slides the thumbs superiorly to contact the inferior slopes of the PSISs (Fig. 5.33).

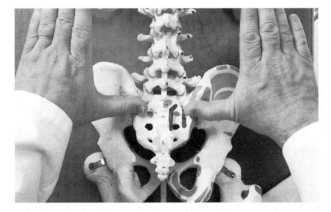

Figure 5.33 Locating the posterior superior iliac spine (PSIS) bilaterally.

5. The practitioner establishes the level of the two PSISs to determine whether one innominate is more superior or inferior than the other.

Sacral Sulcus

• The sacral sulcus is examined as follows:
1. The patient is prone on the examination table.
2. The practitioner stands at the side of the table with his or her dominant eye over the midline.
3. The practitioner places his or her thumbs on the most prominent aspects of the PSISs. The practitioner then curls the thumbs medially and anteriorly until the pads of the thumbs contact the sacral base (Fig. 5.34).
4. The practitioner establishes the depth of the two sides of the sacral sulcus to determine whether the sacrum is rotated in any direction.

Inferior Lateral Angles of the Sacrum

• The ILAs of the sacrum are examined as follows:
1. The patient is prone on the examination table.
2. The practitioner stands at the side of the table with his or her dominant eye over the midline.
3. The practitioner palpates the sacral hiatus at the inferior aspect of the sacrum.
4. The practitioner then places his or her thumbs on the midline at the sacral hiatus and then moves the thumbs laterally equal distances until the posterior aspects of the ILAs are contacted (Fig. 5.35).

Determining the Position of L5 Relative to S1

• The examination is performed as follows:
1. The patient is prone on the examination table.
2. The practitioner stands at the side of the table with his or her dominant eye over the midline.
3. The practitioner places his or her thumb pads on the most posterior aspects of the PSISs and then curls the thumbs medially, approximately 30 degrees superiorly, and then anteriorly until the thumbs contact the transverse processes of L5.
4. The practitioner assesses the depth of the L5 transverse processes relative to the coronal plane (see Fig. 5.19).

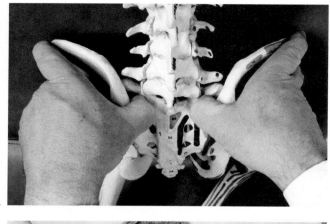

A

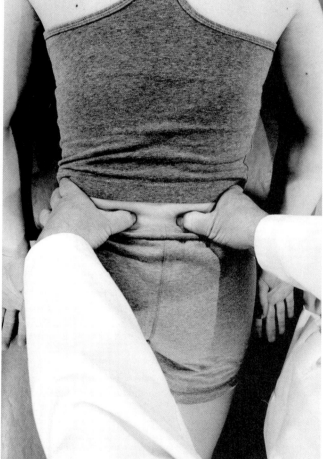

B

Figure 5.34 **A**, Locating the sacral sulcus bilaterally. **B**, Palpating the sacral sulcus bilaterally.

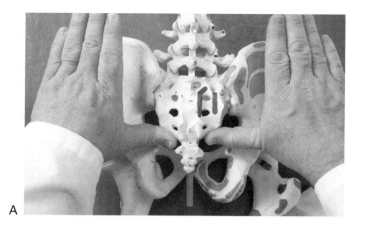

A

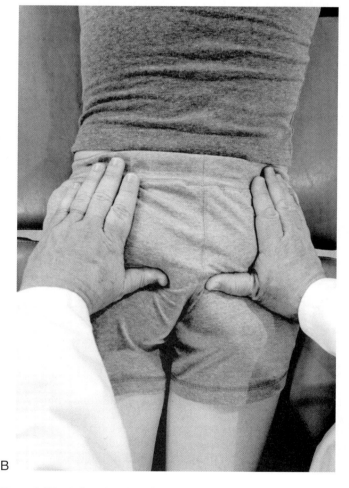

B

Figure 5.35 **A**, Locating the inferior lateral angles (ILAs) bilaterally. **B**, Palpating the ILAs bilaterally.

Pelvic Somatic Dysfunction Diagnosis

Standing Flexion Test

- The standing flexion test (Fig. 5.36) screens for iliosacral somatic dysfunction, defined functionally as somatic dysfunction of the innominate or lower extremity. It is part of

the 12-step structural examination (see Chapter 3) and is performed as follows:

1. The patient stands with his or her feet comfortably apart and weight evenly distributed to the lower extremities.
2. The practitioner sits or kneels behind the patient and places his or her thumbs on the inferior slopes of the patient's PSISs.

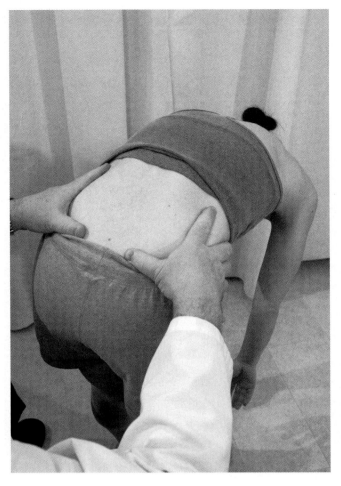

Figure 5.36   The standing flexion test.

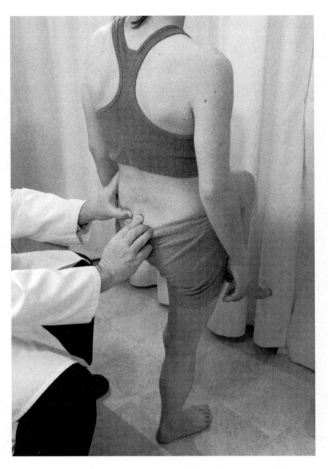

Figure 5.37   The Trendelenburg (stork) test.

3. The patient is then asked to bend forward from the waist with the arms hanging loosely and to attempt to touch the floor.
4. The practitioner observes whether the PSISs move symmetrically (i.e., normal motion) or one PSIS is more superior or ventral than the other at the end of the forward bending motion (i.e., positive test result).

• A positive standing flexion test result indicates a somatic dysfunction in the innominate region or in the lower extremity on the side of the positive test result.

Trendelenburg Test or Sacroiliac Joint Motion Test

• The Trendelenburg or sacroiliac joint motion test (Fig. 5.37) screens for gluteus medius weakness that is often present in patients with chronic LBP and in those with sacral (S1) nerve impingement. It tests the strength of the gluteus medius of the weight-bearing leg. It can also indicate sacroiliac joint dysfunction.
1. The patient is standing.
2. The practitioner is seated behind the patient.

3. The practitioner places a thumb or finger pad on the PSIS on one side and places a finger pad in the midline of the sacrum at the level of the PSIS.
4. On the side being examined, the patient is instructed to flex the hip fully.

• The normal result is for the opposite gluteus medius muscle to contract and the pelvis on the side being examined to elevate. If the opposite gluteus medius muscle is weak, the pelvis on the unsupported side stays level or moves inferiorly, indicating a positive test result.

• If the ipsilateral quadratus lumborum or latissimus dorsi muscles are hypertonic, a situation commonly found in conjunction with lumbar and pelvic somatic dysfunctions, the unsupported ilium may not be able to stay level or may drop and give a false-negative test result.

• Some manual practitioners use this test, which is also called the stork test, to assess sacroiliac joint mobility, based on the fact that it is more common to have quadratus or latissimus dorsi muscle hypertonicity and sacroiliac joint motion dysfunction than to have gluteus medius weakness or sacral nerve dysfunction. If the unsupported ilium does not drop, they assume it is because of sacroiliac joint dysfunction.

Seated Flexion Test

- The seated flexion test (Fig. 5.38) screens for sacroiliac somatic dysfunction, defined functionally as somatic dysfunction of the sacrum or lower lumbar spine. It is performed as follows:
  1. The patient sits with his or her feet flat on the floor and the knees comfortably apart.
  2. The practitioner sits or kneels behind the patient and places his or her thumbs on the inferior slopes of the patient's PSISs.
  3. The patient is then asked to bend forward from the waist with the arms hanging loosely between the knees.
  4. The practitioner observes whether the PSISs move symmetrically (i.e., normal motion is a negative test result) or one PSIS is more superior or ventral than the other at the end of the forward bending motion (i.e., abnormal motion is a positive test result).
- A positive standing flexion test result indicates a somatic dysfunction in the sacral region or in the lower lumbar vertebrae on the side of the positive test result.

Hamstring Tension Test

- The hamstring tension test (Fig. 5.39) determines if the hamstring muscles (i.e., semitendinosus, semimembranosus, and biceps femoris) are hypertonic.

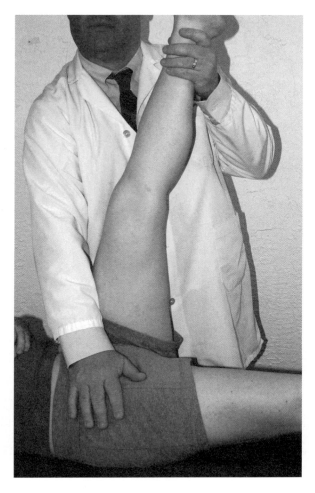

Figure 5.39   The hamstring tension test.

1. The patient is supine on the examination table with his or her legs fully extended.
2. The examiner stands on either side of the table.
3. The examiner grasps one of the patient's ankles with one hand while placing the finger pads of the other hand on the opposite ASIS.
4. The examiner then lifts the extended leg until motion is first felt at the opposite ASIS, gaining an appreciation for the length of the hamstring muscle group on that side.
5. This maneuver is repeated on the opposite side.

- Asymmetry of motion indicates excessive tightness in the hamstring muscles on the side with the lesser range of motion.
- A tight hamstring group of muscles may cause a false-positive standing flexion test result by tethering the ilium so that it does not move superiorly or anteriorly with the ipsilateral dysfunctional sacroiliac joint when the patient bends forward.

Assessment of Leg Length

- This test determines the relative leg lengths by assessing medial malleoli levelness.
  1. The patient is supine with the knees flexed and the feet flat on the examination table (Fig. 5.40A).

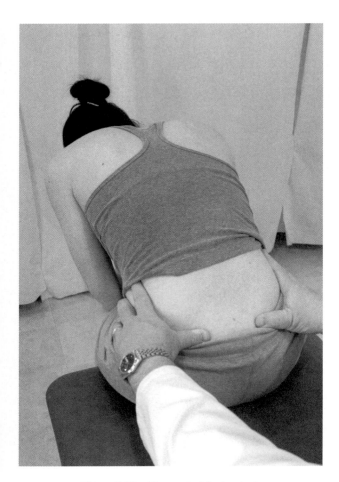

Figure 5.38   The seated flexion test.

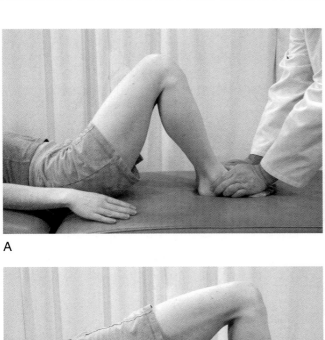

A

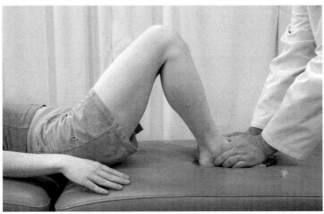

B

C

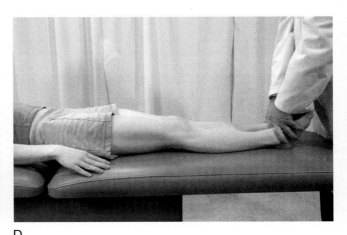

D

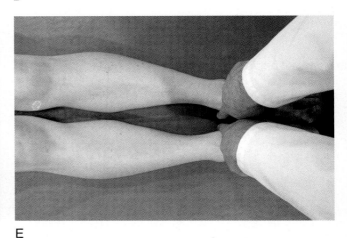

E

Figure 5.40   Determining leg lengths. **A**, Starting position. **B**, Pelvis raised. **C**, Pelvis centered on the table. **D**, Legs extended. **E**, Observation of apparent leg length.

2. The practitioner stands at the foot of the table facing the patient.
3. The practitioner asks the patient to raise his or her buttocks so they are off the examination table (see Fig. 5.40B).
4. The patient then drops the buttocks to the table and extends both lower extremities fully (see Fig. 5.40C).

5. The practitioner places his or her thumbs on the inferior surfaces of the medial malleoli, with the other fingers over the anterolateral aspects of the patient's ankles (see Fig. 5.40D).
6. The practitioner places a slight but equal amount of inferior traction on the patient's lower extremities.
7. The practitioner observes whether the leg lengths appear equal or unequal (see Fig. 5.40E).

- A positive test result indicates the presence of a short leg. Any leg-length inequality is named according to the side of the positive standing or seated flexion test result.
  1. If the left medial malleolus appears more superior than the right, and the patient has a positive standing or seated flexion test result on the left, the patient is said to have a short left leg.
  2. If neither the standing or seated flexion test result is positive, any leg-length discrepancy may be documented as the shorter-appearing leg.

Interpretation of Tests and Examination of Appropriate Landmarks

- The combination of a positive standing flexion test result on one side or the other and a negative seated flexion test result indicates the presence of an iliosacral (innominate) somatic dysfunction. Certain anatomic landmarks can help to determine the exact type of somatic dysfunction present. These anatomic landmarks are as follows:
  1. Pubic symphysis heights
  2. ASISs
  3. PSISs
- Similarly, the combination of a negative standing test result and a positive seated test result on one side or the other indicates the presence of a sacroiliac (sacral) somatic dysfunction. Several anatomic landmarks of interest here:
  1. Depth of the sacral sulcus
  2. ILAs of the sacrum
  3. Position of L5 relative to S1
  4. At least one of the following: the change in sacral sulcus depth with backward bending of the lumbar spine or the amount of stiffness palpable in the lumbosacral area (see "Motion Tests").
- Sometimes, the standing and seated flexion test results both are positive. In such circumstances the practitioner determines which flexion test is *more* positive (i.e., which test shows greater superior or anterior excursion of the PSIS). The more positive flexion test result determines the primary somatic dysfunction (i.e., iliosacral or sacroiliac), and that one is treated first. The pelvis can then be re-evaluated to determine whether the secondary dysfunction is still present. If so, it can then be treated.

Motion Tests

In addition to locating and evaluating the previously described landmarks, two diagnostic motion tests are necessary to confirm the presence of certain sacroiliac somatic dysfunctions. These motion tests are the backward-bending test and the lumbar spring test.

Backward-Bending Test

- The backward-bending test (Fig. 5.41) assesses for the ability of the sacral base to nutate or flex forward in response to active hyperextension of L5. It is performed as follows:
  1. The patient is prone on the examination table.
  2. The practitioner stands at the side of the table with his or her dominant eye over the patient's midline.
  3. The practitioner places his or her thumbs in the sacral sulcus bilaterally.
  4. The patient is asked to rise up on his or her elbows, assuming a position of trunk extension.

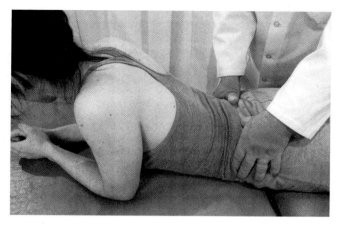

Figure 5.41 The backward-bending test: assessing the depth of the sacral sulcus with the patient in extension.

  5. The practitioner assesses the depth of the sacral sulcus in the coronal plane. The practitioner compares the depth of the sulcus in this position with the depth that occurs with the patient in the prone neutral position.
  6. This test may be applied in a similar fashion to the ILAs. The practitioner's thumbs are placed on the inferior aspects of the ILAs, and the practitioner observes any change in ILA position from the neutral prone position to the trunk extension position (Fig. 5.42).
- Symmetric depth of the sacral sulcus or ILAs on trunk extension indicates a negative test result. Although rare, it is possible to have false-negative tests in cases of bilateral flexed or extended sacrums.
- Asymmetry of depth of the sacral sulcus or ILAs on trunk extension indicates a positive test result.

Lumbar Spring Test

- The lumbar spring test (Fig. 5.43) assesses for the compliance of the lumbosacral spine in response to passive lumbar extension. It is performed as follows:
  1. The patient is prone on the examination table.

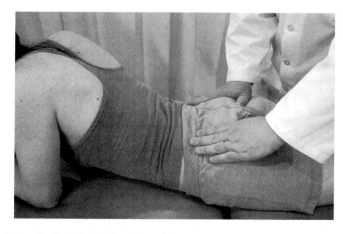

Figure 5.42 The backward-bending test: while palpating the inferior lateral angles (ILAs) for symmetry.

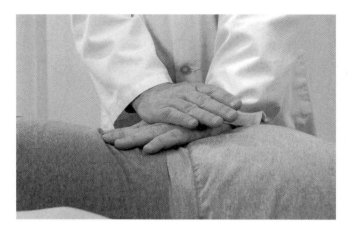

Figure 5.43   The lumbar spring test.

Table 5.6   Pubic symphysis dysfunctions

Positive Standing Flexion Test	Pubic Tubercle Height	Tense, Tender Inguinal Ligament	Diagnosis
Right	Right superior	Right	Superior right
Left	Left superior	Left	Superior left
Right	Right inferior	Right	Inferior right
Left	Left inferior	Left	Inferior left

2. The practitioner stands at the side of the table with his or her dominant eye over the midline.
3. The practitioner places the palm of one hand over the midline of the lumbar region with the heel of the hand over the lumbosacral junction and the fingers extending superiorly over the spinous processes and paravertebral tissues.
4. The practitioner provides a short quick push in an anterior direction with the heel of the hand and evaluates for compliance ("springiness") or resistance of the lumbar spine.

- Compliance of the lumbar spine with no resistance is described as a negative test result.
- Resistance (stiffness) of the lumbar spine to this springing motion is described as a positive test result.

Determination of the Specific Somatic Dysfunction Diagnosis
Iliosacral Somatic Dysfunctions
- A positive standing flexion test result for one side or the other and a negative seated flexion test result bilaterally indicates the presence of iliosacral (i.e., innominate or lower extremity) somatic dysfunction. There are several possible iliosacral somatic dysfunctions:
  1. Superior or inferior pubic symphysis shear
  2. Anterior or posterior innominate bone rotation
  3. Superior or inferior innominate bone shear
  4. Inflare or outflare of the innominate bone
- Diagnosing the specific iliosacral somatic dysfunctions requires examination of the following anatomic landmarks:
  1. Pubic symphysis
  2. ASISs
  3. PSISs
  4. Medial malleoli
- Pubic symphysis somatic dysfunction is named for the side of the positive standing flexion test result.
  1. If the standing flexion test is positive on the left and the pubic tubercle is more superior on the left (possibly along with tenderness and tension in the inguinal ligament on the left), this is a *superior* pubic symphysis shear on the left, not an inferior pubic symphysis shear on the right.

2. The diagnostic criteria for pubic symphysis shears are summarized in Table 5.6.
3. Innominate rotation, shear, or flare somatic dysfunctions are named for the side of the positive standing flexion test result.
4. If the standing flexion test result is positive on the left and the ASIS is superior on the left with the PSIS inferior on the left, this is a left posterior innominate rotation.
5. If the ipsilateral PSIS is instead also superior, this is a superior innominate shear.
6. If the left ASIS is more medial than the contralateral side and the ipsilateral PSIS is more lateral than its counterpart, this is a left inflare innominate.
7. The diagnostic criteria for innominate rotations, innominate shears, and innominate flares are summarized in Table 5.7.

Sacroiliac Somatic Dysfunctions
- A positive seated flexion test result on one side or the other and a negative or less positive standing flexion test result bilaterally indicate the presence of sacroiliac somatic dysfunction. The specific sacroiliac somatic dysfunctions include the following:
  1. Sacral flexion or extension
     Unilateral
     Bilateral
  2. Sacral torsion
     Forward torsion
        Left torsion on the left oblique axis
        Right torsion on the right oblique axis
     Backward torsion
        Left torsion on the right oblique axis
        Right torsion on the left oblique axis
- Diagnosing a specific sacroiliac somatic dysfunction requires examination of the following anatomic landmarks:
  1. Sacral sulcus
  2. ILAs of the sacrum
  3. Position of L5 relative to S1
- The backward-bending test (i.e., prone active extension of the lumbosacral area), and the lumbar spring test (prone passive extension of the lumbosacral area) are useful to confirm the presence or absence of sacral flexions, extensions, or torsions. The diagnostic criteria for sacral flexions and extensions, and sacral torsions are summarized in Table 5.8. An example of how to make a diagnosis of a sacral torsion based on the findings of landmark asymmetry and the motion tests described above is as follows:
  1. The seated flexion test is positive, indicating sacroiliac joint dysfunction (Table 5.8).

Table 5.7   Iliosacral somatic dysfunctions

Positive Standing Flexion Test	Anterior Superior Iliac Spine (ASIS)	Posterior Superior Iliac Spine (PSIS)	Diagnosis
Right	Inferior right	Superior right	Anterior rotation right
Left	Inferior left	Superior left	Anterior rotation left
Right	Superior right	Inferior right	Posterior rotation right
Left	Superior left	Inferior left	Posterior rotation left
Right	Lateral right	Medial right	Outflare right
Left	Lateral left	Medial left	Outflare left
Right	Medial right	Lateral right	Inflare right
Left	Medial left	Lateral left	Inflare left
Right	Superior right	Superior right	Superior shear right
Left	Superior left	Superior left	Superior shear left
Right	Inferior right	Inferior right	Inferior shear right
Left	Inferior left	Inferior left	Inferior shear left

2. The right sacral sulcus is deeper than the left side, indicating a left torsion.
3. The left ILA is more posterior than its counterpart, confirming the left torsion.
4. A positive lumbosacral spring test result indicates noncompliance of the sacral base to forward motion (i.e., it cannot nutate and is counternutated, or extended, at least on one side).
5. A positive backward-bending test result, in which the sacral sulcus and ILA asymmetries become more pronounced, indicates worsening of the torsion with extension of the lumbar spine due to an inability of the sacrum to nutate and L5 to extend.
6. L5 is rotated right, more so during extension (i.e., it is flexed, rotated right, sidebent right).
7. The diagnosis is backward sacral torsion and right rotation on a left oblique axis.

MANUAL TREATMENT PROCEDURES

Five anatomic sites of somatic dysfunction that cause or exacerbate LBP are amenable to manipulation (see Table 5.2):
- Lumbar intervertebral joints
- Myofascial paraspinal soft tissues
- Lumbosacral-pelvic (sacroiliac) joints
- Lumbosacral and lumbopelvic ligaments
- Ilium-pelvic (iliosacral) joints

The following procedures are designed to alleviate these types of somatic dysfunction.

Soft Tissue and Myofascial Release Procedures: Lumbar Spine

Prone Pressure with Counterleverage
- Manipulation is performed as follows:
  1. For prone pressure with counterleverage (Fig. 5.44), the patient is prone on the examination table.
  2. The practitioner stands on either side of the patient.
  3. The practitioner reaches across the patient to contact the opposite ASIS with the fingers of one hand and contacts the paravertebral muscles of that side with the heel of the other hand.
  4. The practitioner lifts the ASIS posteromedially, rotating the lumbar region toward him or her.
  5. The practitioner moves the paravertebral muscles anterolaterally with the other hand.
  6. The practitioner allows the lumbar region to return to a neutral position in relation to the table. The practitioner gently resists the return with one hand while applying opposing torque on the ASIS with the other hand.
  7. This process is repeated in a slow, rhythmic fashion until relaxation of the soft tissues is achieved.

Table 5.8   Sacroiliac somatic dysfunctions

Positive Seated Flexion Test	Sacral Sulcus	Inferior Lateral Angle	L5 Position	Diagnosis
Right	Deep right	Inferior right		Unilateral flexion right
Left	Deep left	Inferior left		Unilateral flexion left
Right	Shallow right	Superior right		Unilateral extension right
Left	Shallow left	Superior left		Unilateral extension left
Right	Deep right	Posterior left	Rotated right, sidebent left	Left on left torsion
Left	Deep left	Posterior right	Rotated left, sidebent right	Right on right torsion
Right	Shallow right	Posterior right	Rotated left, sidebent left	Right on left torsion
Left	Shallow left	Posterior left	Rotated right, sidebent right	Left on right torsion
Bilateral	Deep bilaterally	Posterior bilaterally		Bilateral flexion
Bilateral	Shallow bilaterally	Anterior bilaterally		Bilateral extension

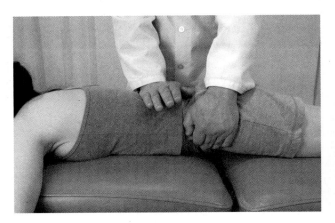

Figure 5.44   Prone pressure with the counterleverage technique.

Lumbosacral Direct Decompression: Prone

- Manipulation is performed as follows:
  1. For lumbosacral direct decompression (Fig. 5.45), the patient is prone on the examination table.
  2. The practitioner stands on either side of the patient.
  3. The practitioner places one hand over sacrum with fingers pointing inferiorly.
  4. The other hand is placed with the heel of the hand contacting the L5 vertebra and the fingers pointing superiorly.
  5. Using his or her body weight, the practitioner applies traction between the two hands, moving them apart until release occurs, denoted by increased soft tissue flexibility and compliance, softening of tissues, and increased tissue warmth.

Articulatory Procedures: Lumbar Spine

All of these treatments may be done bilaterally. In some cases, the treatment is directed to a restriction on one side.

Seated Sidebending

- An example is restricted lumbar right sidebending. Manipulation is performed as follows:
  1. For seated sidebending (Fig. 5.46), the patient is seated on the examination table.

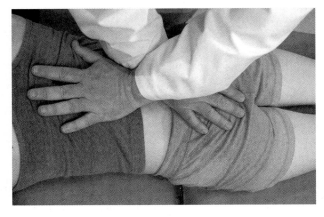

Figure 5.45   Direct lumbosacral decompression.

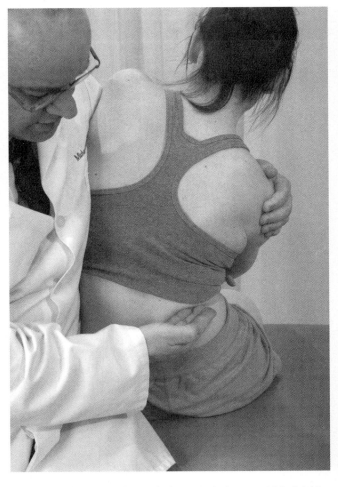

Figure 5.46   Seated lumbar articulatory technique: restricted right sidebending.

  2. The practitioner stands or sits to the left of the patient.
  3. The practitioner's left axilla overlies the patient's left shoulder, and the practitioner's left hand grasps the patient's right shoulder.
  4. The practitioner places the ulnar surface his or her right hand on the right side of the patient's spine, just lateral to the spinous process of the segment to be treated.
  5. The practitioner sidebends the patient to the right, as the practitioner's right hand encourages right sidebending by applying lateral (translatory) pressure toward the left in the lumbar region. The spine is then allowed to return slightly toward neutral.
  6. The sidebending force is directed toward the segment being treated until the desired increase in range of motion is achieved.
  7. This motion is repeated in a rhythmic manner to all segments that need to be treated, sidebending more for the lower lumbar segments.

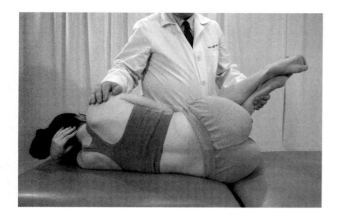

Figure 5.47   Sidelying lumbar articulatory technique: restricted right sidebending.

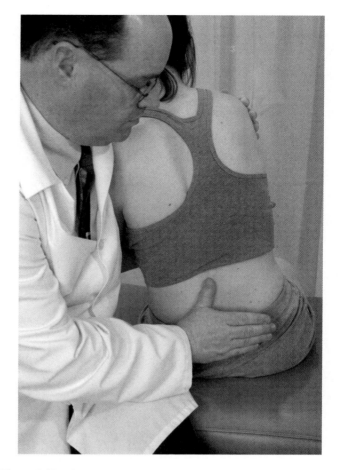

Figure 5.48   Seated lumbar articulatory technique: restricted left rotation.

Sidelying Sidebending
- An example is restricted right sidebending. Manipulation is performed as follows:
  1. For sidelying sidebending (Fig. 5.47), the patient lies in the left lateral recumbent position.
  2. The practitioner stands facing the patient.
  3. The practitioner flexes the patient's knees and hips to 90 degrees.
  4. The practitioner places his or her right hand over the segment being treated to focus the sidebending force at this level.
  5. The practitioner places his or her left hand or forearm under the patient's ankles and lifts them toward the ceiling to induce right sidebending and then brings the legs partially toward neutral.
  6. This motion is repeated in a rhythmic manner to all segments that need to be treated until the desired increase in range of motion is achieved.

Seated Rotation
- An example is restricted left lumbar rotation. Manipulation is performed as follows:
  1. For seated rotation, the patient is seated on the examination table (Fig. 5.48).
  2. The practitioner stands or sits behind and to the patient's left.
  3. The practitioner places his or her left axilla over the patient's left shoulder, and the practitioner's left hand grasps the patient's right shoulder.
  4. The patient grasps the practitioner's left arm.
  5. The practitioner induces left rotation to the lumbar spine by rotating the patient left with his or her left arm and hand.
  6. At the same time, the practitioner places his or her right hand just to the left of the spinous process of the segment being treated and encourages left rotation by applying a lateral force to the spinous process. The spine is then allowed to return slightly toward neutral.
  7. The practitioner repeats the maneuver in a rhythmic manner for all segments, increasing rotation as the lower

lumbar segments are treated, until the desired increase in range of motion is achieved.

Seated Flexion
- Manipulation is performed as follows:
  1. For seated flexion, the patient is seated on the examination table (Fig. 5.49).
  2. The practitioner stands behind and to the left side of the patient.
  3. The practitioner places his or her left axilla over the patient's left shoulder, with his or her left hand on the patient's right shoulder.
  4. The patient grasps the practitioner's arm.
  5. The practitioner places his or her left hand at the level of the lumbar segment to be treated.
  6. Using the left arm, the practitioner leans the patient backward slightly and then flexes the patient forward to the level of the lumbar segment being treated, gapping the joint above.
  7. The practitioner repeats the maneuver in a rhythmic manner for all segments, increasing flexion as the lower lumbar segments are treated, until the desired increase in range of motion is achieved.

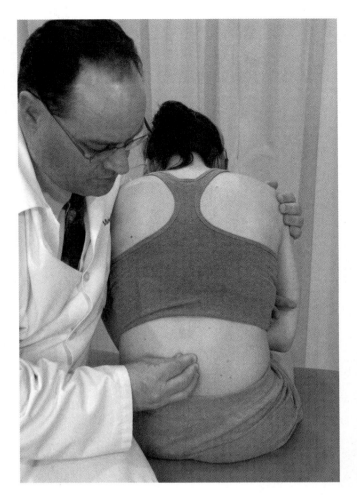

Figure 5.49　Seated lumbar articulatory technique: restricted flexion.

Sidelying Flexion
- Manipulation is performed as follows:
  1. For sidelying flexion, the patient lies in the left or right lateral recumbent position (Fig. 5.50).
  2. The practitioner stands facing the patient.
  3. The practitioner flexes the patient's knees and rests them against his or her thighs.
  4. The practitioner induces flexion in the patient's lumbar spine by using his or her hand to flex the patient's thighs. The practitioner uses one hand to monitor the gapping of the joint space at the segment being treated.
  5. This motion is repeated in a slow, rhythmic manner for all segments, increasing flexion as the upper lumbar segments are treated, until the desired increase in range of motion is achieved.

Seated Extension
- Manipulation is performed as follows:
  1. The patient is seated on the examination table (Fig. 5.51).
  2. The operator stands behind and to the right side of the patient.

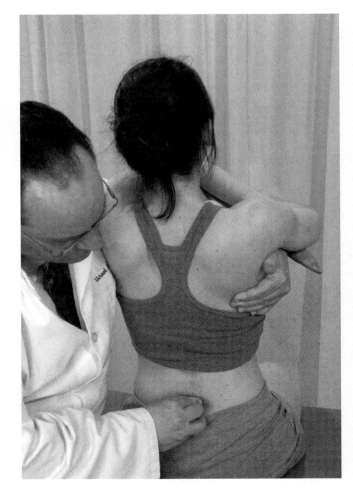

Figure 5.51　Seated lumbar articulatory technique: restricted extension.

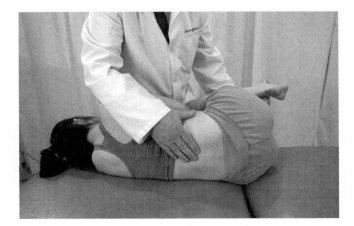

Figure 5.50　Sidelying lumbar articulatory technique: restricted flexion.

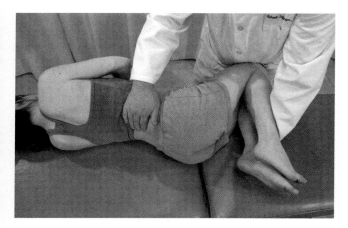

Figure 5.52   Sidelying lumbar articulatory technique: restricted extension.

3. The patient is instructed to cross his or her arms in front, with each hand grasping the opposite shoulder.
4. Using his or her right hand on the patient's elbows, the practitioner leans the patient forward slightly.
5. The practitioner's left hand stabilizes the lumbar spine at the level of the segment being treated.
6. The practitioner then uses his or her right hand to lift the patient's elbows and induce lumbar extension and then allows the spine to return slightly toward neutral.
7. The practitioner accentuates this extension with his or her left hand, applying an anterior force at the level of the segment being treated.
8. This motion is repeated in a slow, rhythmic manner for all segments, increasing extension as the lower lumbar segments are treated, until the desired increase in range of motion is achieved.

Sidelying Extension

• Manipulation is performed as follows:
 1. The patient lies in the right or left lateral recumbent position (Fig. 5.52).
 2. The practitioner stands facing the patient.
 3. The practitioner uses one hand to flex the patient's knees and hips, allowing the lumbar musculature to relax.
 4. The practitioner uses his or her other hand in the lumbar region as a fulcrum, applying an anterior pressure to the segment being treated, inducing a backward-bending lumbar motion, and then allowing the spine to return slightly toward neutral.
 5. This motion is repeated in a slow, rhythmic manner for all segments, increasing extension as the lower lumbar segments are treated, until the desired increase in range of motion is achieved.

Muscle Energy Procedures: Lumbar Spine

L5 in Neutral, Rotated Right, and Sidebent Left

• Diagnosis: L1 through L5 NR_RS_L (apex at L3) (Fig. 5.53)
• Restriction: L1 through L5 NR_LS_R

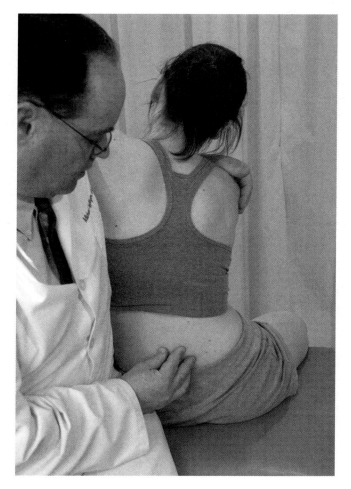

Figure 5.53   Seated lumbar muscle energy technique: L1 through L5; neutral, sidebent right, and rotated left (NS_RR_L).

• Manipulation is performed as follows:
 1. The patient is seated with arms folded.
 2. The practitioner stands or sits on the left side of the patient.
 3. The practitioner's right hand monitors the vertebral segment being treated.
 4. The practitioner places his or her left shoulder under the patient's right axilla, bringing the left arm in front of the patient and placing the left hand on top of the patient's right shoulder.
 5. The practitioner rotates the patient to the left by pulling anteriorly on the patient's left shoulder until a barrier is engaged.
 6. The practitioner sidebends the patient to the right by moving the patient's left shoulder superiorly and right shoulder inferiorly until a barrier is engaged.
 7. The patient is asked to attempt to sidebend to the left against the practitioner's unyielding counterforce offered with the practitioner's left arm.
 8. The patient maintains this effort for 3 to 5 seconds.
 9. This is followed by a complete relaxation for 2 to 3 seconds.

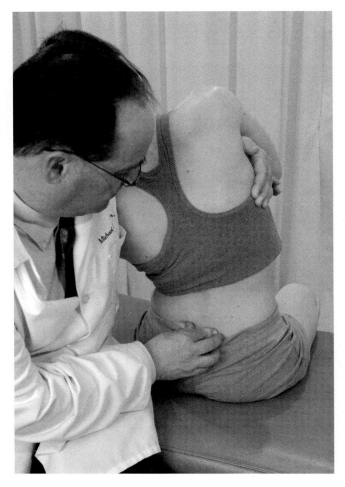

Figure 5.54 Seated lumbar muscle energy technique: L3; flexed, rotated right, and sidebent right (FR$_R$S$_R$).

10. The practitioner then reengages the barrier by further rotating the patient to the left and sidebending the patient to the right.
11. Steps 7 through 10 are repeated three to five times, followed by a final stretch into all planes of restriction.
12. The patient is retested.

L3 in Flexion, Rotated Right, and Sidebent Right
- Diagnosis: L3 FR$_R$S$_R$ (Fig. 5.54)
- Restriction: L3 ER$_L$S$_L$
- Manipulation is performed as follows:
  1. The patient is seated on the examination table with arms folded.
  2. The practitioner stands or sits to the left of the patient.
  3. The practitioner's right hand monitors the vertebral segment being treated.
  4. The practitioner places his or her left axilla over the patient's left shoulder, bringing his or her arm in front of the patient and placing the right hand under the patient's right axilla.

5. The practitioner extends the patient by pushing anteriorly on L3 with his or her left hand until a barrier is engaged.
6. The practitioner rotates the patient to the left by pulling anteriorly on the patient's right shoulder until a barrier is engaged.
7. The practitioner sidebends the patient to the left by moving the patient's left shoulder inferiorly and right shoulder superiorly until a barrier is reached.
8. The patient is asked to push his or her left shoulder toward the ceiling against the practitioner's unyielding counterforce.
9. The patient maintains the effort for 3 to 5 seconds.
10. This is followed by a complete relaxation for 2 to 3 seconds.
11. The practitioner then reengages the barrier by further extending, rotating the patient to the left and sidebending the patient to the left.
12. Steps 8 through 11 are repeated three to five times, followed by a final stretch into all planes of restriction.
13. The patient is retested.

L3 in Extension, Rotated Right, and Sidebent Right
- Diagnosis: L3 ER$_R$S$_R$ (Fig. 5.55)
- Restriction: L3 FR$_L$S$_L$

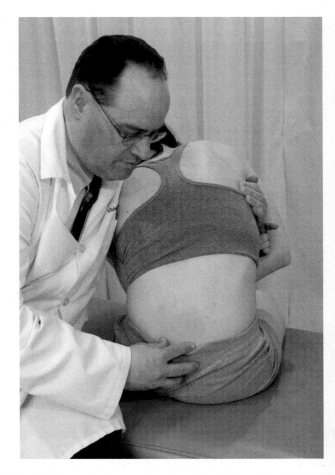

Figure 5.55 Seated lumbar muscle energy technique: L3; extended, rotated right, and sidebent right (ER$_R$S$_R$).

- Manipulation is performed as follows:
  1. The patient is seated on the examination table with arms folded.
  2. The practitioner stands or sits at the right side of the patient.
  3. The practitioner's right hand monitors the vertebral segment being treated.
  4. The practitioner places his or her left axilla over the patient's left shoulder, bringing his or her arm in front of the patient and placing his or her left hand under the patient's right axilla.
  5. Using his or her left arm, the practitioner flexes the patient until a barrier is engaged.
  6. The practitioner rotates the patient to the left by pulling anteriorly on the patient's right shoulder until a barrier is engaged.
  7. The practitioner sidebends the patient to the left by moving the patient's left shoulder inferiorly and right shoulder superiorly until a barrier is reached.
  8. The patient is asked to attempt returning to push his or her left shoulder toward the ceiling against the practitioner's unyielding counterforce.
  9. The patient maintains this effort for 3 to 5 seconds.
  10. This is followed by a complete relaxation for 2 to 3 seconds.
  11. The practitioner then reengages the barrier by further flexing, rotating the patient to the left and sidebending the patient to the left.
  12. Steps 8 through 11 are repeated three to five times, followed by a final stretch into all planes of restriction.
  13. The patient is retested.

L3 in Extension, Rotated Left, and Sidebent Left
- Diagnosis: L3 ER_LS_L (Figs. 5.56 and 5.57)
- Restriction: L3 FR_RS_R
- Manipulation is performed as follows:
  1. The patient lies in the left lateral recumbent position.
  2. The practitioner stands facing the patient.

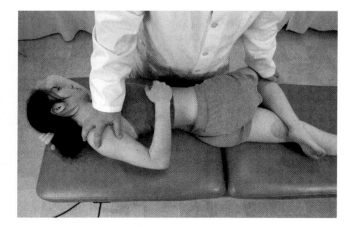

Figure 5.56 Sidelying muscle energy technique for treating the rotational component: L3; extended, rotated left, and sidebent left (ER_LS_L).

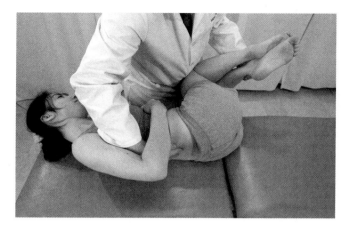

Figure 5.57 Sidelying muscle energy technique for treating the sidebending component: L3, extended, rotated left, and sidebent left (ER_LS_L).

  3. The practitioner monitors the lumbar area with his or her right hand while flexing the patient's knees and hips until the barrier is engaged at L3.
  4. The patient is asked to straighten his or her left leg, and the right foot is placed in the left popliteal space.
  5. The practitioner switches his or her monitoring hand so the left hand palpates the dysfunctional vertebra.
  6. The practitioner pulls the patient's left arm anteriorly and superiorly with the right hand, introducing right rotation and sidebending of the lumbar spine until the barrier is engaged at L3.

The muscle energy component is described subsequently and is broken down into two parts. The first part addresses the rotational component and the second part addresses the sidebending component of L3.

Part I
  7. To treat the rotational component, the practitioner places his or her right hand on the patient's right shoulder.
  8. The patient is asked to push anteriorly with his or her right shoulder against the practitioner's unyielding counterforce.
  9. The patient maintains this effort for 3 to 5 seconds.
  10. This is followed by a complete relaxation for 2 to 3 seconds.
  11. The practitioner then reengages the barrier by further rotating the patient to the right.
  12. Steps 9 through 12 are repeated three to five times, followed by a final stretch.

Part II
  13. To treat the sidebending component, the practitioner flexes both of the patient's hips and knees and lifts the ankles toward the ceiling until the barrier is reached.
  14. The patient is asked to push his or her ankles toward the floor against the practitioner's unyielding counterforce.
  15. The patient maintains this effort for 3 to 5 seconds.
  16. This is followed by a complete relaxation for 2 to 3 seconds.
  17. The practitioner then reengages the barrier by further sidebending the patient to the right.
  18. Steps 15 through 18 are repeated three to five times, followed by a final stretch.
  19. The patient is retested.

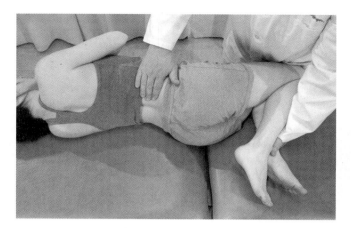

Figure 5.58 Sidelying muscle energy technique for inducing extension in the lumbar spine: L3; flexed, rotated left, and sidebent left (FR$_L$S$_L$).

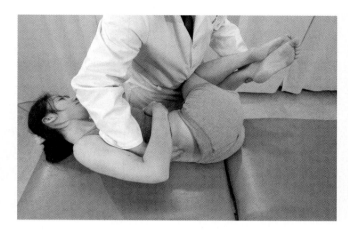

Figure 5.60 Sidelying muscle energy technique for treating the sidebending component: L3; flexed, rotated left, and sidebent left (FR$_L$S$_L$).

L3 in Flexion, Rotated Left, and Sidebent Left

- Diagnosis: L3 FR$_L$S$_L$ (Figs. 5.58 to 5.60)
- Restriction: L3 ER$_R$S$_R$
- Manipulation is performed as follows:
  1. The patient lies in the left lateral recumbent position.
  2. The practitioner stands facing the patient.
  3. The practitioner monitors the lumbar area with his or her right hand while flexing the patient's knees and hips until motion is achieved at L3.
  4. The practitioner then induces extension at L3 by pushing the patient's knees and hips posteriorly.
  5. The patient is asked to straighten his or her left leg, and the right foot is placed in the left popliteal space.
  6. The practitioner switches his or her monitoring hand so that the left hand palpates the dysfunctional vertebra.
  7. The practitioner pulls the patient's left arm anteriorly and superiorly with his or her right hand, introducing right rotation and sidebending of the lumbar spine until the barrier is engaged at L3.

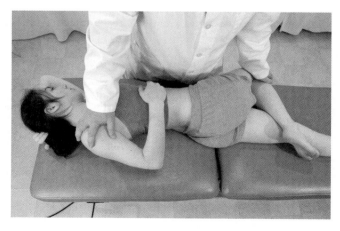

Figure 5.59 Sidelying muscle energy technique for treating the rotational component: L3; flexed, rotated left, and sidebent left (FR$_L$S$_L$).

The muscle energy component is described subsequently and is broken down into two parts. The first part addresses the rotational component and the second part addresses the sidebending component of L3.

Part I

8. To treat the rotational component, the practitioner places his or her right hand on the patient's right shoulder.
9. The patient is asked to push anteriorly with his or her right shoulder against the practitioner's unyielding counterforce.
10. The patient maintains this effort for 3 to 5 seconds.
11. This is followed by a complete relaxation for 2 to 3 seconds.
12. The practitioner then reengages the barrier by further rotating the patient to the right.
13. Steps 10 through 13 are repeated three to five times, followed by a final stretch.

Part II

14. To treat the sidebending component, the practitioner flexes both of the patient's hips and knees and lifts the ankles toward the ceiling until the barrier is reached.
15. The patient is asked to push his or her ankles toward the floor against the practitioner's unyielding counterforce.
16. The patient maintains this effort for 3 to 5 seconds.
17. This is followed by a complete relaxation for 2 to 3 seconds.
18. The practitioner then reengages the barrier by further sidebending the patient to the right.
19. Steps 17 through 20 are repeated three to five times, followed by a final stretch.
20. The patient is retested.

L1 to L5 in Neutral, Rotated Left, and Sidebent Right

- Diagnosis: L1 through L5 NR$_L$S$_R$ (apex at L3) (Figs. 5.61 and 5.62)
- Restriction: L1 through L5 NR$_R$S$_L$
- Manipulation is performed as follows:
  1. The patient lies in the left lateral recumbent position.
  2. The practitioner stands facing the patient.

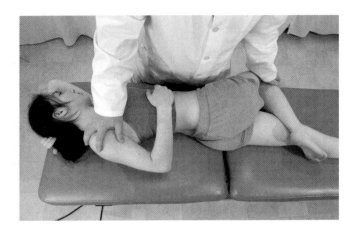

Figure 5.61 Sidelying muscle energy technique for treating the rotational component.: L1 through L5; neutral, rotated left, and sidebent right (NR$_L$S$_R$).

3. The practitioner monitors the lumbar area with his or her right hand while flexing the patient's knees and hips until motion is achieved at L3.
4. The patient is asked to straighten his or her left leg, and the right foot is placed in the left popliteal space.
5. The practitioner switches his or her monitoring hand so the left hand is palpating the dysfunctional vertebra.
6. The practitioner pulls the patient's left arm anteriorly and inferiorly with his or her right hand introducing right rotation and left sidebending of the lumbar spine until motion is achieved at L3.

The muscle energy component is described subsequently and is broken down into two parts. The first part addresses the rotational component, and the second part addresses the sidebending component of L3.

Part I

7. To treat the rotational component, the practitioner places his or her right hand on the patient's right shoulder.

8. The patient is asked to push anteriorly with his or her right shoulder against the practitioner's unyielding counterforce.
9. The patient maintains this effort for 3 to 5 seconds.
10. This is followed by a complete relaxation for 2 to 3 seconds.
11. The practitioner then reengages the barrier by further rotating the patient to the right.
12. Steps 8 through 11 are repeated three to five times, followed by a final stretch.

Part II

13. To treat the sidebending component, the practitioner flexes both of the patient's hips and knees and brings the ankles down off the table until the barrier is reached.
14. The patient is asked to lift his or her ankles toward the ceiling against the practitioner's unyielding counterforce.
15. The patient maintains this effort for 3 to 5 seconds.
16. This is followed by a complete relaxation for 2 to 3 seconds.
17. The practitioner then reengages the barrier by further sidebending the patient to the left.
18. Steps 14 through 17 are repeated three to five times, followed by a final stretch.
19. The patient is retested.

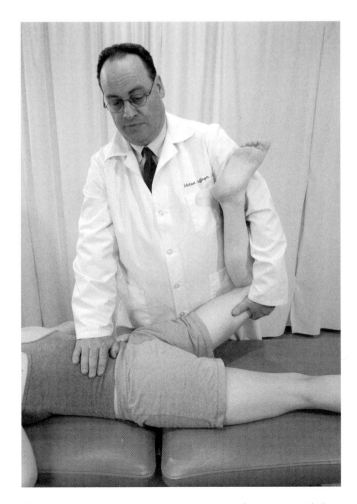

Figure 5.63 Prone muscle energy technique for psoas restriction.

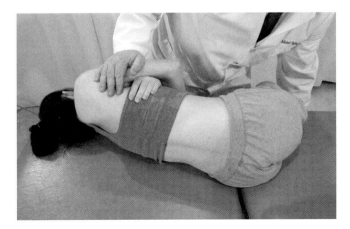

Figure 5.62 Sidelying muscle energy technique for treating the sidebending component: L1 through L5; neutral, rotated left, and sidebent right (NR$_L$S$_R$).

Hypertonic Psoas Muscle

- Diagnosis: hypertonic psoas muscle
- Restriction: hip restriction in extension (Fig. 5.63)
- Manipulation is performed as follows:
  1. The patient is prone on the examination table.
  2. The practitioner stands on the side of the dysfunctional psoas muscle.
  3. The practitioner flexes the patient's knee to 90 degrees.
  4. The practitioner then grasps the patient's leg just above the knee with one hand, and with the other hand, the practitioner stabilizes the patient's lumbar region.
  5. The practitioner extends the patient's leg, stretching the psoas muscle until the barrier is engaged.
  6. The patient is instructed to pull his or her leg toward the table against the practitioner's unyielding counterforce.
  7. The patient maintains this effort for 3 to 5 seconds.
  8. This is followed by a complete relaxation for 2 to 3 seconds.
  9. The practitioner then further extends the patient's leg until the next barrier is engaged.
  10. Steps 6 through 9 are repeated three to five times.
  11. The patient is retested.

Muscle Energy Procedures: Pelvis

Forward Sacral Torsion

- Diagnosis: forward sacral torsion (Fig. 5.64)
- Example: left on left sacral torsion (i.e., sacral base is rotated toward the left on a left oblique axis)
- Restriction: Right sacral base is restricted in extension or counternutation.
- Manipulation is performed as follows:
  1. The patient is prone on the examination table.
  2. The practitioner stands to the right side of the patient.
  3. The practitioner flexes the patient's knees to 90 degrees and rolls the patient onto his or her left hip, keeping the patient's chest and upper trunk flat on the table.
  4. The practitioner monitors the L5 vertebra with his or her left hand.

5. The practitioner uses his or her right hand on the patient's posterior right shoulder to induce trunk rotation to the left until motion at L5 is palpated.
6. The practitioner uses his or her right hand to monitor the lumbosacral junction.
7. With his or her left hand, the practitioner extends the patients lower legs off the table and sidebends the legs toward the floor until motion is felt at the lumbosacral junction.
8. The patient is then instructed to attempt to raise both feet toward the ceiling against the practitioner's unyielding counterforce.
9. The patient maintains the effort for 3 to 5 seconds.
10. This is followed by a complete relaxation for 2 to 3 seconds.
11. The practitioner engages the next motion barrier by sidebending the lower legs further toward the floor.
12. Steps 8 through 11 are repeated three to five times, followed by a final stretch.
13. The patient is retested.

Backward Sacral Torsion

- Diagnosis: backward sacral torsion (Fig. 5.65)
- Example: right on left sacral torsion (i.e., sacral base is rotated toward the right on a left oblique axis)
- Restriction: The right sacral base is restricted in flexion or nutation.
- Manipulation is performed as follows:
  1. The patient lies in the left lateral recumbent position.
  2. The practitioner stands facing the patient.
  3. The practitioner monitors the patient's lumbosacral junction with his or her left hand.
  4. The practitioner pulls the patient's left arm anteriorly and inferiorly, introducing left sidebending and right rotation of the lumbar spine until motion at L5 is palpated.
  5. The practitioner introduces extension of both of the patient's legs with his or her left hand while the right hand monitors the left sacral base until the base begins to move anteriorly.
  6. The practitioner places the patient's right leg over the edge of the table, flexing the patient's hip to 90 degrees.

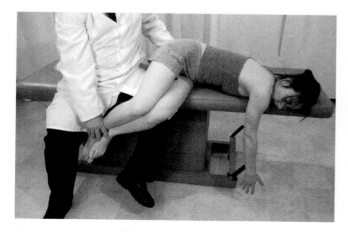

Figure 5.64 Muscle energy technique for left on left sacral torsion.

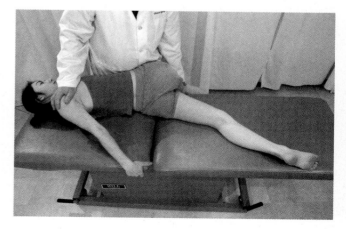

Figure 5.65 Muscle energy technique for right on left sacral torsion.

7. The practitioner places his or her left hand against the lateral aspect of the patient's distal right femur.
8. The patient is instructed to attempt to raise his or her right leg toward the ceiling against the practitioner's unyielding counterforce.
9. The patient maintains this effort for 3 to 5 seconds.
10. This is followed by a complete relaxation for 2 to 3 seconds.

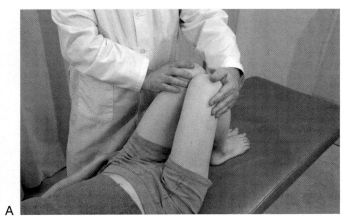

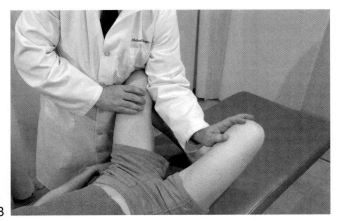

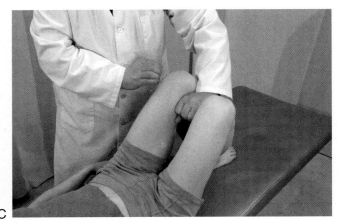

Figure 5.66 Muscle energy technique for pubic symphysis restriction. **A**, Resisting abduction. **B**, Resisting adduction of the legs using the forearm. **C**, Resisting adduction using the fist.

11. The practitioner engages the next motion barrier by moving the patient's right leg further toward the floor.
12. Steps 8 through 11 are repeated three to five times, followed by a final stretch into the restriction.
13. The patient is retested.

Pubic Symphysis Dysfunction
- Diagnosis: pubic symphysis dysfunction (Fig. 5.66)
- Manipulation is performed as follows:
  1. The patient is supine on the examination table.
  2. The practitioner stands at either side of the patient.
  3. The patient flexes the hips and knees leaving his or her feet together and flat on the table.

Part I
  4. The practitioner holds the patient's knees together.
  5. The patient is instructed to abduct his or her knees against the practitioner's unyielding counterforce (see Fig. 5.66A).
  6. This effort is maintained for 3 to 5 seconds.
  7. This is followed by a complete relaxation for 2 to 3 seconds.
  8. Steps 5 through 7 are repeated three to five times.

Part II
  9. The patient is instructed to abduct his or her knees, and the practitioner places his or her forearm or fist between them.
  10. The patient is instructed to adduct his or her knees against the practitioner's unyielding counterforce (see Fig. 5.66B and C).
  11. This effort is maintained for 3 to 5 seconds.
  12. This is followed by a complete relaxation for 2 to 3 seconds.
  13. Steps 10 through 12 are repeated three to five times.
  14. The patient is retested.

- Part I uses isometric contraction of the abductors for reciprocal inhibition of the adductors to decrease their tone; part II uses the adductors to pull on the pubic bones from their attachments on the inferior pubic rami to level the pubic symphysis.

Superior Innominate Shear
- Diagnosis: superior innominate shear (Fig. 5.67)
- Example: right superior innominate shear (this is a positional diagnosis, and therefore no particular motion restriction is

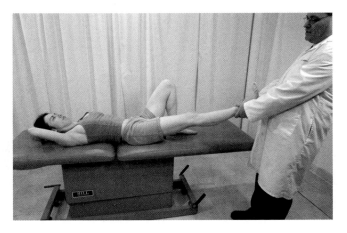

Figure 5.67 Muscle energy technique for right superior innominate shear.

assigned because motion in all directions is not possible due to the lack of proper articulation of the iliosacral joint; the innominate is superior to the sacral articular surfaces).
• Manipulation is performed as follows:
  1. The patient is supine on the examination table with his or her feet extending to the end of the table.
  2. The practitioner stands at the end of the table and grasps the patient's right leg just proximal to the ankle with both hands.
  3. The practitioner abducts the patient's right leg 10 to 15 degrees to gap the sacroiliac joint.
  4. The practitioner internally rotates the patient's abducted right leg to provide slight compression of the right sacroiliac joint.
  5. The practitioner applies inferior traction to the patient's right leg while the patient performs a series of deep inhalation and exhalation efforts.
  6. The patient attempts to flex his or her left hip, pulling the right leg superiorly against the practitioner's unyielding counterforce.
  7. Steps 5 and 6 are repeated three to five times.
  8. The patient is retested.
• Having the patient hop on the affected leg with an extended knee to move the hip superiorly can often reduce the inferior innominate shear, and manual procedures usually are unnecessary.
• The innominates can also be anteriorly or posteriorly rotated (Fig. 5.68).

Anterior Innominate Rotation
• Diagnosis: anterior innominate rotation (Fig. 5.69)
• Example: left anterior innominate rotation
• Restriction: restriction of the left innominate in posterior rotation
• Manipulation is performed as follows:
  1. The patient is supine on the examination table.
  2. The practitioner stands at the left side of the supine patient.
  3. The practitioner fully flexes the patient's left hip and knee.
  4. The thenar eminence of the practitioner's left hand contacts the patient's left ischial tuberosity with the fingers extending toward the PSIS.

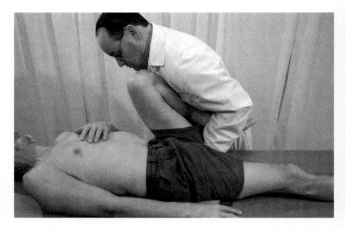

Figure 5.69   Muscle energy technique for left anterior innominate rotation.

  5. The practitioner flexes, externally rotates, and abducts the patient's left leg with his or her right hand.
  6. The practitioner exerts a superior and lateral force on the patient's left ischial tuberosity.
  7. The patient is instructed to attempt to extend his or her leg against the practitioner's unyielding counterforce.
  8. This contraction is held for 3 to 5 seconds, followed by complete relaxation for 2 to 3 seconds.
  9. The practitioner reengages the barrier by increasing the posterior rotation of the left innominate.
  10. Steps 5 through 7 are repeated three to five times, followed by a final stretch into the resistance.
  11. The patient is retested.

Posterior Innominate Rotation
• Diagnosis: posterior innominate rotation (Fig. 5.70)
• Example: left posterior innominate rotation
• Restriction: left innominate anterior rotation restriction
• Manipulation is performed as follows:
  1. The patient is supine on the examination table.
  2. The practitioner stands at the left side of the patient.

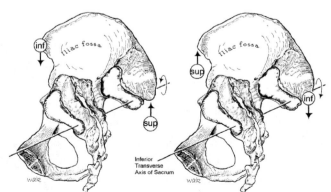

Figure 5.68   Comparison of anterior and posterior innominates.

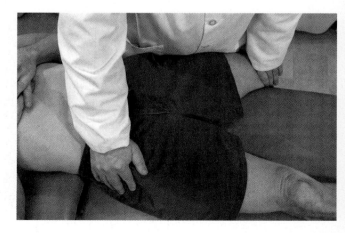

Figure 5.70   Muscle energy technique for left posterior innominate rotation.

3. The patient is positioned on the left side of the table until the left sacral border is at the edge of the table.

4. The patient's left lower extremity is extended off the table and held between the practitioner's knees.

5. The practitioner places his or her left hand over the patient's right ASIS region for stability.

6. The practitioner's right hand contacts the patient's left distal femur above the patella.

7. The patient is instructed to raise his or her left leg toward the ceiling against the practitioner's unyielding counterforce.

8. This effort is maintained for 3 to 5 seconds, followed by complete relaxation for 2 to 3 seconds.

9. The practitioner engages a new barrier by extending the patient's leg further toward the floor.

10. Steps 7 through 9 are repeated three to five times, followed by a final stretch into the restriction.

11. The patient is retested.

Functional (Indirect) Technique for Lumbosacral Somatic Dysfunction

- Indications
  1. Diagnosis of lumbar or sacral somatic dysfunction
  2. Patients who cannot lie down

3. Works well in the third-trimester pregnant patient and the postpartum patient

- Treatment
  1. The patient is seated.
  2. The practitioner sits in front of the knees of the seated patient.
  3. The practitioner gently grasps the patient's distal femurs bilaterally and uses the palms to cup the patient's knees.
  4. The practitioner introduces a compressive force toward the patient's hip joints one side at a time, observing the relative tightness or looseness of the lumbar-pelvic tissues (Fig. 5.71A and B).
  5. The practitioner determines which side is more compliant to the compressive force. The patient's right side in this series of pictures is more compliant.
  6. The practitioner maintains compression toward the compliant right hip and asks the patient to flex at the waist while retesting compression toward the right hip joint (see Fig. 5.71C).
  7. To maintain the balance of forces, the practitioner pulls the patient's left proximal tibia toward him or her using the four finger pad contact on the posterior aspect of the tibia.
  8. To compare, the practitioner asks the patient to extend backward and retests compression toward the compliant hip (see Fig. 5.71D).

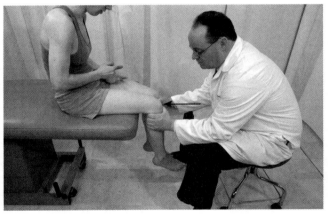

A

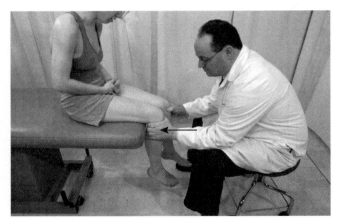

B

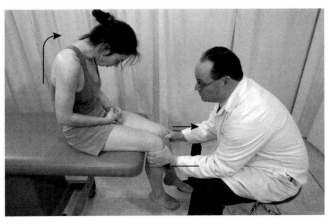

C

Figure 5.71   Seated functional technique for the lumbosacral spine. **A**, The practitioner compresses the left hip. **B**, The practitioner compresses the patient's right hip. **C**, The patient flexes her spine while the practitioner compresses the right hip.

Continued

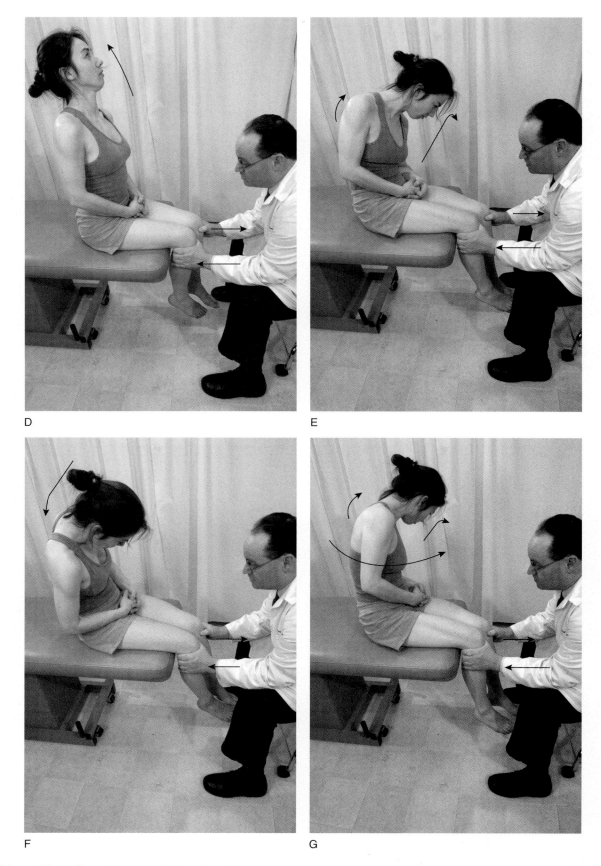

Figure 5.71, cont'd D, The patient extends her spine while the practitioner compresses the right hip. **E**, The patient is slightly flexed and sidebends left while the practitioner compresses the right hip. **F**, The patient is slightly flexed and sidebends right while the practitioner compresses the right hip. **G**, The patient is slightly flexed, slightly sidebends left, and rotates left while the practitioner compresses the right hip.

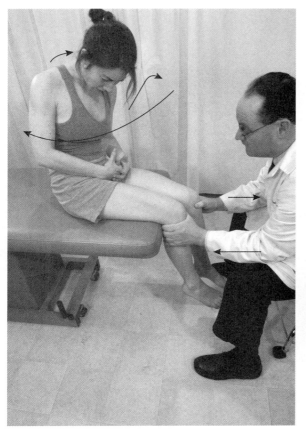

H

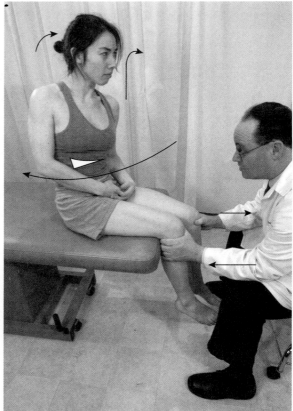

I

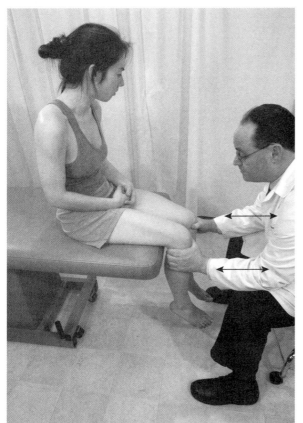

J

Figure 5.71, cont'd   H, The patient is slightly flexed, slightly sidebends left, and rotates right while the practitioner compresses the right hip. I, The patient slightly flexes, slightly sidebends left, rotates right, and inhales while the practitioner compresses the right hip. J, The practitioner rechecks the right and left hips with the compliance test. After these manipulations, both should be equally compliant.

9. The practitioner determines whether flexion or extension made the hip more compliant, or loose, and has the patient maintain that posture. In the example depicted in the figures, the patient's right hip is more compliant when the patient flexes than extends. She is asked to maintain a slightly flexed spine while testing the other spinal motions one at a time.

10. The same procedure is repeated for sidebending with the patient maintaining the compliant posture (flexed in this case) (see Fig. 5.71E and F).

11. The practitioner determines to which direction of sidebending the compressive force toward the right hip joint has less resistance. In this case, sidebending left enabled more compliance in the right hip.

12. While maintaining the positions of ease in slight flexion and slight left sidebending, the patient is asked to rotate left and then right to determine which direction facilitates ease of the hip compression (see Fig. 5.71G and H). In this case, right rotation enabled more compliance.

13. The practitioner determines in which phase of respiration—inhalation or exhalation—there is more ease of hip compression.

14. The practitioner stacks, or combines, all the spinal motions of ease at one time, adding at the very end the phase of respiration that facilitates compliance of passive hip compression. In this case, the patient's right hip is most compliant to compression when she flexes, sidebends left, rotates right, and inhales (see Fig. 5.71I). The patient need not use a full range of motion. Initiating the motion in the directions that facilitate ease or compliance is sufficient.

15. When the patient finishes the phase of respiration that facilitates ease and compliance of hip compression (inhalation in this case), the patient is asked to return to a resting sitting position, and left and right hip compressions are retested (see Fig. 5.71J).

16. There should be ease in either direction. If not, the procedure can be repeated without harm.

Lumbar and Pelvic Strain and Counterstrain

Anterior Lumbar Counterstrain Points

The anterior lumbar counterstrain points are shown in Figure. 5.72.

Anterior Lumbar 1
- Location: 2 to 3 cm medial to the ASIS (Fig. 5.73A)
- Treatment position: see Figure 5.73B
- Manipulation is performed as follows:
  1. The patient is supine.
  2. The practitioner stands on same side as the tender point.
  3. The practitioner places one foot on the treatment table and rests the patient's lower extremities over the practitioner's femur.
  4. The practitioner flexes the patient's hips to about 135 degrees.
  5. The practitioner pulls the patient's knees and ankles slightly toward the tender point until the maximum position of comfort is reached.
  6. The practitioner holds this position for 90 seconds.

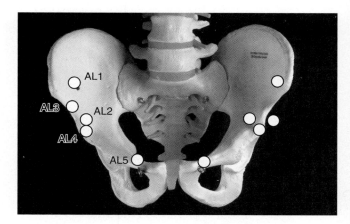

Figure 5.72   Anterior lumbar counterstrain tender points AL1 through AL5.

7. The practitioner slowly returns the patient to a neutral, resting supine position.

8. The practitioner rechecks the severity of the tender point.

- The anterior L2 (AL2), L3 (AL3), and L4 (AL4) counterstrain points are located very close to each other. As a result, the treatment positions for these three counterstrain points are similar. Figure 5.74 shows the location of and treatment position for AL2 as an example of the treatment positioning for these three counterstrain points.

Anterior Lumbar 2
- Location: on the medial aspect of the AIIS (see Fig. 5.74A)
- Treatment position: see Figure 5.74B
- Manipulation is performed as follows:
  1. The patient is supine.
  2. The practitioner stands on side opposite the tender point.
  3. The practitioner places one foot on the treatment table and rests the patient's lower extremities over the practitioner's femur.
  4. The practitioner flexes the patient's hips to about 135 degrees.
  5. The practitioner pulls the patient's knees and ankles slightly toward himself or herself until the maximum position of comfort is reached.
  6. The practitioner holds this position for 90 seconds.
  7. The practitioner slowly returns the patient to a neutral, resting supine position.
  8. The practitioner rechecks the severity of the tender point.

Anterior Lumbar 3 and 4
- Locations: AL3 on the lateral aspect of the AIIS and AL4 on the inferior aspect of the AIIS
- Manipulation is performed as follows:
  1. The patient is supine.
  2. The practitioner stands on side opposite the tender point.
  3. The practitioner places one foot on the treatment table and rests the patient's lower extremities over the practitioner's femur.
  4. The practitioner flexes the patient's hips to about 90 degrees.

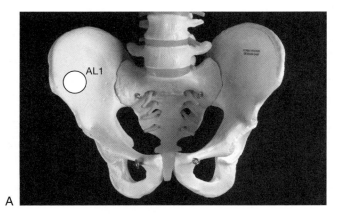

A

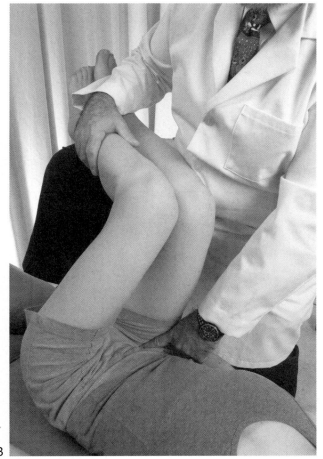

B

Figure 5.73 **A**, Location of the right anterior lumber 1 (AL1) counterstrain point. **B**, Treatment position for the right AL1 counterstrain point.

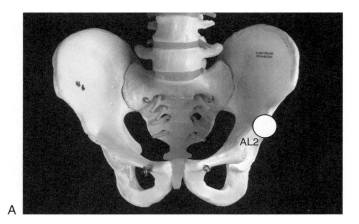

A

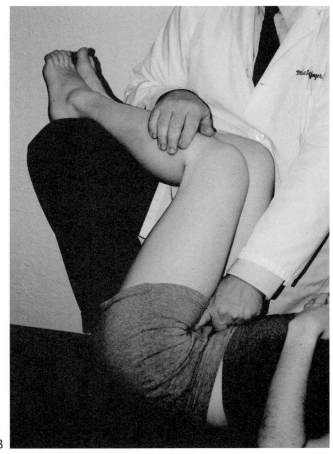

B

Figure 5.74 **A**, Location of the left anterior lumbar 2 (AL2) counterstrain point. **B**, Treatment position for the left AL2 counterstrain point.

5. The practitioner pulls the patient's ankles slightly toward himself or herself while the knees remain in the midline until the maximum position of comfort is reached.
6. The practitioner holds this position for 90 seconds.
7. The practitioner slowly returns the patient to neutral, resting supine position.
8. The practitioner rechecks the severity of the tender point.

Anterior Lumbar 5
- Location: on the anterior pubic bone approximately 1 cm lateral to the pubic symphysis (Fig. 5.75A)
- Treatment position: see Figure 5.75B
- Manipulation is performed as follows:
  1. The patient is supine.
  2. The practitioner stands on side opposite the tender point.

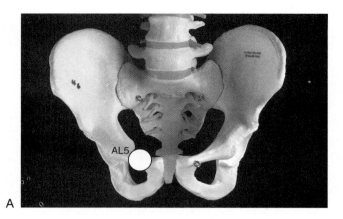

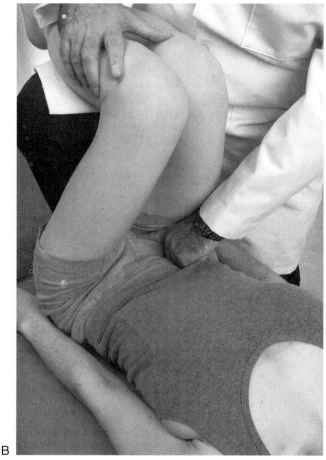

Figure 5.75 **A**, Location of the right anterior lumbar 5 (AL5) counterstrain point. **B**, Treatment position for the right AL5 counterstrain point.

3. The practitioner places one foot on the treatment table and rests the patient's lower extremities over the practitioner's femur.
4. The practitioner flexes the patient's hips to about 90 degrees.
5. The practitioner pulls the patient's knees slightly toward himself or herself while the ankles remain in the midline until the maximum position of comfort is reached.

6. The practitioner holds this position for 90 seconds.
7. The practitioner slowly returns the patient to neutral, resting supine position.
8. The practitioner rechecks the severity of the tender point.

Posterior Lumbar Counterstrain Points

Posterior lumbar counterstrain points are shown in Figure 5.76. The posterior lumbar (PL) counterstrain points PL1 through PL5 are all located and treated similarly. The PL3 counterstrain point location and its treatment position are described as an example for these five counterstrain points.

Posterior Lumbar 1 through 5

- Location: on the spinous process of each corresponding vertebra, L1 through L5 (Fig. 5.77A shows the location of PL3 as an example)
- Treatment position: see Figure 5.77B (for PL3 as an example)
- Manipulation is performed as follows:
  1. The patient is prone.
  2. The practitioner diagnoses the rotational component of the corresponding vertebra. The practitioner then stands

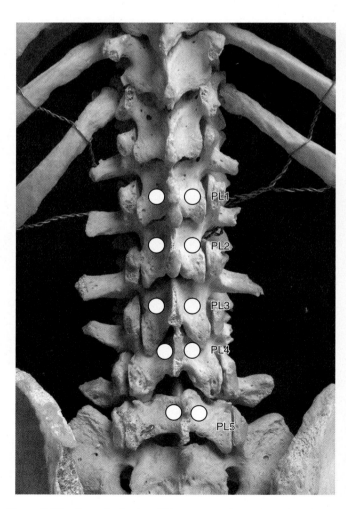

Figure 5.76 Posterior lumbar (PL) counterstrain tender points PL1 through PL5.

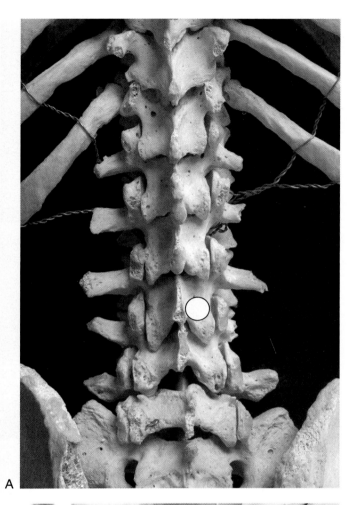

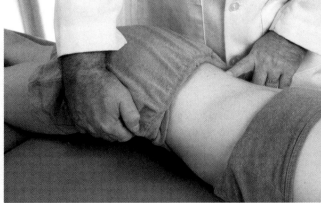

Figure 5.77 **A**, Location of the right posterior lumbar 3 (PL3) counterstrain point. **B**, Treatment position for the right PL3 counterstrain point.

on the side opposite the posterior transverse process. The practitioner grasps the opposite ASIS and raises the pelvis toward himself or herself approximately 45 degrees until the maximum position of comfort is reached.
3. The practitioner holds this position for 90 seconds.

4. The practitioner slowly returns the patient to neutral, resting prone position.
5. The practitioner rechecks the severity of the tender point.

Posterior Pelvis Counterstrain Points
The posterior pelvis counterstrain points are shown in Figure 5.78.

Upper Pole Lumbar 5
- Location: on the superomedial surface of the PSIS (Fig. 5.79A)
- Treatment position: see Figure 5.79B
- Manipulation is performed as follows:
  1. The patient is prone.
  2. The practitioner extends the patient's ipsilateral leg and externally rotates the hip, adding adduction or abduction as needed.
  3. The practitioner holds this position for 90 seconds.
  4. The practitioner slowly returns the patient to neutral, resting prone position.
  5. The practitioner rechecks the severity of the tender point.

Lower Pole Lumbar 5
- Location: on the inferior surface of the PSIS (Fig. 5.80A)
- Treatment position: see Figure 5.80B
- Manipulation is performed as follows:
  1. The patient is prone.
  2. The practitioner flexes the patient's hip and knee to 90 degrees off the side of the table and adducts and internally rotates the hip as needed until the maximum position of comfort is reached.
  3. The practitioner holds this position for 90 seconds.
  4. The practitioner slowly returns the patient to neutral, resting prone position.
  5. The practitioner rechecks the severity of the tender point.

Piriformis
- Location: midway between the greater trochanter and ILA, in the belly of the piriformis muscle (Fig. 5.81A)
- Treatment position: see Figure 5.81B

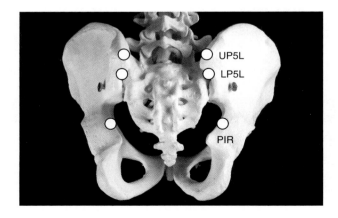

Figure 5.78 Posterior pelvis counterstrain tender points upper pole lumbar 5 (UPL5), lower pole lumbar 5 (LPL5), and piriformis (PIR).

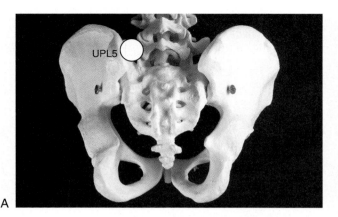

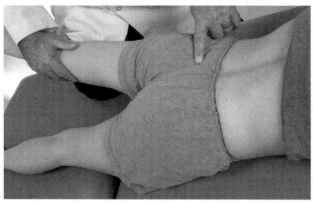

Figure 5.79 **A,** Location of the left upper pole lumbar 5 (UPL5) counterstrain point. **B,** Treatment position for the left UPL5 counterstrain point.

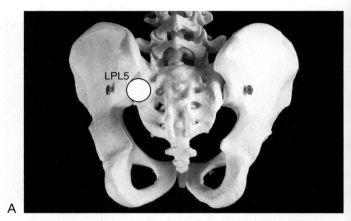

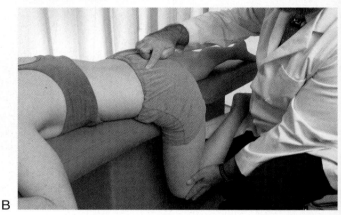

Figure 5.80 **A,** Location of the left lower pole lumbar 5 (LPL5) counterstrain point. **B,** Treatment position for the LPL5 counterstrain point.

- Manipulation is performed as follows:
  1. The patient is prone.
  2. The patient's thigh on the affected side is suspended over the side of the table.
  3. The practitioner flexes the patient's hip to 90 to 135 degrees and then adds abduction and external rotation of the femur until the maximum position of comfort is reached.
  4. The practitioner holds this position for 90 seconds.
  5. The practitioner slowly returns the patient to neutral, resting prone position.
  6. The practitioner rechecks the severity of the tender point.

ADJUNCT TREATMENTS

- Surgical consultation is indicated in cases of disc herniation with radiculopathy to the lower extremity, intractable leg pain, footdrop, progressive neurologic deficits, or a change in bowel or bladder control.
- Acupuncture has shown conflicting results in RCTs.
- Back schools, bed rest, traction, corsets, electrical stimulation, most exercises, and oral or injected medications have not been shown to prevent initial or recurrent episodes of LBP or prevent

acute LBP from becoming chronic. However, they are popular options that are still used by practitioners and patients.[2,39]
- Psychosocial and behavioral issues should also be addressed as part of the management plan because they play a significant role in the prevention, prognosis, and rehabilitation of patients with mechanical LBP.[2,3,39,54]

EDUCATION

- Proper posture and ergonomics are essential (i.e., no twisting and lifting while bending forward with knees extended).
- Objects should be held close to the body, because held any distance away from the body increases the amount of force (i.e., load) and strain on the lumbar spine.
- When reaching for objects above head level, the object should be kept directly in front at all times to avoid twisting the spine while holding it.
- When reaching for objects below waist level, the person should bend the knees and keep the back extended before standing up

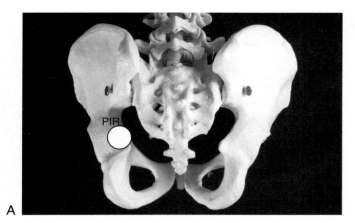

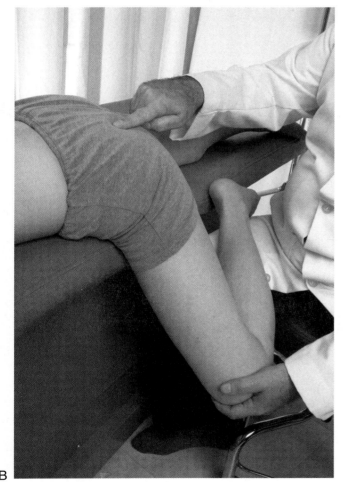

Figure 5.81 **A,** Location of the left piriformis (PIR) counterstrain point. **B,** Treatment position for the PIR counterstrain point.

with the object to diminish the amount of load placed on the lumbar spine.

- Patient information brochures and recommendations for content or educational instructions to patients with LBP for primary care practitioners are available on the internet and in journal articles.[55]

EXERCISES

- Exercises have been helpful for patients with acute LBP, especially if they are designed for each patient's needs,[56] if they match the patient's directional preference,[57] and if they centralize the pain.[58]
- Exercise for patients with chronic LBP is thought to prevent debilitation of the musculoskeletal system from inactivity.
- There is limited evidence that back exercises are superior to manipulation for LBP after disc herniation surgery (grade A evidence).[19]
- Exercises for patients with LBP are primarily designed to relieve and prevent recurrence of pain by restoring and maintaining lumbar and trunk muscle strength and lower extremity muscle flexibility. All exercises are designed to improve motion and function of the lumbar spine. They can help promote proper postural mechanics during activities of daily living. Some exercises are designed to help centralize the back pain, and others relieve the pain completely.
- The practitioner can design an exercise regimen for each patient based on the clinical situation, taking into account the practitioner's and patient's preferences and goals. The CD contains printable exercise handouts for patients.
- Exercises to improve lumbar spine mobility and strength, abdominal strength, and some lower extremity stretches are presented here, with several more strengthening and stretching exercises available on the CD accompanying this book.

Exercises to Improve Mobility of the Lumbar Spine

For this set of exercises, you lie supine (face up) on your back on an exercise mat on the floor with your feet flat and knees bent. The number of repetitions and sets is gradually increased as your endurance develops.

Pelvic Tilt with a Flat Back
- The exercise is performed as follows:
  1. Push your the back toward the floor, and flatten it on the floor. This is done by tilting your pelvis toward your trunk by tightening your abdominal muscles (Fig. 5.82A). Do not lift your pelvis off the floor during this exercise.
  2. Hold this position for 10 seconds.
  3. Relax your abdominal muscles, and return to the starting position.
  4. Repeat steps 1 through 3 for 3 sets of 3 repetitions.

Pelvic Tilt with an Arched Back
- The exercise is performed as follows:
  1. Lift your back away from the floor, and arch your back. This is done by tilting your pelvis toward your knees using the low back muscles (see Fig. 5.82B).
  2. Hold this position for 10 seconds.
  3. Relax the low back muscles, and return to the starting position.
  4. Repeat steps 1 through 3 for 3 sets of 3 repetitions.

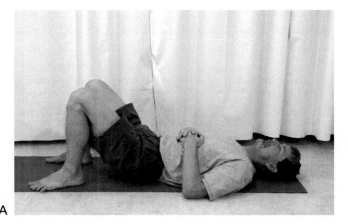

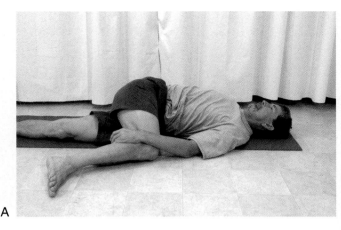

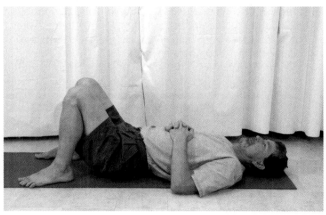

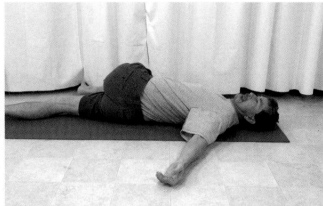

Figure 5.82 **A,** Pelvic tilt with a flat back. **B,** Pelvic tilt with an arched back.

Figure 5.83 **A,** one-leg hip roll to the left. **B,** one-leg hip roll to the right.

One-Leg Hip Roll

- The exercise is performed as follows:
  1. Lie down on your back on an exercise mat on the floor (Fig. 5.83).
  2. Bring your right knee across your hips to the opposite side toward the floor using your left hand to hold it so that your right hip is 90 degrees to your body. Keep your shoulders on the floor.
  3. The ipsilateral arm can be used for balance, stretching it out at 90 degrees to your body (see Fig. 5.83).
  4. Hold this position for 5 to 10 seconds.
  5. Return to the starting position.
  6. Repeat this exercise with the opposite leg.
  7. Repeat steps 1 through 6 for 2 sets.
  8. This exercise can also be performed on a bed or sturdy treatment table (see Fig. 5.83C to E).

Both-Legs Hip Roll

- The exercise is performed as follows:
  1. Lie on your back with your feet flat and knees bent on an exercise mat on the floor (Fig. 5.84).
  2. Rotate both knees to one side as far as possible, allowing the feet to come off the floor, but the knees continue to rotate to one side toward the floor. Move as far as you can.

3. Hold this position for 5 seconds.
4. Return to the starting position.
5. Repeat this exercise on the opposite side.
6. Repeat steps 1 through 5 until you have performed 2 sets of 2 repetitions.

Sphinx Pushup

- The exercise is performed as follows:
  1. Lie face down on a mat with your arms away to your sides, elbows bent, beside your face (Fig. 5.85).
  2. Slowly push up on your arms, supported by your elbows; look forward while you rise, and extend your back.
  3. Hold this position for 5 to 10 seconds.
  4. Return to the starting position.
  5. Repeat steps 1 through 4 for 2 sets of 3 repetitions.

Scared Cat

- The exercise is performed as follows:
  1. Begin on your hands and knees on a mat on the floor (Fig. 5.86).
  2. Arch your back upward toward the ceiling and put your head down toward the floor to round your back like an angry cat.
  3. Hold this position for 10 seconds.

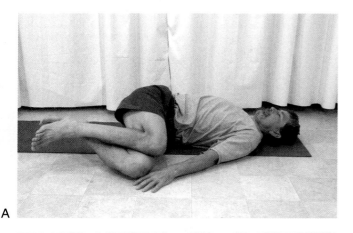

A

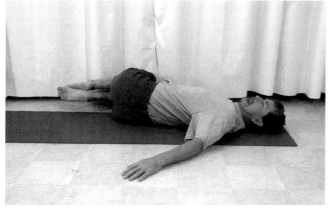

B

Figure 5.84 **A**, Both-legs hip roll to the left. **B**, Both-legs hip roll to the right.

4. Return to the starting position.
5. Repeat steps 1 through 4 for 3 sets.

Downward-Arched Back
- The exercise is performed as follows:
  1. Begin on your hands and knees on a mat on the floor (Fig. 5.87).
  2. Arch your back by raising your head and pushing your abdomen downward toward the floor.

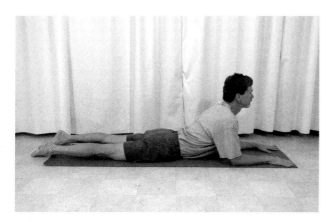

Figure 5.85   Sphinx pushup.

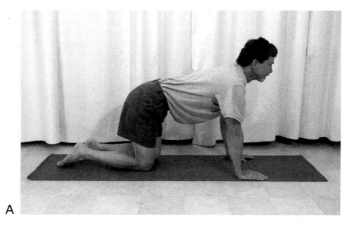

A

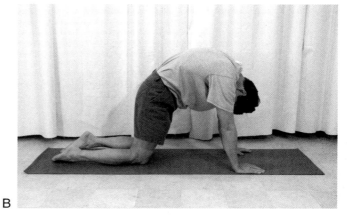

B

Figure 5.86   **A**, Scared cat starting position. **B**, Scared cat with an arched back.

3. Hold this position for 5 seconds.
4. Return to the starting position.
5. Repeat steps 1 through 4 for 2 sets of 2 repetitions.

Exercise to Strengthen Low Back Muscles

These exercises are performed lying in a prone position on an exercise mat on the floor.

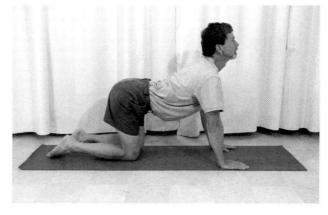

Figure 5.87   Downward arched back.

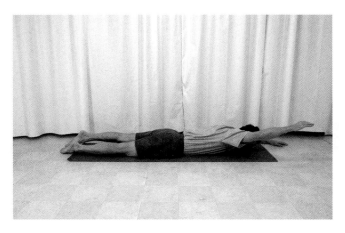

Figure 5.88   Single-arm raise.

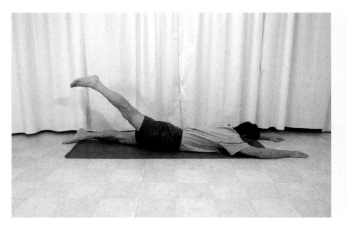

Figure 5.90   Single-leg raise.

Single-Arm Raise
- The exercise is performed as follows:
  1. Lie face down on an exercise mat on the floor (Fig. 5.88).
  2. Raise one arm straight in front of you.
  3. Hold this position for 5 seconds.
  4. Return to the starting position.
  5. Repeat this exercise with the opposite arm.
  6. Repeat steps 1 through 5 for 2 sets.

Single-Arm High Raise
- The exercise is performed as follows:
  1. Lie face down on an exercise mat on the floor (Fig. 5.89).
  2. Raise one arm upward.
  3. Hold this position for 5 seconds.
  4. Return to the starting position.
  5. Repeat this exercise with the opposite arm.
  6. Repeat steps 1 through 5 for 2 sets of 2 repetitions.

Single-Leg Raise
- The exercise is performed as follows:
  1. Lie face down on an exercise mat on the floor (Fig. 5.90).
  2. Raise one leg upward.

3. Hold this position for 5 seconds.
4. Return to the starting position.
5. Repeat this exercise on the opposite side.
6. Repeat steps 1 through 5 for 2 sets of 2 repetitions.

Opposite Leg and Arm Raise
- The exercise is performed as follows:
  1. Lie face down on an exercise mat on the floor (Fig. 5.91).
  2. Raise one leg and the opposite arm simultaneously.
  3. Hold this position for 5 seconds.
  4. Return to the starting position.
  5. Repeat this exercise on the opposite side
  6. Repeat steps 1 through 5 for 2 sets of 2 repetitions.

Exercises for Strengthening Weak Abdominal Muscles

For this set of exercises, you lie on your back supine on an exercise mat on the floor with your feet flat and knees bent. The amount of hold time, repetitions, and sets is gradually increased as your strength develops.

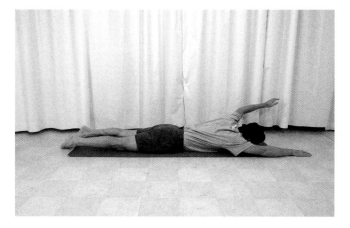

Figure 5.89   Single-arm high raise.

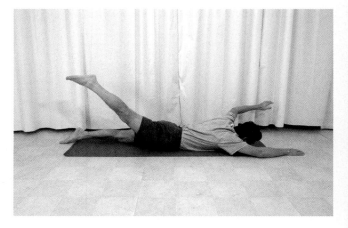

Figure 5.91   Opposite leg and arm raise.

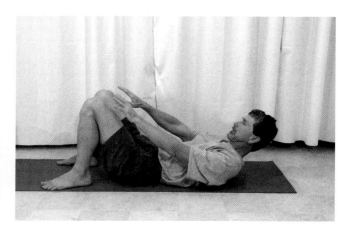

Figure 5.92   Curls.

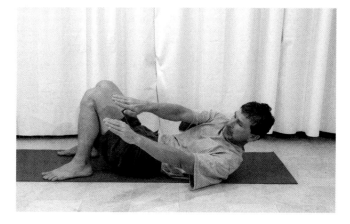

Figure 5.94   Lateral curls.

Curls
- The exercise is performed as follows:
  1. Slowly reach with both hands toward your knees so that your head and upper back come off the mat (Fig. 5.92).
  2. Hold this position for 5 seconds.
  3. Relax the abdominal muscles, and return to the starting position.
  4. Repeat steps 1 through 3 for 2 sets of 3 repetitions.

Curls for Weaker Abdominal Muscles
- The exercise is performed as follows:
  1. Lift your head and shoulders off the mat without using your arms. Your arms can be crossed over your chest (Fig. 5.93).
  2. Repeat steps 2 through 4 for regular curls.

Lateral Curls
- The exercise is performed as follows:
  1. Slowly reach with both hands to one side of your knees so that your head and upper back come off the mat (Fig. 5.94).
  2. Hold this position for 5 seconds.

  3. Relax your abdominal muscles, and return to the starting position.
  4. Repeat this exercise on the opposite side.
  5. Repeat steps 1 through 4 for 2 sets of 3 repetitions.

Core Stability Basic Exercise
- The following exercise can be done in any position:
  1. Tighten the abdominal muscles around the umbilicus (i.e., navel or belly button) and pull them toward your back.
  2. Hold for 30 seconds or as long as is comfortable.
  3. Relax the abdominal muscles.
  4. Repeat as often as possible throughout the day and gradually increase the holding time.

Exercises to Stretch the Leg Muscles

For this set of exercises, you lie on your back on an exercise mat on the floor with your feet flat and knees bent. The length and duration of the stretch are gradually increased as your flexibility improves.

Hamstring Stretches
- Stage 1 of the exercise is performed as follows:
  1. Bring one knee toward your chest using both hands over your knee (Fig. 5.95).
  2. Hold this position for 5 to 10 seconds.
  3. Return to the starting position.
  4. Repeat this exercise with the opposite leg.
  5. Repeat steps 1 through 4 until for 3 sets of 3 repetitions.
- Stage 2 of the exercise is performed as follows:
  1. Bring both knees to your chest assisted by both hands. The hands can be in front or behind the knees—whatever is more comfortable (Fig. 5.96).
  2. Hold this position for 5 to 10 seconds.
  3. Return to the starting position.
  4. Repeat steps 1 through 3 for 3 sets of 3 repetitions.
- Stage 3 of the exercise is performed as follows:
  1. Bend one knee and support it from underneath with both hands (Fig. 5.97A).

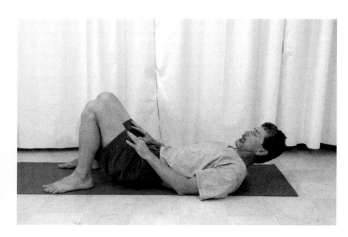

Figure 5.93   Curls for weaker abdominal muscles.

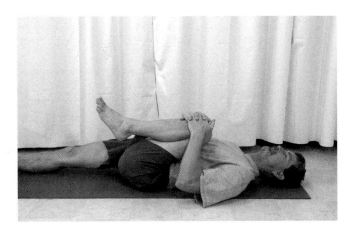

Figure 5.95 Stage 1 hamstring stretch.

2. Gradually straighten out your leg so that it is at 90 degrees to your body. A stretch should be felt in the back of your leg. To increase the stretch, point your toes toward your head (see Fig. 5.97B).
3. Hold this position for 5 to 10 seconds.
4. Return to the starting position.
5. Repeat this exercise with the opposite leg.
6. Repeat steps 1 through 5 until for 3 sets of 3 repetitions.

Piriformis Stretch

- The exercise is performed as follows:
  1. Lie on your back on an exercise mat on the floor (Fig. 5.98).
  2. Bring your right knee toward your left shoulder using your right hand. The knee can be pushed toward the midline, and your ankle can be pulled toward your left hip. A stretching sensation should be felt in the outside of your right hip.
  3. Hold this position for 5 to 10 seconds.
  4. Return to the starting position.
  5. Repeat this exercise with the opposite leg.
  6. Repeat steps 1 through 5 until for 3 sets of 3 repetitions.

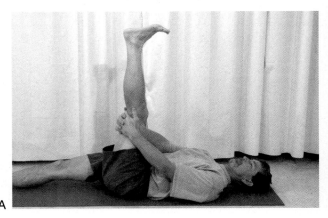

A

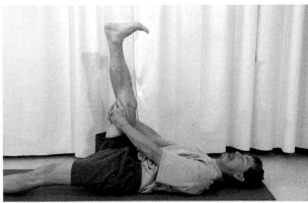

B

Figure 5.97 **A,** Stage 3 left hamstring stretch. **B,** Stage 3 right hamstring stretch.

CONTROVERSIES

- Should all physicians be taught palpatory musculoskeletal (including spinal) diagnosis and manipulative treatment as part of their training, or should they decide individually whether they want to study and learn it as an adjunctive skill obtained in postgraduate training?

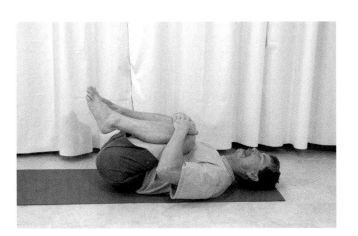

Figure 5.96 Stage 2 hamstring stretch.

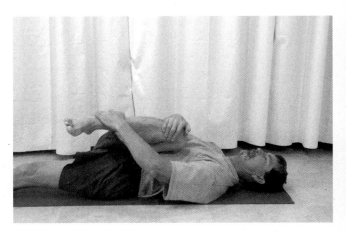

Figure 5.98 Piriformis stretch.

- Should all patients be offered spinal manipulation for acute LBP as an option or as a standard of care?
- An RCT by a health maintenance organization (HMO) in Southern California randomized patients to care with an MD alone or with the addition of a PT or to a DC. The study demonstrated higher expenses for DC or PT care compared with MD care alone, with no additional benefit in measurable outcomes at 18 months' follow-up. However, patients were most satisfied with chiropractic care.[7]
- The cost-effectiveness of manual treatment compared with traditional medical care alone was not demonstrated in this HMO environment; results may be different with fee for service, other insurance plans, or patients covered under worker's compensation. Osteopathic physicians (DO) have long maintained that their combined care of medications plus manual treatment cuts costs by limiting the need for PT or DC care.[47]

OPPORTUNITIES FOR RESEARCH

The following questions should be addressed in regard to manipulation for patients with LBP:

- What are the biologic mechanisms of efficacy of manual therapy?
- What is the safety and efficacy of various manual treatment procedures?
- What is the incidence and prevalence of lumbar, sacral, and pelvic somatic dysfunction in the general population, in the military population, and in the work environment?
- What is the natural course in patients who have suffered trauma (e.g., motor vehicle accidents, falls) compared with those who did not have a history of trauma?
- Which is most beneficial: standard medical care with or without exercise versus standard care plus manipulation with or without exercise?
- Can benefit from manipulation be predicted from the patient's history and physical examination results?
- Can early spinal manipulation treatment of soldiers with acute LBP decrease the time to resolution of symptoms and increase function and earlier return to duty?
- Should the U.S. Department of Defense guidelines for the evaluation and treatment of low back pain and guidelines for spinal manipulation utilization by military personnel be updated since manual treatment is now widely available and utilized on military bases since the 1999 guidelines were published?[59]
- What is the optimal number of treatments for patients with acute and chronic LBP?
- What is the cost-effectiveness of this form of therapy?

REFERENCES

1. Hurwitz EL, Morgenstern H: Correlates of back problems and back-related disability in the United States. J Clin Epidemiol 50:669-681, 1997.
2. Hurwitz EL, Shekelle PG: Epidemiology of low back syndromes. In Morris CE (ed): Low Back Syndromes: Integrated Clinical Management. New York, McGraw-Hill, 2005.
3. National Research Council and the Institute of Medicine: Musculoskeletal Disorders and the Workplace: Low Back and Upper Extremities. Panel on Musculoskeletal Disorders and the Workplace, Commission on Behavioral and Social Sciences and Education. Washington, DC, National Academy Press, 2001.
4. Guo HR, Tanaka S, Halperin WE, et al: Back pain prevalence in US industry and estimates of lost workdays. Am J Public Health 89:1029-1035, 1999.
5. Wheeler AH: Diagnosis and management of low back pain and sciatica. Am Fam Physician 52:1333-1341, 1995.
6. Mein E: Low back pain and manual medicine: A look at the literature. In Stanton D (ed): Manual Medicine. Physical Medicine and Rehabilitation Clinics of North America. New York, WB Saunders, 1996, pp 715-729.
7. Kominski GF, Heslin KC, Morgenstern H, et al: Economic evaluation of four treatments for low back pain: Results from a randomized controlled trial. Med Care 43:428-435, 2005.
8. Deyo RA, Weinstein JN: Low back pain. N Engl J Med 344:363-370, 2001.
9. Jones HJ: Somatic dysfunction. In Ward RC (ed): Foundations for Osteopathic Medicine, 2nd ed. Philadelphia, Lippincott Williams & Wilkins, 2003, pp 1153-1161.
10. Patterson MM, Wurster RD: Neurophysiologic mechanisms of integration and disintegration. In Ward RC (ed): Foundations for Osteopathic Medicine, 2nd ed. Philadelphia, Lippincott Williams & Wilkins, 2003, pp 120-136.
11. Willard FW: Nociception, the neuroendocrine immune system, and osteopathic medicine. In Ward RC (ed): Foundations for Osteopathic Medicine, 2nd ed. Philadelphia, Lippincott Williams & Wilkins, 2003, pp 137-156.
12. Peng B, Hou S, Wu W, et al: The pathogenesis and clinical significance of a high-intensity zone (HIZ) of lumbar intervertebral disc on MR imaging in the patient with discogenic low back pain. Eur Spine J 15:583-587, 2006.
13. Peng B, Wu W, Hou S, et al: The pathogenesis of discogenic low back pain. J Bone Joint Surg Br 87:62-67, 2005.
14. Dugan SA, Frost D, Sullivan KP: An active and cost-conservative approach to the management of low back pain. J Clin Outcomes Manage 8:38-47, 2001.
15. Al-Eisa E, Egan D, Wassersug R: Fluctuating asymmetry and low back pain. Evol Hum Behav 25:31-37, 2004.
16. Seffinger MA, Najm WI, Mishra SI, et al: Reliability of spinal palpation for diagnosis of back and neck pain: A systematic review of the literature. Spine 29:E413-E425, 2004.
17. Goldstein M (ed): The Research Status of Spinal Manipulative Therapy. NINCDS monograph no. 15, DHEW publication (NIH) no. 76-998. Bethesda, U.S. Department of Health, Education, and Welfare, 1975.
18. Bigos SJ, Bowyer OR, Braen GR, et al: Acute Low Back Problems in Adults: Assessment and Treatment. Clinical practice guideline no. 14. Public Health Services, Agency for Health Care Policy and Research publication no. 95-0643. Rockville, MD, U.S. Department of Health and Human Services, December 1994.
19. Bronfort G, Haas M, Evans RL, et al: Efficacy of spinal manipulation and mobilization for low back pain and neck pain: A systematic review and best evidence synthesis. Spine J 4:335-356, 2004.
20. Bronfort G: Spinal manipulation: Current state of research and its indications. Neurol Clin 7:91-111, 1999.
21. Buerger AA, Greenman PE (eds): Empirical Approaches to the Validation of Spinal Manipulation. Springfield, IL, Charles C Thomas, 1985.
22. Koes BW, Assendelft WJ, van der Heijden GJ, et al: Spinal manipulation for low back pain: An updated systematic review of randomized clinical trials. Spine 21:2860-2873, 1996.
23. Kuchera ML, DiGiovanna EL, Greenman PE: Efficacy and complications. In Ward RC (ed): Foundations for Osteopathic Medicine, 2nd ed. Philadelphia, Lippincott Williams & Wilkins, 2003, pp 1143-1152.
24. Shekelle PG, Adams AH, Chassin MR, et al: Spinal manipulation for low-back pain. Ann Intern Med 117:590-598, 1992.
25. Shekelle PG: Spine update: Spinal manipulation. Spine 19:858-861, 1994.
26. Tobis JS, Hoehler F: Musculoskeletal Manipulation. Springfield, IL, Charles C Thomas, 1986.
27. van Tulder MW, Goossens M, Waddell G, et al: Conservative treatment of chronic low back pain. In Nachemson AL, Jonsson E (eds): Neck and Back Pain: The Scientific Evidence of Causes, Diagnosis, and Treatment. Philadelphia, Lippincott Williams & Wilkins, 2000, pp 271-304.
28. van Tulder MW, Koes BW, Bouter LM: Conservative treatment of acute and chronic nonspecific low back pain: A systematic review of randomized controlled trials of the most common interventions. Spine 22:2128-2156, 1997.
29. Bigos SJ: Lower back pain. Perils, pitfalls, and accomplishments of guidelines for treatment of back problems. Neurol Clin 17:179-192, 1999.
30. Koes B, Tulder MV, Ostelo R, et al: Clinical guidelines for the management of low back pain in primary care: An international comparison. Spine 26:2504-2514, 2001.
31. Assendelft WJJ, Morton SC, Yu EI, et al: Spinal manipulative therapy for low back pain: A meta-analysis of effectiveness relative to other therapies. Ann Intern Med 138:871-881, 2003.
32. Assendelft WJJ, Morton SC, Yu E I, et al: Spinal manipulative therapy for low-back pain: The Cochrane Database Syst Rev (1):CD000447, 2004; dol.
33. Institute for Clinical Systems Improvement: Adult Low Back Pain Guidelines, 10th ed, 2004. Available at http://www.icsi.org/knowledge/detail.asp?catID=29&itemID=149/ Accessed August 12, 2005.
34. Licciardone JC: The unique role of osteopathic physicians in treating patients with low back pain. J Am Osteopath Assoc 104(Suppl 8):S13-S18, 2004.
35. Licciardone J, Brimhall AK, King LN: Osteopathic manipulative treatment for low back pain: A systematic review and meta-analysis of randomized controlled trials. BMC Musculoskelet Disord 6:43, 2005. Available at http://www.biomedcentral.com/1471-2474/6/43/ Accessed August 14, 2005.

36. Ernst E, Harkness E: Spinal manipulation: A systematic review of sham-controlled, double-blind, randomized clinical trials. J Pain Symptom Manage 22:879-889, 2001.
37. Cherkin DC, Sherman KJ, Deyo RA, Shekelle PG: A review of the evidence for the effectiveness, safety, and cost of acupuncture, massage therapy, and spinal manipulation for back pain. Ann Intern Med 138:898-906, 2003.
38. Ferreira ML, Ferreira PH, Latimer J, et al: Efficacy of spinal manipulative therapy for low back pain of less than three months' duration. J Manipulative Physiol Ther 26:593-601, 2003.
39. Hansson TH, Hansson EK: The effects of common medical interventions on pain, back function, and work resumption in patients with chronic low back pain: A prospective 2-year cohort study in six countries. Spine 25:3055-3064, 2000.
40. Aure OF, Nilsen JH, Vasseljen O: Manual therapy and exercise therapy in patients with chronic low back pain: A randomized, controlled trial with 1-year follow-up. Spine 28:525-531, 2003.
41. Childs JD, Fritz JM, Flynn TW, et al: A clinical prediction rule to identify patients with low back pain most likely to benefit from spinal manipulation: A validation study. Ann Intern Med 141:920-928, 2004.
42. Childs JD, Fritz JM, Piva SR, et al: Clinical decision making in the identification of patients likely to benefit from spinal manipulation: A traditional versus an evidence-based approach. J Orthop Sports Phys Ther 33:259-272, 2003.
43. Fritz JM, Childs JD, Flynn TW: Pragmatic application of a clinical prediction rule in primary care to identify patients with low back pain with a good prognosis following a brief spinal manipulation intervention. BMC Fam Pract 6:29, 2005; electronic version can be found online at: http://www.biomedcentral.com/141-2296/6/29.
44. Harvey E, Burton AK, Moffetgt JK, Breen A: Spinal manipulation for low back pain: A treatment package agreed by the UK chiropractic, osteopathy and physiotherapy professional associations. Man Ther 8:46-51, 2003.
45. UK BEAM Trial Team: United Kingdom back pain exercise and manipulation (UK BEAM) randomised trial: Effectiveness of physical treatments for back pain in primary care. BMJ 329:1377, 2004.
46. UK BEAM Trial Team: United Kingdom back pain exercise and manipulation (UK BEAM) randomised trial: Cost effectiveness of physical treatments for back pain in primary care. BMJ 329:1381, 2004.
47. Andersson, GB, Lucente T, Davis AM, et al: A comparison of osteopathic spinal manipulation with standard care for patients with low back pain. N Engl J Med 341:1426-1431, 1999.
48. Strickland C: Spinal manipulation effective for low back pain. J Fam Pract 52:925-929, 2003.
49. Curtis P, Carey TS, Evans P, et al: Training primary care physicians to give limited manual therapy for low back pain. Spine 25:2954-2961, 2000.
50. Haldeman S, Kohlbeck FJ, McGregor M: Risk factors and precipitating neck movements causing vertebrobasilar artery dissection after cervical trauma and spinal manipulation. Spine 24:785-794, 1999.
51. Powell FC, Hanigan WC, Olivero WC: A risk/benefit analysis of spinal manipulation therapy for relief of lumbar or cervical pain. Neurosurgery 33:73-78, commentary 78-79, 1993.
52. Swenson R, Haldeman S: Spinal manipulative therapy for low back pain. J Am Acad Orthop Surg 11:228-237, 2003.
53. Senstad O, Leboeuf-Yde C, Borchgrevink C: Frequency and characteristics of side effects of spinal manipulation therapy. Spine 22:435-441, 1997.
54. Waddell G: The Back Pain Revolution. New York, Churchill Livingstone, 2004.
55. Atlas SJ, Deyo RA: Evaluating and managing acute low back pain in the primary care setting. J Gen Intern Med 16:120-131, 2001.
56. Greenman PE: Principles of Manual Medicine, 3rd ed. Philadelphia, Lippincott Williams & Wilkins, 2003.
57. Long A, Donelson R, Fung T: Does it matter which exercise? A randomized control trial of exercise for low back pain. Spine 29:2593-2602, 2004.
58. Aina A, May S, Clare H: The centralization phenomenon of spinal symptoms: A systematic review. Man Ther 9:134-143, 2004.
59. Guideline Working Group, Veterans Health Administration, Department of Veterans Affairs, and Health Affairs, Department of Defense: Low Back Pain or Sciatica in the Primary Care Setting. Evidence-Based Clinical Practice. Office of Quality and Performance publication 10Q-CPG/LBP-99. Washington, DC, Veterans Health Administration and Department of Defense, November 1999.

Assendelft WJ, Koes BW, van der Heijden GJ, et al: The effectiveness of chiropractic for treatment of low back pain: An update and attempt at statistical pooling. J Manipulative Physiol Ther 19:499-507, 1996.
Atchison JW: Manipulation for the treatment of occupational low back pain. Occup Med 13:185-97, 1998.
Blomberg S, Svardsudd K, Tibblin G: A randomized study of manual therapy with steroid injections in low back pain: Telephone interview follow-up of pain, disability, recovery and drug consumption. Eur Spine J 3:246-254, 1994.
Boesler D, Warner M, Alpers A, et al: Efficacy of high-velocity low-amplitude manipulative technique in subjects with low-back pain during menstrual cramping. J Am Osteopath Assoc 93:203-214, 1993.
Bogduk N, McGuirk B: Medical Management of Acute and Chronic Low Back Pain. An Evidence-Based Approach. Pain Research and Clinical Management, vol 13. New York, Elsevier, 2002.
Bronfort G, Goldsmith CH, Nelson CF, et al: Trunk exercise combined with spinal manipulative or NSAID therapy for chronic low back pain: A randomized, observer-blinded clinical trial. J Manipulative Physiol Ther 19:570-582, 1996.
Carey TS, Garrett J, Jackman A, et al: The North Carolina back pain project: The outcomes and costs of care for acute low back pain among patients seen by primary care practitioners, chiropractors, and orthopedic surgeons. N Engl J Med 333:913-917, 1995.
Cherkin DC, DeyoRA, Battié M, et al: A comparison of physical therapy, chiropractic manipulation, and provision of an educational booklet for the treatment of patients with low back pain. N Engl J Med 339:1021-1029, 1998.
Connolly JF, Dehaven KE, Mooney V: Primary care management of musculoskeletal disorders. J Musculoskeletal Med 15:28-38, 1998.
Deyo RA, Rainville J: What can the history and physical examination tell us about low back pain? JAMA 268:760-765, 1992.
Dvorák J, Dvor·k V: Diagnostics. In Gilliar WG, Greenman PE (trans, eds): Manual Medicine. New York, Thieme, 1984.
Erhard RE, Delitto A, Cibulka MT: Relative effectiveness of an extension program and a combined program of manipulation and flexion and extension exercises in patients with acute low back syndrome. Phys Ther 74:1093-1100, 1994.
Fredericks CM, Saladin LK (eds): Pathophysiology of the Motor System. Philadelphia, FA Davis, 1996.
Gilliar WG, Kuchera ML: Neurologic basis of manual medicine. In Stanton D (ed): Manual Medicine. Physical Medicine and Rehabilitation Clinics of North America. New York, WB Saunders, 1996, p 693.
Greenman PE: Syndromes of the L-spine, pelvis and sacrum. In Stanton D (ed): Manual Medicine. Physical Medicine and Rehabilitation Clinics of North America. New York, WB Saunders, 1996, p 773.
Grieve GP: Common Vertebral Joint Problems. New York, Churchill Livingstone, 1981.
Haas M, Jacobs GE, Raphael R, et al: Low back pain outcome measurement assessment in chiropractic teaching clinics: Responsiveness and applicability of two functional disability questionnaires. J Manipulative Physiol Ther 18:79-87, 1995.
Haldeman SD: Spinal manipulation: When, how, and who? Bull Hosp Joint Dis 55:135-137, 1996.
Herzog W, Scheele D, Conway PT: Electromyographic responses of back and limb muscles associated with spinal manipulative therapy. Spine 24:146-153, 1999.
Hoffman KS, Hoffman L: Effects of adding sacral base leveling to osteopathic manipulative treatment of back pain: A pilot study. J Am Osteopath Assoc 94:217-228, 1994.
Khalil TM, Abdel-Moty EM, Rosomoff RS, et al: Ergonomics in Back Pain. A Guide to Prevention and Rehabilitation. New York, Van Nostrand Reinhold, 1993.
Koes BW: The second international forum for primary care research on low back pain. Spine 23:1991, 1998.
Leboeuf-Yde C, Hennius B, Rudberg E, et al: Side effects of chiropractic treatment: A prospective study. J Manipulative Physiol Ther 20:511-515, 1997.
MacDonald RS, Bell CMJ: An open controlled assessment of osteopathic manipulation in nonspecific low-back pain. Spine 15:346-370, 1990.
McIntyre IN, Broadhurst NA: Effective treatment of low back pain in pregnancy. Aust Fam Physician 54:456, 1996.
Östgaard HC, Zetherström G, Roos-Hansson E, et al: Reduction of back and posterior pelvic pain in pregnancy. Spine 19:894-900, 1994.
Patel AT, Ogle AA: Diagnosis and management of acute low back pain. Am Fam Physician 61:1779-1786, 2000.
Pope MH, Phillips RB, Haugh LD, et al: A Prospective randomized three-week trial of spinal manipulation, transcutaneous muscle stimulation, massage and corset in the treatment of subacute low back pain. Spine 19:2571-2577, 1994.
Schiötz EH, Cyriax J: Manipulation. Past and Present. London, William Heinemann Medical Books, 1975.
Shekelle PG, Hurwitz EL, Coulter I, et al: The appropriateness of chiropractic spinal manipulation for low back pain: A pilot study. J Manipulative Physiol Ther 18:265-270, 1995.
Von Korff M, Saunders K: The course of back pain in primary care. Spine 21:2833-2839, 1996.
Ward RC (ed): Foundations for Osteopathic Medicine. Philadelphia, Lippincott Williams & Wilkins, 2003.

SUGGESTED READING

Adams MA, Bogduk N, Burton K, et al: The Biomechanics of Back Pain. New York, Churchill Livingstone, 2002.
American Osteopathic Association: Glossary of osteopathic terminology. In American Osteopathic Association Yearbook and Directory of Osteopathic Physicians. Chicago, American Osteopathic Association, 2006. Available at www.osteopathic.org

CHAPTER **6**

Mechanical Neck and Upper Back Pain

- The pain is of musculoskeletal origin, typically in the posterior cervical region; it may also include the upper back.
  It is characterized by the presence of muscle spasm, decreased range and quality of motion, and pain worse with movement and better with rest.
- There is a lack of organic or systemic pathology to account for the pain.

EPIDEMIOLOGY

Age

- The age range is 9 to 102 years.[1-4]
- The incidence peaks between 20 and 40 years when the pain is related to motor vehicle accidents.[5]
- The incidence peak in the general population is between 30 and 59 years.[1,6]

Gender

- Females present with complaints of neck and upper back pain more than males.

Prevalence

- The point prevalence is 8% to 24%; the lifetime rate is 71%.[1-3,7]
- Neck pain is one of the most common complaints of patients seen by primary care practitioners worldwide.[8]
- Mechanical neck disorder is the most common cause of neck pain.[9]
- It is the second most common reason for which patients seek manual medical treatment (low back pain is the first).
- Neck pain is the most frequently reported symptom in connection with whiplash injury.[10]

1. Neck pain can result from 66% to 82% of rear end collisions and from 56% of side-impact collisions.[10] (Whiplash is a total-body injury, although people associate it most with neck symptoms.)
2. Seventy percent of patients with neck pain after rear-end traffic collisions are female drivers.[5]
3. For female drivers involved in collisions, the likelihood of neck pain increases as head restraint height decreases below the head's center of gravity.[5]
4. Reported neck pain decreases for older female drivers, drivers in less severe crashes, and female drivers in heavier cars.[5]

- Neck somatic dysfunction was the most commonly reported somatic dysfunction in patients seen by 10 osteopathic practitioners board certified in neuromusculoskeletal medicine and osteopathic manipulative medicine over a 6-month period.[11]
- Age- and gender-standardized annual incidence is 14.6%; less than 1% develop disabling neck pain.[1]
- Fifty-four percent of individuals surveyed have experienced neck pain within a 6-month period.[12,13]

Natural Clinical Course

- Neck pain is a chronic, episodic condition characterized by persistent, recurrent, or fluctuating pain and disability.[1]
- Only about one third of patients with neck pain experience complete resolution.[1]
- About one half of patients with an acute episode have persistent neck pain at 12 months.[6]
- After whiplash injury, neck pain along with headache persists for up to 2 years in 29% to 90% of patients (depending on the study), and neck pain alone can persist at 10 years in 74% of patients.[10] Even 17 years after a motor vehicle accident, 55% experience neck pain.[14]

Effect on Society

- Neck pain correlates with substantial medical consumption, absenteeism from work, and disability.[15]

- In the Netherlands, the total cost of neck pain in 1996 was estimated to be $686 million. The share of these costs was about 1% of total health care expenditures and 0.1% of the gross domestic product (GDP) in 1996. Direct costs were $160 million (23%). The total number of sick days related to neck pain were estimated to be $1.4 million, with a total cost of $185.4 million.[15]
- Neck pain from strain or sprain of the paraspinal soft tissues accounts for the greatest number of primary care visits to an out patient clinic or emergency room of all musculoskeletal nonskin laceration soft tissue injuries.[16]
- Permanent medical disability occurs in about 10% of patients involved in rear-end motor vehicle collisions. Although 79% may return to work within 1 month, 6% are unable to return to work at 1 year.[10]
- A higher severity of pain at onset and a history of previous attacks seem to be associated with a worse prognosis. However, localization (i.e., radiation to the arms or neurologic signs) and radiographic findings (i.e., degenerative changes in the discs and joints) are not associated with a worse prognosis.[17]

Risk Factors

- Risks for developing neck pain can be categorized as comorbid conditions that are found most commonly in patients with neck pain or work-related risk factors, non–work-related risk factors, whiplash-related risk factors, and characteristics of patients with radicular neck pain (Tables 6.1 to 6.4).
- Somatic dysfunction in the upper back, low back, and shoulder can also predispose a person to develop mechanical neck pain (see "Pathophysiology").

FUNCTIONAL ANATOMY

Cervical Spine

The cervical spine has seven vertebrae (Figs. 6.1 to 6.3). The most superior is the atlas, designated as the first cervical vertebra (C1). It is a ringlike structure with anterior and posterior arches supported by intervening lateral masses that consist of articular surfaces and a modified transverse process (Fig. 6.4).

The atlas articulates with the occiput superiorly. This joint is designated in this text as the occipitoatlantal (OA) joint. It has several unique features. It has elliptical, bilateral, concave superior facets that converge anteriorly with a medial and inferior inclination to articulate with the convex surfaces of the occipital condyles. The atlas supports and enables the head to glide like a ball, nodding forward (i.e., nutation or flexion) and backward (i.e., counternutation or extension) as if to signal "yes" (Fig. 6.5).

The second cervical vertebra (C2) is called the axis (Fig. 6.6) The atlas' articulation with the axis is unique. This joint is called the atlantoaxial (AA) joint (Fig. 6.7). Unlike all other vertebrae, the atlas lacks a vertebral body. In its place, the odontoid process of the second cervical vertebra (called the dens for *toothlike*) fills the void and articulates on the posterior surface of the anterior arch of the atlas, held firmly in place by two cruciate ligaments

Table 6.1 Comorbid conditions associated with neck pain

Associated Comorbidities	Studies
Autonomic failure	Bleasdale-Barr and Mathias, 1998[23]
Cardiovascular disease	Côté et al, 2000[12,13]
	Hartvigsen et al, 2004[2]
Concentration problems	Hoving et al, 2002[26]
Digestive system disease	Côté et al, 2000[12,13]
	Hartvigsen et al, 2004[2]
Dizziness	Hoving et al, 2002[26]
Headaches	Côté et al, 2000[12,13]
	Ståhl et al, 2004[4]
Low back pain	Côté et al, 2000[12,13]
	Hartvigsen et al, 2004[2]
	Hill et al, 2004[6]
Occipitoatlantal osteoarthritis	Zapletal et al, 1996[24]
Orthostatic hypotension	Bleasdale-Barr and Mathias, 1998[23]
Shoulder pain	Andersen et al, 2003[21]
	Borg et al, 2004[20]
	Bot et al, 2005[8]
	Grooten et al, 2004[19]
	Hartvigsen et al, 2004[2]
	Hill et al, 2004[6]
	Siivola et al, 2004[18]
	Ståhl et al, 2004[4]
	Vogt et al, 2003[7]
	Walker-Bone et al, 2004[3]
Temporomandibular joint syndrome	Ciancaglini et al, 1999[22]
Trapezius muscle ischemia	Larsson et al, 1999[25]
Nausea	Hoving et al, 2002[26]

Table 6.2 Work environment–related risk factors for development of neck pain

Work Risk Factors	Studies
Hand-arm vibration	Ariëns et al, 2000[27]
High and low skill discretion	Ariëns et al, 2001[28,29]
High quantitative job demands	Ariëns et al, 2001[28,29]
	Andersen et al, 2003[21]
Low job control	Ariëns et al, 2001[28,29]
	Andersen et al, 2003[21]
Low job satisfaction	Ariëns et al, 2001[28,29]
Low social (coworker) support	Ariëns et al, 2001[28,29]
Neck flexion (>20 degrees)	Ariëns et al, 2001[28,29]
	Andersen et al, 2003[21]
Sitting at work >95% of the working time	Ariëns et al, 2001[28,29]
Sustained arm postures	Ariëns et al, 2000[27]
Twisting or bending of the trunk	Ariëns et al, 2000[27]
Use of arm force	Ariëns et al, 2000[27]
Workplace design	Ariëns et al, 2000[27]

Table 6.3 Non–work-related risk factors for development of neck pain

Non–work-Related Risk Factors	Studies
Cycling	Hill et al, 2004[6]
Ergonomic factors involved with driving	Krause et al, 1997[30]
Female	Krause et al, 1997[30]
	Hill et al, 2004[6]
History of motor vehicle accident	Bunketorp et al, 2005[14]
Older age	Hill et al, 2004[6]
Previous low back pain	Hill et al, 2004[6]
Previous neck injury	Hill et al, 2004[6]
	Guez et al, 2003[32]
Psychological distress	Hill et al, 2004[6]
	Siivola et al, 2004[18]
Static postures (children)	Murphy et al, 2004[33]
Unemployed	Hill et al, 2004[6]
Very slow or very rapid arm motion speed	Lauren et al, 1997[31]

Table 6.4 Factors associated with radiating neck pain

Characteristics of Patients with Cervical Radiculopathy	Studies
Dental-facial problems	Friedman and Nelson, 1996[35]
Duration of work with a hand above shoulder level	Viikari-Juntura et al, 2001[34]
Female	Viikari-Juntura et al, 2001[34]
Mental stress	Viikari-Juntura et al, 2001[34]
Middle age	Viikari-Juntura et al, 2001[34]
Other musculoskeletal pains	Viikari-Juntura et al, 2001[34]
Overweight	Viikari-Juntura et al, 2001[34]
Smoking	Viikari-Juntura et al, 2001[34]

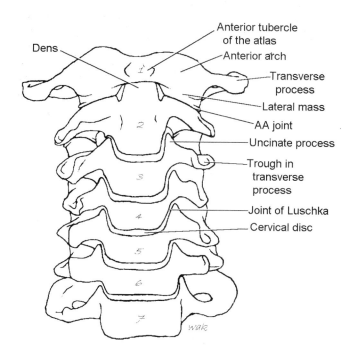

Figure 6.2 Posterior cervical spine.

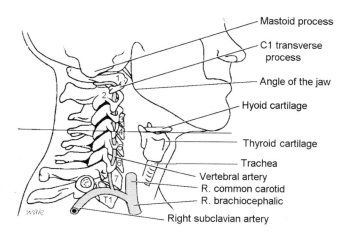

Figure 6.1 Lateral head and neck and cervical spine anatomic relationships.

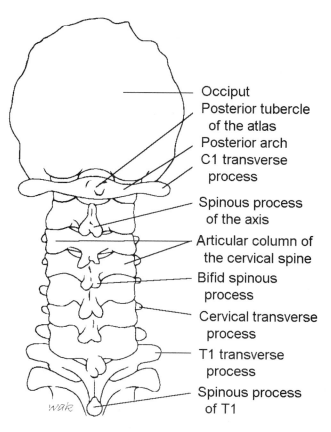

Figure 6.3 Anterior cervical spine.

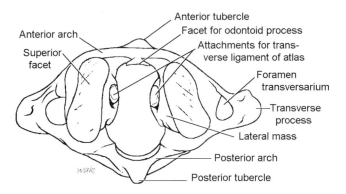

Figure 6.4   Atlas: superior view.

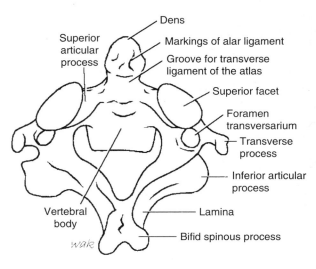

Figure 6.6   Axis: superior view.

and the odontoid ligament, which attaches the dens to the occiput. The atlas rotates, along with the head, left and right, pivoting around the dens of the second cervical vertebra, as if to signal "no" (Fig. 6.8). There also are bilateral inferior facets that articulate with C2.

The vertebral body of C2 is modified superiorly to form the odontoid process to articulate with the atlas (Fig. 6.9). The inferior facets of C2 are similar to those of C3 through C7; they are inclined at approximately 45 degrees, with their surfaces facing inferiorly and anteriorly. The approximating superior facets of C3, as well as the rest of the cervical vertebrae, face superiorly and posteriorly, angled at approximately 45 degrees (Fig. 6.10).

The cervical spine has a few more anatomic peculiarities. There is another synovial joint that enables articulation between the cervical vertebrae. It is bilateral on the lateral surface of each vertebral body of the C3 to C7 area, forming a lip, called an

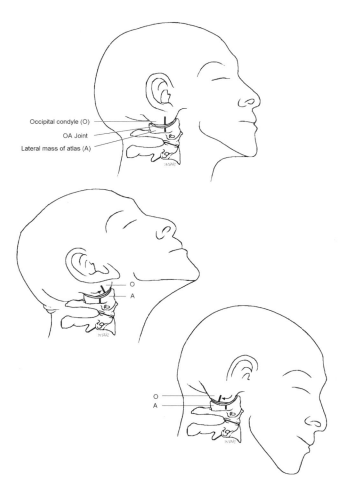

Figure 6.5   Occipitoatlantal (OA) joint in neutral, extension (counternutation), and flexion (nutation) positions.

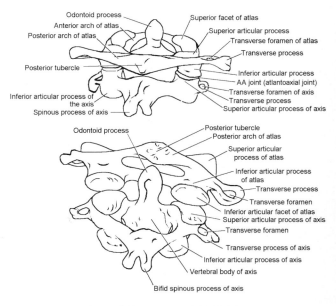

Figure 6.7   Atlantoaxial (AA) joint.

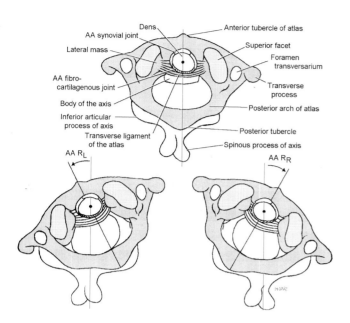

Figure 6.8   Atlantoaxial (AA) rotation.

uncinate process, that functions to add support to the cervical spine and help prevent disc herniation (Fig. 6.11).

The cervical vertebral transverse processes are unique in that they encase and protect the vertebral artery, which angulates three times at 90 degrees around the atlas as it ascends into the cranium through the foramen magnum (Figs. 6.12 and 6.13).

The muscular attachments to the cervical spine enable flexion and extension when acting bilaterally and sidebending and rotation when acting unilaterally (Figs. 6.14 to 6.17). They integrate neck motion with thoracic, rib, and upper extremity motions. These muscles also stabilize the cervical spine and head during upper extremity and trunk movements. The scalene muscles assist in elevating the first and second ribs during deep inhalation. The suboccipital muscles adjust the level of the occiput to the horizon to ensure the visual and vestibular systems function

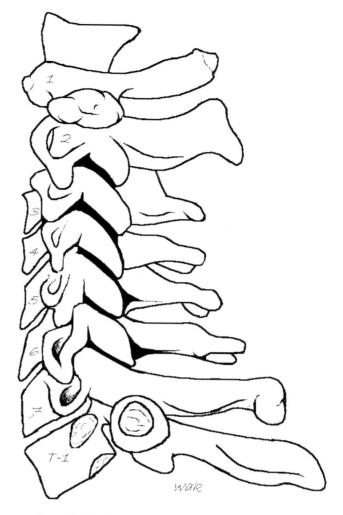

Figure 6.10   Lateral cervical spine view of facet angles.

optimally (Fig. 6.18). The obliquus capitis superior sidebends the head, whereas the obliquus capitis inferior rotates the atlas and head around the odontoid process of C2 such that the face turns toward the side of the contraction. Unilateral contraction of the semispinalis capitis rotates the head and face to the opposite side of the contracting muscle. The rotatores and multifidi muscles

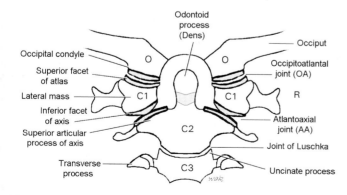

Figure 6.9   Occipitoatlantal and atlantoaxial joints: coronal section view.

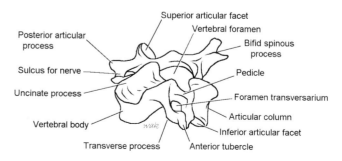

Figure 6.11   Typical cervical vertebra; notice the uncinate process.

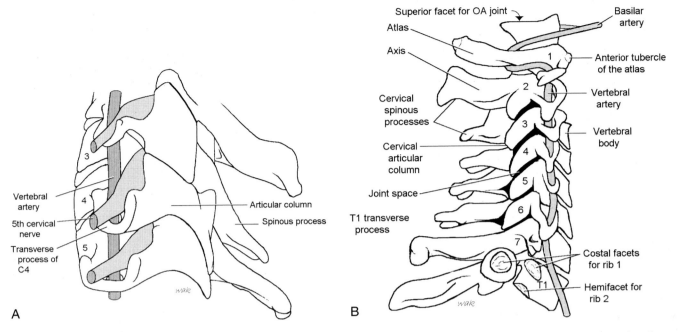

Figure 6.12   **A,** The vertebral artery traverses the cervical spine encased within the transverse processes. **B,** The vertebral artery makes three 90-degree bends as it wraps around the atlas on its way into the foramen magnum.

are responsible for segmental motion (Fig. 6.19). Because their origins are inferior and lateral to their insertions, unilateral contraction of these muscles rotates the body of the superior vertebra of the unit toward the side opposite of the contracting muscle; contraction of a right rotatores or multifidi muscle rotates the superior vertebra toward the left.

Thoracic Spine

The thoracic spine anchors the origins to muscles that stabilize and extend the cervical spine. Typically, when a patient has a mechanical neck disorder, the thoracic region's spinal muscles and joints need to be evaluated and treated in addition to those in the cervical region. The thoracic spine consists of 12 vertebra (Fig. 6.20). Their structure is similar to the lumbar vertebrae in that they have vertebral bodies anteriorly with intervertebral fibrocartilaginous discs, posterior arches that surround the spinal column and meninges, and spinous and transverse processes that emanate from the pedicles. Their superior articular facets differ

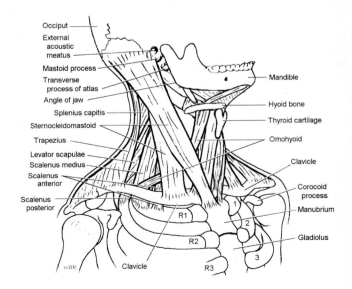

Figure 6.14   Anterior cervical muscles. With permission from Simons DG, Travell JG, Simons LS: Myofascial Pain and Dysfunction, Vol. I: Upper Half of the Body, Second Edition, Baltimore, Williams and Wilkins, 1999:515.

Figure 6.13   Superior view of the anatomic relationship between the atlas and the vertebral and basilar arteries (a.).

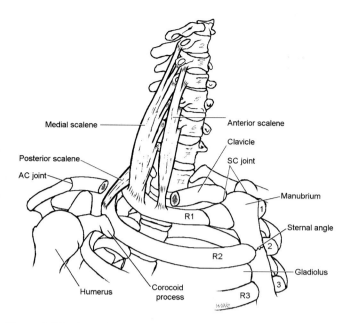

Figure 6.15 Scalene muscles. AC, acromioclavicular; SC, sternocleidomastoid. With permission from Simons DG, Travell JG, Simons LS: Myofascial Pain and Dysfunction, Vol. I: Upper Half of the Body, Second Edition, Baltimore, Williams and Wilkins, 1999:507.

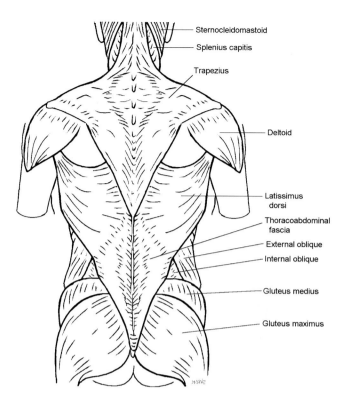

Figure 6.17 Superficial posterior cervical muscles. With permission from Simons DG, Travell JG, Simons LS: Myofascial Pain and Dysfunction, Vol. I: Upper Half of the Body, Second Edition, Baltimore, Williams and Wilkins, 1999:435.

in orientation; they face posteriorly in the coronal plane. They also have articular facets on their bodies and transverse processes to accommodate a rib on each side (Fig. 6.21) (see Chapter 2). There are costovertebral ligaments to stabilize the rib articulations in addition to intervertebral ligaments common amongst all the vertebrae (Fig. 6.22).

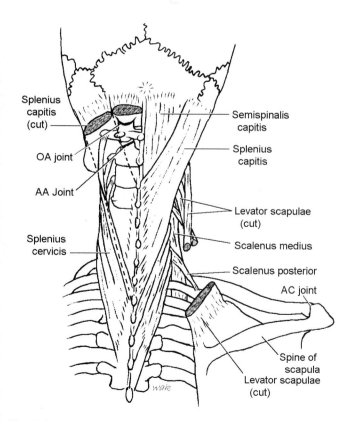

Figure 6.16 Posterior cervical muscles. AA, atlantoaxial; AC, acromioclavicular; OA, occipitoatlantal. With permission from Gray's Anatomy 35th British Edition, Saunders Co., Philadelphia, 1973:533.

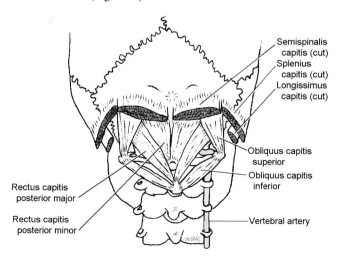

Figure 6.18 Suboccipital muscles. With permission from Simons DG, Travell JG, Simons LS: Myofascial Pain and Dysfunction, Vol. I: Upper Half of the Body, Second Edition, Baltimore, Williams and Wilkins, 1999:474.

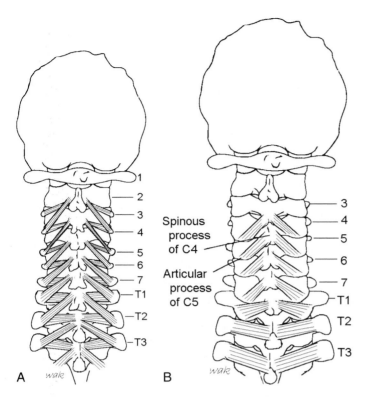

Figure 6.19   **A,** Cervical rotatores muscles. **B,** Cervical multifidi muscles.

Pathophysiology

- In the United States, almost 85% of neck pain may be attributed to chronic stresses and strains or acute or repetitive neck injuries.[9]
- Tables 6.1 to 6.4 list comorbidities, work-related factors, and non–work-related factors. Tables 6.5 and 6.6 delineate factors related to radiating neck pain and whiplash injuries.
- In general, somatic dysfunction involving the OA and AA joints usually causes head pain and somatic dysfunction of C2 to C7 joints causes neck pain.
- Using a diagnostic double-blind, placebo-controlled protocol with local anesthetic blocks to determine the prevalence of cervical zygapophyseal joint pain among patients with chronic neck pain (>3 months' duration) after whiplash injury, researchers found that in 50% of those with dominant headache, the C2-C3 zygapophyseal joint was the pain generator; overall, the pain generator in 60% of patients was C2-C3 or below.[36]
- In more than one third of patients with chronic (>6 months) refractory neck pain, symptoms were reproducibly alleviated by fluoroscopically guided joint anesthetic injections.[37]
- Cervical facet pain is typically a unilateral, dull aching pain with occasional referral into the occipital or trapezial region, depending on the facet joint involved (Table 6.7).
- The pain referral zones for facet pain overlap with myofascial and disc pain patterns, making it difficult to ascertain the exact level of the pain generator.

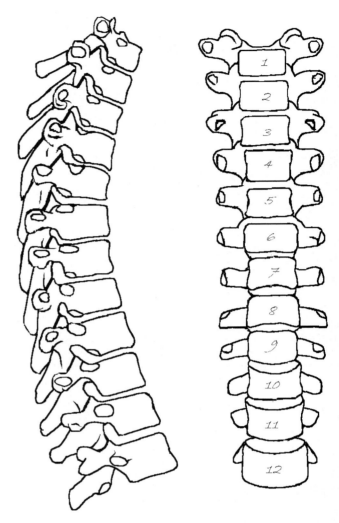

Figure 6.20   Lateral and anterior thoracic spine.

- In some patients, neck pain and head pain are associated with trigeminal nerve activity from dental-facial problems, activation of the cervical branches of the trigeminal nerve, or influence of the trigeminal nerve on the thalamic pain receptor field in the brain.[35]

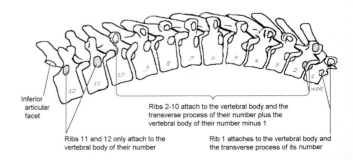

Figure 6.21   Thoracic spine lateral view shows the facets and demifacets for the articulation of the ribs.

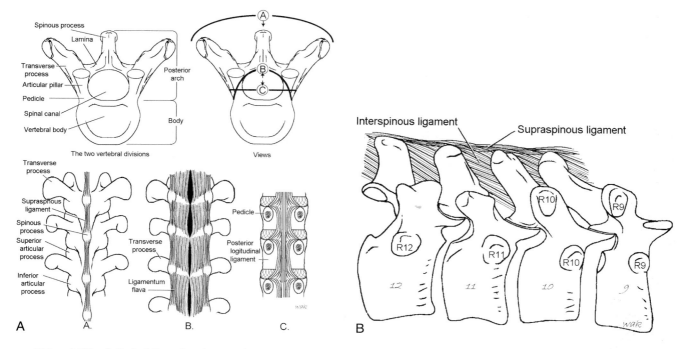

Figure 6.22   A, Typical thoracic spine vertebra and ligamentous attachments. **B,** Interspinous and supraspinous ligaments. R, rib.

- Thoracic, shoulder, and low back somatic dysfunction and pain and depressive symptoms are potential causative or complicating factors in patients with chronic mechanical neck disorders and pain.[1-3,38]
- Thoracic somatic dysfunction is a significant predictor of neck and shoulder pain and of hand weakness symptoms.[38-41]

DIFFERENTIAL DIAGNOSIS

Several musculoskeletal, neurologic, and systemic conditions can be related to neck pain. Because the pain generators may be located in the muscles, ligaments, capsules, periosteum, intervertebral discs, and dura, all pathologic processes affecting these structures—degenerative, infectious, inflammatory, neoplastic, and congenital diseases; major trauma, fractures, dislocations,

Table 6.6   Characteristics of patients with neck pain after automobile accidents

Characteristics	Studies
Sex: female	Chapline et al, 2000[5]
Age: 20 to 40 years old	Chapline et al, 2000[5]
Head restraint height below the head's center of gravity	Chapline et al, 2000[5]
Increased severity of collision	Chapline et al, 2000[5]
Lightweight cars	Chapline et al, 2000[5]

Table 6.5   Whiplash-associated symptoms accompanying neck pain

Symptoms (%)	Studies
Headache (82)	Bilkey, 1996[10]
Vertigo (50)	Bilkey, 1996[10]
Cognitive disturbances (55)	Bilkey, 1996[10]
Visual disturbances (38)	Bilkey, 1996[10]
Low back pain (35)	Bilkey, 1996[10]
Interscapular pain (20)	Bilkey, 1996[10]

Table 6.7   Cervical facet (zygapophyseal) joint referred pain patterns

Cervical Spine Facets	Referred Pain
C1-2	Posterior auricular area in the distribution of the greater occipital nerve
C2-3, C3-4	Paraspinal and trapezial areas
C4-5, C5-6	Trapezial area
C5-6, C6-7	Trapezial and periscapular areas
C1-2	Posterior auricular area in the distribution of the greater occipital nerve

From Narayan P, Haid RW: Treatment of degenerative cervical disc disease. Neurol Clin 19:217-229, 2001.

Table 6.8   Differential diagnosis of neck pain

Diagnosis	Characteristics	Gold Standard Tests
Unilateral Neck Pain		
Acute pharyngitis	Erythematous pharynx; exudates; jugulodigastric lymphadenopathy	Streptococcus screen and Culture
Carotidynia	Tender carotid	Carotid ultrasound
Dental disease	Tooth or gingival pain, tenderness, swelling	Dental radiographs
Dissecting carotid aneurysm	Tender carotid, bruit on auscultation	Carotid ultrasound
Lymphadenitis, mononucleosis	Enlarged, tender lymph nodes; enlarged liver and spleen (i.e., mononucleosis)	Ebstein-Barr virus antibodies (i.e., mononucleosis)
Myositis	Very tender muscles in several body regions	Complete blood cell count, erythrocyte sedimentation rate
Peritonsillar abscess	Tonsil protruding anteriorly or medially	Aspiration
Submandibular gland disease	Tender, mass palpable	Ultrasound
Temporomandibular joint (TMJ) pathology	Tender TMJ, deviation of jaw on opening, decreased movement	Computed tomography
Thyroiditis	Palpable thyroid, may be tender	Thyroid-simulating hormone, thyroxine (T_4), triiodothyronine (T_3)
Torticollis	Contracture of sternocleidomastoid muscle	Cervical radiographs, magnetic resonance imaging (MRI)
Tumor of tongue	Palpable mass	MRI, tissue biopsy
Vertebral artery rupture	Ophthalmologic and cerebellar neurologic deficits	Ultrasonography, MRI angiogram
Bilateral Neck Pain		
Cervical fracture	Muscle splinting, history of trauma	Cervical spine radiographs
Meningitis	Nuchal ligament rigidity, fever, malaise	Spinal tap
Spinal cord injury	If C3-5: diaphragm paralysis; neurologic deficits below neck	Cervical spine MRI

and spinal cord injuries; and neurovascular diseases—must be considered in the differential diagnosis of neck pain.[9]

A word of caution is in order. Not all neck pain after seemingly mild or moderate whiplash injury is related to soft tissue sprain. There is a case report of a patient with headache and neck pain after whiplash injury who had pain that was out of proportion to his apparent injury. He subsequently developed cerebellar infarction due to vertebral artery dissection.[42]

Some neurologic conditions, such as atypical facial pain, trigeminal and glossopharyngeal neuralgia, reflex sympathetic dystrophy, neurogenic inflammation, headaches, and systemic disorders, such as osteoarthritis, rheumatoid arthritis, and rheumatoid-related conditions, such as dermatomyositis, temporal arteritis, Lyme disease, and fibromyalgia, are less common causes of neck pain (Table 6.8).

HISTORY

- Typically, patients complain of pain in the posterior cervical region or upper back, or both.
- Patients have difficulty moving the neck; the pain is worse with movement and better with rest.
- The examiner should elicit any trauma or injury history, especially motor vehicle accidents.
- The examiner should ask about congenital or acquired spinal or muscular conditions.

- Any surgical history should be documented.
- The examiner should inquire about the presence of any of the associated factors of mechanical neck pain listed in Tables 6.1 through 6.7.
- The examiner should perform a review of systems to help identify any underlying systemic conditions.

PHYSICAL FINDINGS

Physical examination findings found to be most reliable are listed in Tables 6.9 and 6.10. The standard examination entails a general visual screening of the cervical region and then active and passive range and quality of motion assessments, followed by a palpatory examination of all structures of the neck, including

Table 6.9   Physical findings for patients with chronic neck pain

Physical Findings	Studies
Decreased range of motion	Hagen et al, 1997[44]
Measurable decrease in standing balance	McPartland et al, 1997[43]
Somatic dysfunction	McPartland et al, 1997[43]
Trigger points	Dyrehag et al, 1998[45]

Table 6.10   Reliable physical examination tests for patients complaining of neck pain*

Pain in response to digital pressure on bone or muscle
Tests for regional range of motion
Spurling's maneuver for cervical radiculopathy

*Neck pain (kappa values > 0.4) based on a systematic review of the reliability of spinal palpatory findings.

From Seffinger MA, Najm WI, Mishra SI, et al: Reliability of spinal palpation for diagnosis of neck or back pain: A systematic review of the literature. Spine 29:413-425, 2004.

assessment of tender points that may be amenable to manual treatment. Asymmetry of musculoskeletal structural landmarks, altered quantity or quality of active or passive neck motion, and tissue texture abnormalities, including tenderness and temperature variations (i.e., *a*symmetry of structural position, altered *r*ange of motion, and *t*issue texture abnormalities or tenderness [ART]), lead the practitioner to consider a mechanical neck disorder or cervical somatic dysfunction diagnosis. Observing for pharyngeal and tonsil inflammation, glandular hypertrophy or tenderness, and lymphadenopathy can alert the practitioner to internal organic problems that can also be an underlying cause of the somatic findings by means of viscerosomatic reflexes. Findings of ART in the thoracic, low back, and shoulder regions that indicate somatic dysfunction are often associated with findings of ART in the cervical region.

Physician practitioners typically auscultate the carotid arteries with a stethoscope, listening in particular for bruits that indicate a compromised vascular lumen (i.e., from cholesterol buildup or an aneurysm). A neurologic examination can show deficits in the case of cervical peripheral nerve impingement with radiculopathy or spinal cord impingement from a herniated cervical disc.

LABORATORY AND RADIOGRAPHIC FINDINGS

Routine laboratory and radiographic evaluations are unnecessary if the history and physical examinations are consistent with mild sprain or strain of the neck musculoskeletal tissues. In acute whiplash or any trauma, it is prudent to obtain cervical radiographs to rule out vertebral fracture or dislocation. Patients with chronic mechanical neck pain refractory to manual treatments plus exercise require further diagnostic imaging to rule out less common causes underlying persistent neck pain. Radiographic evaluations correlated with chronic mechanical neck pain are listed in Table 6.11.

MANUAL MEDICINE

Best Evidence

- For mechanical neck pain after whiplash injury, successful mobilization or manipulation procedures of the cervical spine quiet, or render silent, the mechanoreceptors and nociceptors of the cervical facet or zygapophyseal joints (Table 6.12).
- Cervical spine manipulation and mobilization provides at least short-term benefits for some patients with acute neck pain and headaches (grade A evidence).[47]
- For patients with subacute or chronic neck pain, spinal manipulation is more effective compared with muscle relaxants or usual medical care. Effectiveness is enhanced when used in combination with other supportive modalities such as exercise and ergonomic adjustments (grade A evidence).[48,49]
- Spinal manipulation provides short-term relief for patients with tension-type headache (grade A evidence).[50,51]
- A retrospective, outcomes-based analysis of chiropractic management of patients with uncomplicated mechanical neck pain showed statistically significant reductions in standard measures of disability (48.4% reduction) and pain (53.8% reduction).[52] Treatment consisted of spinal manipulation, various soft tissue techniques, home-care instructions, and ergonomic and return-to-activity advice, including rehabilitative exercises. Patients received an average of 12 treatments over a 4-week period.
- Mobilization or manipulation plus exercise have short-term and long-term benefits for subacute or chronic mechanical neck disorders with or without headache (grade A evidence)[51] However, the evidence did not favor manipulation or mobilization alone or in combination with various other physical medicine agents; when compared with one another, neither was superior. There was insufficient evidence available to draw conclusions about neck disorder with radicular findings.[50,51]
- Based on data obtained from the Work Loss Data Institute's *Disorders of the Neck and Upper Back*,[53] the 2004 edition of the National Guidelines Clearinghouse (www.ngc.gov) recommends up to 4 weeks of manual therapy for workers with job-related acute neck pain not due to damaged tissue injury (i.e., neck muscle strain or whiplash as a mechanism of injury with no radicular signs or symptoms).
- Depending on the mechanism and severity of injury (i.e., tissue damage) and patient's pain and anxiety, the upper back and neck can be evaluated and treated by manipulative medicine with the nonforceful, indirect procedures within 2 days of onset of the mechanical neck pain from a whiplash-type injury.

Table 6.11   Cervical radiographic findings associated with mechanical neck pain*

Procedure	Findings	Pain Characteristics	Studies
Magnetic resonance imaging	Atrophy of rectus capitis posterior major and minor muscles, fatty infiltration	Chronic neck pain	McPartland et al, 1997[43]
Computed tomography	Occipitoatlantal osteoarthritis	Suboccipital neck pain	Zapletal et al, 1996[24]

Table 6.12   Evidence-based medicine recommendations

Evidence Level*	Recommendation	Studies
A	Cervical spine manipulation and mobilization is useful in providing at least short-term benefits for some patients with acute mechanical neck pain and associated headaches.	Hurwitz et al, 1996[47]
A	Spinal manipulation should be used to treat patients with subacute or chronic neck pain because it is more effective than muscle relaxants or usual medical care. Effectiveness is enhanced when used in combination with other supportive modalities such as exercise and ergonomic adjustments.	Gross et al, 1996[48] Fiechtner and Brodeur, 2000[49]
A	Spinal manipulation is useful for patients with tension-type headache as it provides short-term relief.	Gross et al, 1996[48] Fiechtner and Brodeur, 2000[49]
A	Mobilization or manipulation, or both, plus exercise should be used for patients with subacute or chronic mechanical neck disorders with or without headache to provide both short-term and long-term maintained benefits.	Gross et al, 2004[51]

*Evidence levels: A, randomized, controlled trials, meta-analyses, and well-designed systematic reviews; B, case-control or cohort studies, retrospective studies, and certain uncontrolled studies; C, consensus statements, expert guidelines, usual practice, and opinion.

- In the acute phase of injury (24 to 48 hours), if disruption of neurologic, vascular, or bony tissues occurred, manipulation would not be an appropriate modality other than application of compressive forces to prevent further damage from edema.
- However, after the acute phase, while soft tissues are healing, some procedures are still considered safe, such as tender point (i.e., "find a position of diminished or no pain and hold") treatment with strain/counterstrain technique or indirect functional or myofascial release techniques.
- Occasionally, the practitioner may have to wait 2 to 6 weeks before being able to manipulate the tissues. Typically, gentle, nonforceful, and non–pain-generating range of motion and isometric exercises are used during this time to facilitate proper healing of the tissues.
- It is desirable to mobilize the joints as soon as it is reasonably safe to prevent further stiffness, muscle atrophy, and abnormal pain cycles.
- Economically, manual therapy (i.e., spinal mobilization) has been more effective and less costly for treating mechanical neck pain than physiotherapy modalities or care by a general practitioner.[54]
- Thoracic manipulation has analgesic effects in patients with mechanical neck pain.[41]

Risks

- The primary risk is using manual procedures identified in the literature is hyperextension coupled with rotation of the upper cervical spine because of concern regarding potential occlusion of the vertebral artery (see "Controversies").
- Caution should be exercised with patients with primary or secondary bone, neural, or muscular disease, as is true for any region.
- Contraindications to manual medical treatment of mechanical cervical spine disorders are listed in Table 6.13.

Benefits

- Primary benefits
  1. Increased range of motion
  2. Decreased pain
  3. Improved activities of daily living
  4. Return to work (i.e., shortened disability time)
- Secondary benefits
  1. Reduced reliance on medication for pain relief
  2. Improved postural efficiency

Practice Recommendations

- The American Osteopathic Association (AOA) and the American Academy of Osteopathy (AAO) fully support the use of osteopathic manipulative procedures for cervical somatic dysfunction. They have developed position papers that reflect their critical review of the literature and that provide recommendations for further research and practice (Appendix 6.1).
- The American Academy of Family Physicians has offered a manipulative medicine for mechanical upper back and neck pain introductory seminar at their annual scientific assembly since 1995 and has approved it as an evidence-based continuing

Table 6.13   Contraindications to manual medicine for mechanical neck pain

Acute cervical vertebral fracture
History of acute trauma, before diagnosis is established
Metabolic or neoplastic bone disease
Treatment refused by patient
Primary muscle or joint disease
Vertebral or carotid artery dissection

medical education course for its members since implementing that form of designation in 2004.

- The National Guidelines Clearinghouse, Cochrane Reviews, Work Loss Data Institute, Clinical Evidence (published by the *British Medical Journal*), and associations of chiropractors, osteopaths, and physical therapists worldwide recommend manual treatment for mechanical neck pain.

MANUAL DIAGNOSTIC PROCEDURES

- The ICD-9 diagnostic code for cervical somatic dysfunction is 739.1
- The ICD-9 diagnostic code for thoracic somatic dysfunction is 739.2

Patients complaining of neck pain with or without upper back pain should be evaluated standing, seated, prone, and supine. The musculoskeletal screening and scanning (cervical and upper thoracic regional) examinations (see Chapter 3) should be performed. These regions will likely show asymmetric landmarks and restriction of motion. Positive findings on the cervical or upper thoracic regional examinations lead the practitioner to investigate the possibility of segmental somatic dysfunction. Examination of the patient in the standing and seated positions is performed as part of the structural examination described in Chapter 3. Key positive findings in that examination that lead to the segmental examinations described in this chapter include the following:

- Asymmetric horizontal levels of the tips of the mastoid processes, inferior tips of ears, shoulders, or scapulae (standing posterior postural screen)
- Decreased cervical lordosis or thoracic kyphosis (lateral postural examination)
- Thoracic or cervical scoliosis (scoliosis screening test)
- Decreased upper thoracic or cervical flexion, extension, sidebending, or rotation (active and passive motion tests)

The thoracic spine is commonly evaluated in conjunction with the cervical spine when a patient complains of neck pain. As can be appreciated by reviewing the functional anatomy section, many of the muscles that govern neck motions have their origin in the upper thoracic spine. Upper thoracic somatic dysfunction usually creates compensatory cervical dysfunction, and vice versa.

After the patient is evaluated while standing during the musculoskeletal screening and regional scanning procedures, he or she usually is asked to sit for further regional and segmental evaluations. The upper thoracic region is easily evaluated with the patient in the seated position. Because the patient is asked to lie supine after sitting and the cervical segmental evaluation and treatments are performed with the patient supine on the treatment table, the diagnostic procedures for a patient complaining of mechanical neck pain begin with the evaluation and treatment of the upper thoracic spine with the patient seated, followed by evaluation of the cervical spine with the patient supine.

Thoracic Spine Anatomic Landmarks

- Some useful thoracic cage landmarks may be located in the following manner:
  1. The first thoracic vertebra has a prominent spinous process that is easily palpable when the patient flexes his or her cervical spine. C7 typically moves into flexion with the rest of the cervical spine, leaving the T1 spinous process projecting posteriorly. The remaining thoracic vertebrae may then be located by palpating the spinous processes of the next 11 vertebrae.
  2. The spine of each scapula is approximately at the level of the spinous process of T3.
  3. T5 is at the midscapular level.
- Another useful way of identifying the thoracic vertebrae involves using what is commonly called the *rule of threes* (Fig. 6.23). The spinous processes of T1, T2, and T3 project directly posteriorly; the tip of the spinous process of each vertebra is at the level of the transverse process of the associated vertebra.
  1. The spinous processes of T4, T5, and T6 project slightly inferiorly; the tip of the spinous process of each vertebra is located approximately one half of the way (about 0.5 inch) between the transverse process of each vertebra and the one immediately below it.
  2. The spinous processes of T7, T8, and T9 project inferiorly at a more acute angle so that the tips of these spinous processes are located at the level of the transverse processes of each vertebra and the one immediately below it (about 1 inch).

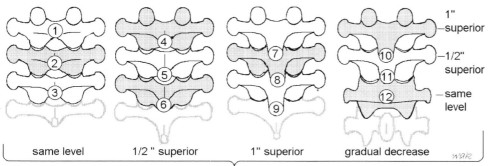

same level   1/2 " superior   1" superior   gradual decrease

1"
—superior
—1/2"
superior
—same
level

Distance to level of transverse processes from spinous process

Figure 6.23 The *rule of threes* commonly is used to identify the level of the thoracic transverse processes from the easily identifiable spinous process of the same or an adjacent vertebra.

3. The spinous process of T10 is located similarly to those of T7 to T9 (about 1 inch below the level of its transverse processes).
4. The spinous process of T11 is located similarly to those of T4 to T6 (about 0.5 inch below the level of its transverse processes).
5. The spinous process of T12 is located similarly to those of T1 to T3 (level with its transverse processes).

The longissimus muscles run bilaterally along the spine, longitudinally alongside the thoracic spinous processes about a thumb's breadth in width, and provide a medial border landmark for palpation of the transverse processes. To locate the transverse processes of a thoracic vertebra, first locate the spinous process, and roll your thumb tips over the longissimus muscles from medial to lateral, which feel like 1-inch-thick ropes, and press anteriorly until bony resistance is encountered (Fig. 6.24).

Thoracic Somatic Dysfunction Diagnosis: Segmental Examination

Examination
- Segmental examination of upper thoracic spine (T1 to T4) can be performed as follows:
  1. The patient is seated on a stool or treatment table.
  2. The practitioner stands behind the patient.

3. The practitioner palpates for soft tissue abnormalities.
4. Segmental motion testing is performed using active motion.
5. Segmental motion testing is performed using passive motion.
- Palpation for soft tissue abnormalities in the thoracic region entails the following:
  1. Using the back part of his or her hands, the practitioner feels for heat radiation from about 1 inch above the patient's skin surface bilaterally along the spine, noticing changes from segment to segment or between groups of segments (Fig. 6.25). A change in temperature sensation indicates alteration of blood flow due to inflammation or ischemia. Increased heat is felt over the midline and on the left side between T3 and T5 due to the heart.
  2. The practitioner then feels the paraspinal soft tissues with his or her finger pads, using the thumb and index or middle fingers, one segment at a time, assessing tissue texture abnormalities, such as dry or moist skin, numbness or tenderness, swelling or ropy, and firm textures (Fig. 6.26A).
  3. Tenderness is assessed by digital pressure over the paraspinal soft tissues and alongside the spinous processes (see Fig. 6.26B and C) and anteriorly along the midline of the sternum (see Fig. 6.26D).
  4. Tender points may or may not be related to a particular segmental spinal dysfunction that has other soft tissue abnormalities or motion restriction.
  5. Regardless of where a segmental somatic dysfunction is found, the entire region needs to be assessed for tender

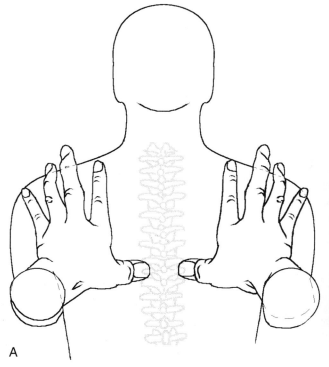

A

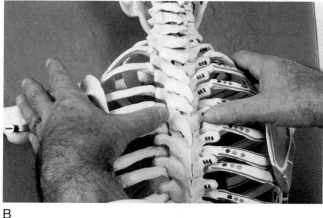

B

Figure 6.24   A, Depiction of palpating the transverse processes of a thoracic vertebra. **B,** Oblique view of palpation of the transverse processes of a thoracic vertebra on a skeleton model.

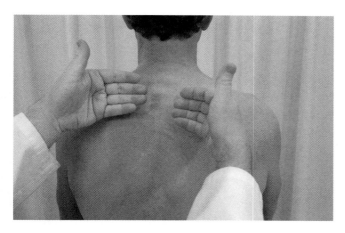

Figure 6.25   The practitioner assesses temperature variations overlying the thoracic paraspinal soft tissues, looking for asymmetries and comparing side to side and each successive vertebral level.

points and three of the most tender points selected for treatment with strain/counterstrain procedures.

6. Select the three most tender points in the region to later treat with strain/counterstrain manual procedures (see "Procedure").

7. Palpate all anatomic structures in the thoracic spinal region for orientation and evaluation of any abnormalities.

8. Some practitioners find it helpful to run two fingers down the spine along either side of the spinous processes to assess alignment and to elicit a *red reflex*, which is a cutaneous vasodilation response to digital pressure. The vasodilatory response is often altered at dysfunctional spinal segments and provides an indication for where to look for spinal somatic dysfunction (Fig. 6. 27).

9. An area that has persistent red streak marks for 3 minutes, which is about how long it takes for normal skin to return to normal color after the provocative test, is considered to have an abnormal autonomic and local vasodilator response due to spinal sensitization or facilitation.

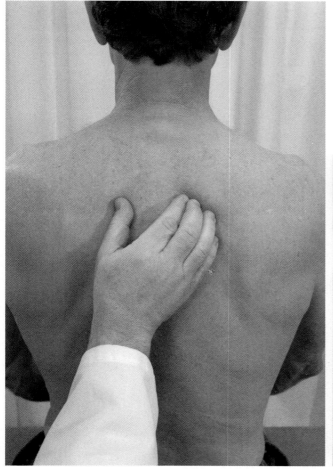

A

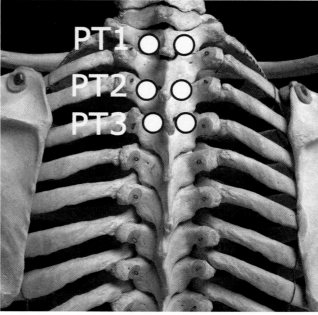

B

Figure 6.26   A, Assessment of tissue texture in the upper thoracic paraspinal soft tissues. **B,** Assessment of the posterior thoracic region along the T1 to T3 spinous processes for tender points that can be treated with counterstrain.

Continued

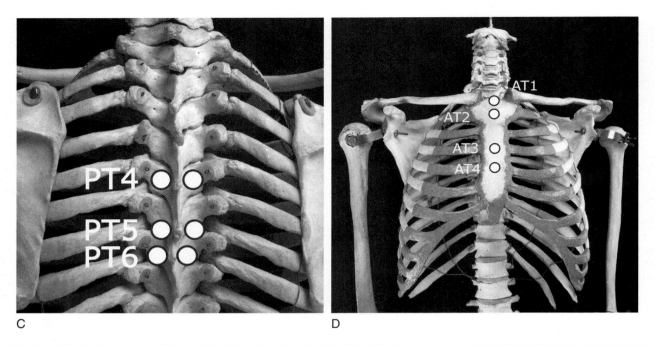

Figure 6.26, cont'd   C, Assessment of the posterior thoracic region along the T4 to T6 spinous processes for tender points that can be treated with counterstrain. **D,** Assessment of the anterior thoracic region along the midline of the sternum for tender points that can be treated with counterstrain.

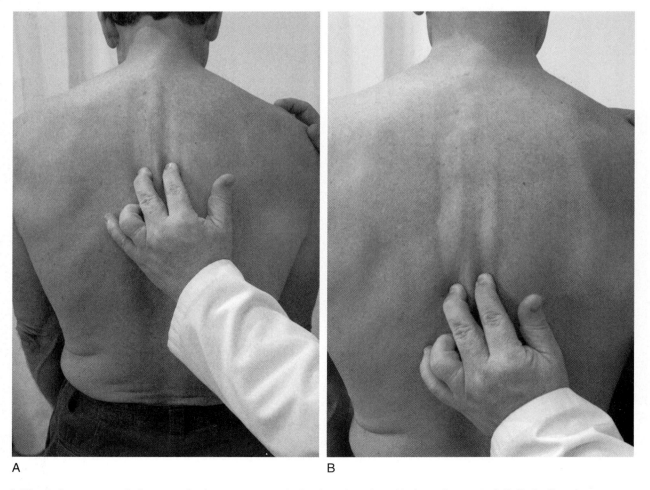

Figure 6.27   A, Assessment of alignment of spinous processes in the thoracic region with the patient seated. **B,** Red reflex response assessment of the thoracic spine with the patient seated.

- Segmental motion testing using active motion entails the following:
  1. The practitioner finds an area along the spine that demonstrates tissue texture or vascular abnormalities and tests for motion asymmetry one segment at a time in that area, typically testing three or more successive segments (Fig. 6.28A to C).
  2. The practitioner places the thumbs on the transverse processes of each vertebra in the region where dysfunction is suspected and observes whether there is a more posterior transverse process on one side compared with its contralateral side.
  3. The practitioner continues to monitor these transverse processes as the patient actively flexes and extends the spine at that level (see Fig. 6.28D and E).
  4. The side of the more posterior transverse process in neutral, flexed, or extended positions is identified.

- Segmental motion testing using passive motion entails the following:
  1. The practitioner places the pads of the thumb and index finger (or the index and middle fingers) of one hand over the posterior aspects of the transverse processes of the vertebra being examined.
  2. Using the other hand, the practitioner moves the patient's head passively into flexion until motion is felt at the segment being palpated.
  3. The practitioner notices whether the posterior transverse process has become more or less symmetric in the horizontal plane.
  4. The patient's head is moved passively into extension until motion is felt at the segment being palpated.
  5. The practitioner observes whether the posterior transverse process has become more or less symmetric in the horizontal plane.

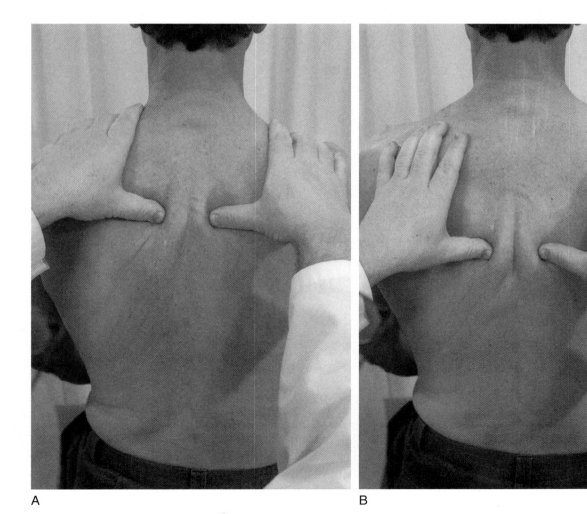

A

B

Figure 6.28   **A,** Assessing an area of tissue texture changes starting with the superior of three successive thoracic transverse processes with the patient seated. **B,** Assessing the middle of three successive thoracic transverse processes with the patient seated.

Continued

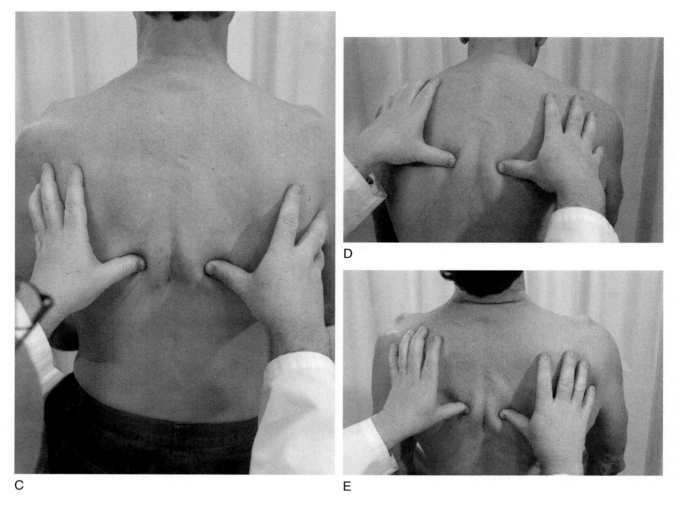

C

D

E

Figure 6.28, cont'd   C, Assessing the inferior of three successive thoracic transverse processes with the patient seated. **D,** The most dysfunctional segment in the group is identified. It is characterized by having the most motion restriction, lack of compliance to digital pressure, or the most posterior transverse process on one side in the neutral position. It is then assessed in the flexed position. **E,** The dysfunctional segment is also assessed in the extended position.

Interpretation

Using this approach, it is possible to have any one of the following structural diagnoses.

- If the transverse processes become more symmetric with the thoracic spine flexed, the vertebra is described as being flexed, rotated, and sidebent to the same directions (according to Fryette's principle II). This is its position of ease.
  1. If the posterior transverse process was on the right, the vertebra is said to be rotated to the right and therefore sidebent to the right.
  2. In this case, the vertebra is described as being flexed, rotated right, and sidebent right.
- If the transverse processes become more symmetric with the thoracic spine extended, the vertebra is described as being extended and rotated and sidebent in the same directions (according to spinal motion principle II).

  1. If the posterior transverse process was on the right, the vertebra is said to be rotated to the right and therefore sidebent to the right.
  2. In this case, the vertebra is described as being extended, rotated right, and sidebent right.
- If the greatest symmetry of the transverse processes is found in the neutral position, the vertebral segments (typically three or more) in this area exhibit fullness of the paraspinal soft tissues and are described as being neutral and rotated and sidebent in opposite directions (according to spinal motion principle I).
  1. If the posterior transverse processes become more asymmetric or do not change in terms of how much asymmetry they have compared with the neutral position, the practitioner should suspect a group somatic dysfunction and check the vertebra above and below for the same findings.

2. If the posterior transverse processes of the group are on the right, the group is rotated to the right and sidebent left.

3. The central vertebra in the group is the one to be treated.

Examples

Consider the following clinical scenario. The practitioner observes paravertebral fullness from T2 to T4 on the right side of the patient, with the most fullness (i.e., the most posterior transverse process) at T3. Motion designations are abbreviated by E for extended, F for flexed, N for neutral, R for rotated, S for sidebent, and subscripted L and R for the left and right sides.

1. Example: The transverse processes become more symmetric when the patient's thoracic spine is in the flexed position. The T3 structural diagnosis is T3 FR_RS_R.

2. Example: The transverse processes become more symmetric when the patient's thoracic spine is in the extended position. The T3 structural diagnosis is T3 ER_RS_R.

3. Example: The transverse processes are most symmetric when the patient's thoracic spine is in the neutral position. The structural diagnosis is: T2 to T4 NR_RS_L, and T3 would be the focus of treatment.

Myofascial tension in the paraspinal soft tissues is assessed with the patient prone and using medial to lateral force at 90 degrees to the direction of the myofascial fibers being assessed. Paraspinal soft tissue around each thoracic segment can be evaluated for abnormal response (i.e., sensitization or facilitation of spinal cord segments) to adjacent regional passive movements.

1. The patient is seated.

2. The practitioner stands behind the patient.

3. The paraspinal soft tissue is monitored with the thumb pad and index finger pad of one hand while the other hand introduces passive head and neck movements in one direction at a time, such as sidebending right (Fig. 6.29).

4. If passive motion in a particular direction, such as sidebending right, causes the monitored paraspinal soft tissues to bind, grab, or tighten but to release, loosen, or soften when the head and neck are moved in the opposite direction, that segment is considered to be dysfunctional and can be treated with functional procedures.

Cervical Spine Anatomic Landmarks

• Performing a structural examination requires being able to locate and palpate certain anatomic landmarks. A useful method of finding the cervical vertebral landmarks is as follows:

1. To locate C1, palpate the transverse processes between the mastoid process and the posterior border of the mandible on each side.

2. To locate C2, palpate the transverse processes just below and medial to the tips of the mastoid processes. There is a prominent spinous process that is easily palpable when the head is nutated (i.e., flexed). It is the first bony prominence palpable in the midline inferior to the occiput.

3. To locate C3 to C6, place the tips of second, third, fourth, and fifth fingers along the transverse processes just below the mastoid processes, and the fingertips then rest approximately at the level of C3, C4, C5, and C6.

4. To locate C7, the examiner places a thumb or finger on what is believed to be the C7 spinous process, and the patient is instructed to extend his or her neck and look toward the ceiling. If the spinous process being palpated is C7, the vertebra will translate forward. If no movement occurs, the examiner is palpating the T1 spinous process.

The transverse processes are tender to palpation laterally (Fig. 6.30). When palpating a cervical vertebra, the practitioner places the finger pads of the probing fingers just lateral to the spinous processes and posterior and medial to the lateral spiny tips of the transverse processes and contacts the pedicles (Fig. 6.31). The articular processes and facets form the articular column, which offers a flat tolerable surface for motion testing (Fig. 6.32). Because the pedicles support the facets, they are also referred to as *articular pillars*.

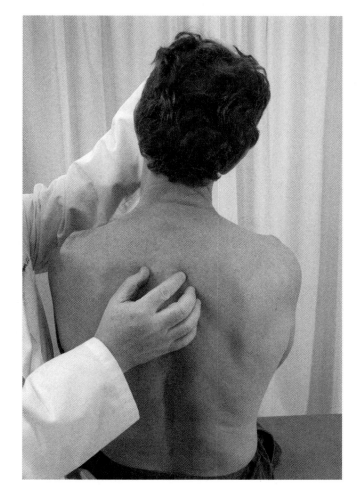

Figure 6.29 Functional assessment of an upper thoracic spine somatic dysfunction. The practitioner's left hand guides the patient's head off midline (i.e., slight passive cervical sidebending to the right) while monitoring the response in the paraspinal soft tissues with the right index finger and thumb pads to identify a facilitated thoracic segment.

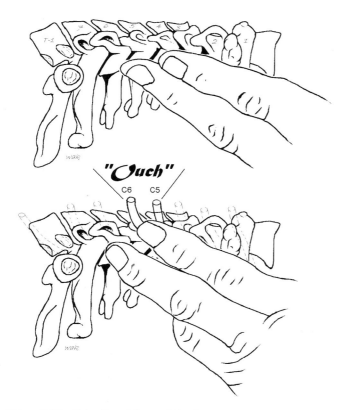

"*Ouch*"

C6 C5

Figure 6.30 Palpation of the pedicles is not tender *(top)*. Palpation of the tips of the cervical transverse processes is very tender *(bottom)*.

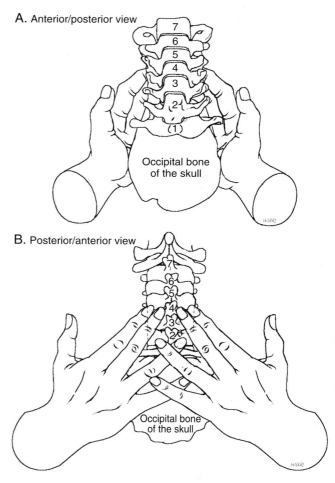

A. Anterior/posterior view

7
6
5
4
3
2
(1)

Occipital bone of the skull

B. Posterior/anterior view

7
6
5
4
3
2

Occipital bone of the skull

Figure 6.31 **A,** Palpating the articular pillars lateral to the spinous processes and posterior to the transverse processes. **B,** Palpating the articular pillars: anterior view *(top)* and posterior view *(bottom)*.

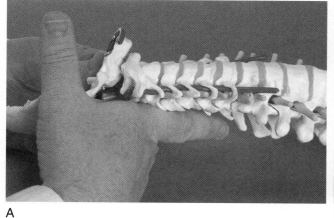

A

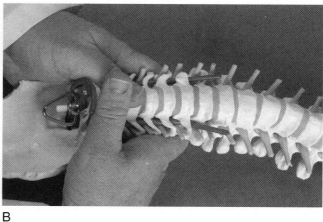

B

Figure 6.32 **A,** Finger contact position for motion testing a cervical spine vertebra using passive lateral translation in the assessment of sidebending compliance. Using a broad contact with the palmar aspect of the proximal phalanx of the index finger is more tolerable to the patient than using the fingertips. **B,** Translating from right to left, which is similar to testing for right sidebending compliance. Notice that the contact point is on the posterior articular pillar.

Cervical vertebrae are approximately one finger's width apart (the patient's own finger width). The spinous processes of the C3 to C5 region are anterior to the spinous processes of C2 and C6; with the patient supine, the practitioner can locate these three vertebra by palpation (Fig. 6.33).

- Position: The patient is supine, and the practitioner sits at the head of the table.
- The procedure is performed as follows:
  1. The practitioner's palm of one hand is placed upward, and the second to fourth finger pads are placed on the bifid tips of the spinous processes of C2 and C6 so that the medial aspect of the distal fourth finger is in contact with the inferior portion of the spinous process of C2 and the lateral aspect of the index finger is in contact with the superior edge of the C6 spinous process.
  2. The vertebral body of C4 is at the level of the third finger and in the same horizontal plane as the thyroid cartilage.

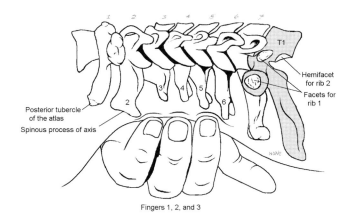

Figure 6.33 Palpating the spinous processes with the patient supine to identify the cervical vertebrae.

Cervical Somatic Dysfunction Diagnosis: Segmental Examination

- The examination can be performed as follows:
  1. The patient is supine on the treatment table.
  2. The practitioner is seated at head of table.
  3. The practitioner palpates with a light touch, using only as much pressure as needed to locate and move the structures being evaluated.
  4. Passive segmental motion testing is performed.
- Palpation entails the following:
  1. The practitioner assesses for paraspinal soft tissue tension at each spinal level and selects the level that has the greatest amount of tension, as determined by resistance to compressive, sliding, pulling, or pushing forces from digital palpation (Fig. 6.34).
  2. The practitioner assesses for tenderness along the anterior and posterior surfaces of the pedicles and along the paraspinal muscles. He or she assesses for tender points: anteriorly along the anterior surfaces of the cervical transverse processes and the clavicular and sternal insertion points of the sternocleidomastoid muscles; laterally between the mastoid processes and the ascending rami of the mandible; and posteriorly along the occiput and the lateral aspects of the spinous processes (Fig. 6.35).
  3. The practitioner selects the three most tender points in the region to later treat with strain/counterstrain manual procedures (see "Procedures").
  4. All anatomic structures in the neck are palpated for orientation and evaluation of any abnormalities.
- Passive segmental motion testing entails the following:
  1. After determining the spinal level with the greatest amount of abnormal tissue feel or tenderness, the practitioner identifies the restrictive motion barrier sensation by testing sidebending motion using lateral translation to minimize tilting of the head and movement off of midline (Figs. 6.36 and 6.37).
  2. The OA joint has a small range of sidebending mobility and can be tested using a lateral translation test.

3. The AA joint is tested only in rotation with the rest of the cervical spine flexed to limit any rotational movements from the other cervical joints.
4. For C3 through C7, although the uncinate processes limit sidebending, with practice, this method can become very efficient with minimal motion or discomfort.
5. After the resistance to sidebending is determined, the flexion or extension component of the restrictive barrier can be easily identified, and rotation, which is coupled with sidebending, can be inferred to make the complete diagnosis in all planes and directions of motion.

Occipitoatlantal Segmental Diagnosis

Examination
- The procedure can be done as follows:
  1. The patient is supine on the treatment table.
  2. The practitioner is seated at the head of the table.

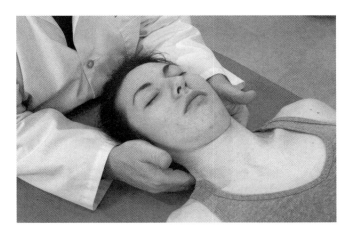

Figure 6.34 Palpating the cervical paraspinal soft tissues for asymmetries, decreased compliance, tissue texture abnormalities, and tenderness.

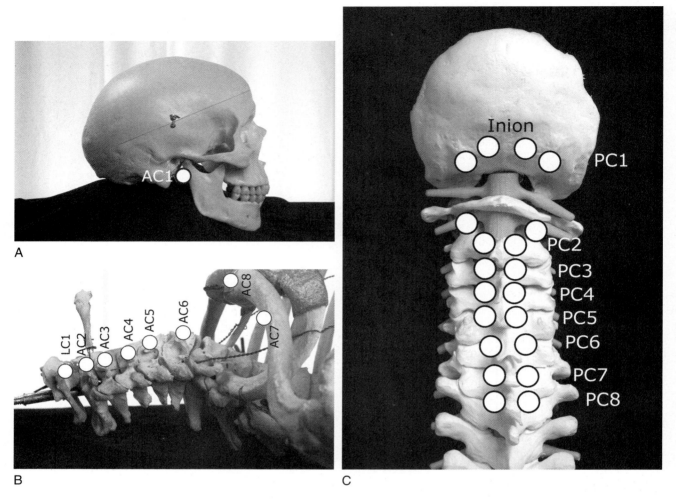

Figure 6.35 **A,** Counterstrain tender points anterior cervical 1 (AC1) and lateral cervical 1 (LC1) are in similar locations. Both are between the mastoid process and mandible bilaterally. To evaluate AC1, the practitioner presses anteriorly toward the ascending ramus of the mandible; for LC1, the practitioner presses medially. **B,** Counterstrain tender points for the anterior cervical spine. The lateral view is depicted to enable appreciation of the location of these points on the anterior surface of the transverse processes. These points are bilateral. **C,** Counterstrain tender points for the posterior cervical (PC) spine.

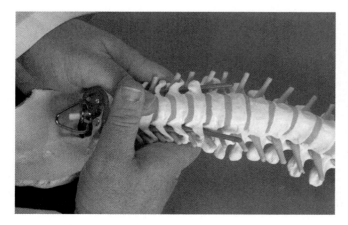

Figure 6.36 Lateral translation of cervical vertebrae to assess sidebending compliance. Notice the contact of the palmar aspect of the proximal index fingers on the posterior aspect of the cervical pedicles.

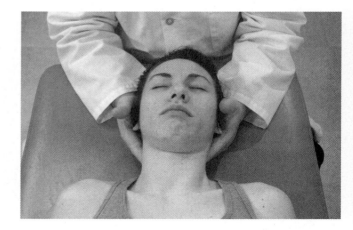

Figure 6.37 Passive right lateral translation of a cervical vertebra to assess left sidebending compliance.

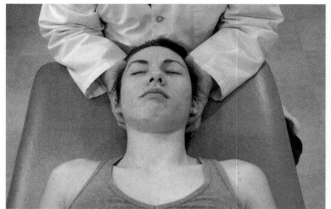
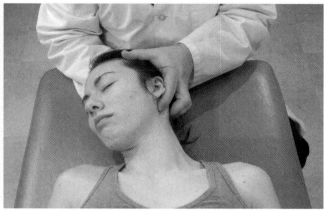

A   B

Figure 6.38   A, Hand position for occipitoatlantal (OA) assessment. **B,** Hand and index finger placement for OA assessment.

3. The practitioner cups the patient's occiput in his or her palms and stabilizes the atlas bilaterally by contacting the lateral tips of the transverse processes of C1 with the tips of his or her index fingers between the patient's mastoid processes and ramus of the mandible bilaterally (Fig. 6.38).

4. The practitioner laterally translates the occiput on the atlas without moving the atlas; if the atlas is felt to move, motion testing is not segmentally localized at the OA joint (Fig. 6.39).

The sidebending motion is less than 5 degrees, so the practitioner must determine on initiation of lateral translation whether there is immediate resistance or compliance.

Translating toward the left is akin to sidebending to the right.

Primarily the movement of C1 on C2 accomplishes rotation of the head, but when the OA joint sidebends, as in a slight head tilt, the head rotates to the opposite side, and rotation at the occiput on the atlas is essentially coupled to the opposite direction of sidebending. For example, if sidebending is restricted to the right, rotation is restricted to the left. (Tilt your head slightly to the left, and notice how easily your head can rotate to the right but not to the left.)

5. After determining to which side the sidebending (i.e., lateral translation) is more resistant, the practitioner retests that same translation of the occiput with the patient's head flexed and then extended (see Fig. 6.39C to H).

6. The practitioner determines in which position, flexed or extended, there is more resistance to lateral translation (i.e., sidebending). For example, if the practitioner found that laterally translating the occiput to the left (i.e., sidebending to the right) was most resistant with the patient's OA joint in neutral position, the practitioner would next test lateral translation to the left again in flexion and then extension to determine in which position there was even more resistance.

Interpretation
- If left lateral translation was most resistant while the patient's head was in an extended position, the restrictive barrier would be defined as resisting extension, sidebending right and, due to the biomechanics by inference, rotating left.
- The most compliant *position of ease* should be when the occiput is flexed, sidebent left, and rotated right.
- The practitioner should recheck translation or sidebending at the OA joint in the flexed position to confirm this concept.
  1. If the occiput resists translation to the left, it resists right sidebending and left rotation. If this is more restricted in extension than flexion, the occiput is resistant to moving into extension, right sidebending, and left rotation. The OA is in a relative position of ease when flexed, sidebent left, and rotated right.
  2. The practitioner can document "OA FS_LR_R" in the objective or physical examination part of the medical record.

Atlantoaxial Segmental Diagnosis

Examination
- The procedure can be done as follows:
  1. The patient is supine on the treatment table.
  2. The practitioner can be seated at the head of the table; however, it may be necessary to stand at the head of the table to assess nasal bone position relative to midline at the restrictive or physiologic barrier.
  3. The patient's neck is flexed fully to limit rotation from other vertebrae, and the practitioner gently rotates the head (AA joint) to the left and then to the right, observing the range and quality of passive motion (Fig. 6.40).

Interpretation
- If the direction of restriction of motion is to the left, the direction to which the head moves farthest and easiest (with most compliance) is to the right, which is the relative position of the AA joint.

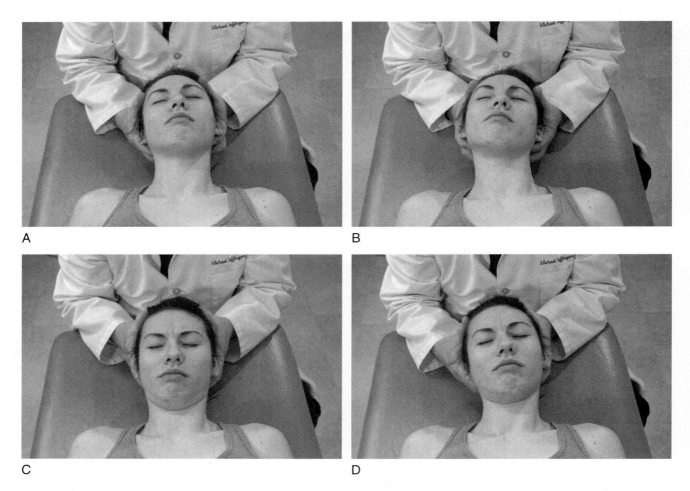

A   B

C   D

Figure 6.39   A, Translating left at the occipitoatlantal (OA) joint sidebends it to the right. **B,** Translating right at the OA joint sidebends it to the left. **C,** Flexing the OA joint. **D,** Translating the OA joint left in flexion.

- Practitioner can document "AA rotated right" in the medical record.

C3 to C7 Segmental Diagnosis

Examination
- The procedure can be done as follows:
  1. Patient is supine on the treatment table.
  2. Practitioner is seated at the head of the table.
  3. To test a vertebral segment for sidebending restriction, the practitioner laterally translates each vertebra from side to side through contact on the pedicles of the vertebrae (Fig. 6.41A and B).
  4. Translation is similar to sidebending.
  5. The practitioner determines in which direction there is restriction to motion.
  6. The practitioner determines in which direction there is most restriction in flexion or extension.
  7. After the direction of restriction is determined in neutral, it is necessary to test only that same direction in flexion

and extension. (i.e., there is no need to retest the compliant translation or sidebending motion in flexion and extension) (see Fig. 6.41C and D).
  8. Options in testing for cervical sidebending restriction are depicted in Figure 6.42.
  9. The practitioner makes a diagnosis of segmental somatic dysfunction based on the direction of restriction of motion.
  10. The practitioner can recheck the diagnosis by repeating the previous steps of this procedure, but this time finding the direction of compliant motion on translation of the vertebrae in neutral and then in flexion and extension.

Interpretation
- If sidebending of C5 is restricted on translating C5 from right to left, which is similar to sidebending it to the right, the practitioner should check translation toward the left (i.e., right sidebending) in flexion and extension to determine which is more restricted. If, for example, it is more restricted in flexion, the restriction of C5 is toward flexion and right sidebending.

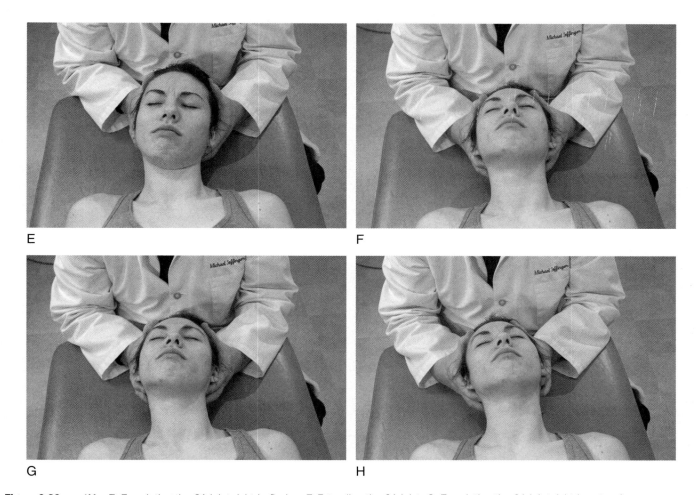

Figure 6.39, cont'd **E,** Translating the OA joint right in flexion. **F,** Extending the OA joint. **G,** Translating the OA joint right in extension. **H,** Translating the OA joint left in extension.

Because rotation is coupled with sidebending to the same side, it is restricted to the right as well.

- The position of the vertebra can be determined by interpolation. The position of ease is opposite to that of restriction: extended, sidebent left, and rotated left. The practitioner can recheck the diagnosis by testing the compliant motions that should be the same as the position of the vertebra, or position of ease.
- The practitioner can document: "C5 ERS left" or "C5 ER_LS_L" in the medical record.

MANUAL TREATMENT PROCEDURES

Upper Thoracic Treatment Procedures

Upper Thoracic Soft Tissue Treatment

- Diagnosis: any thoracic somatic dysfunction (Fig. 6.43)
- The procedure is performed as follows:
  1. The table height should be adjusted such that the patient is lower than the practitioner's hands as they rest along side the practitioner in the standing position.

  2. The patient is prone, with head turned away from the side being treated.
  3. The practitioner is standing on the side and facing the table at the level of the patient's thoracic spine, contralateral to the paraspinal muscles to be treated. For example, to treat the right paraspinal muscles, the practitioner stands on the left side of the table.
  4. The practitioner keeps his or her elbows and wrists locked in extension and contacts the medial border of the contralateral thoracic longitudinal paraspinal muscles with the heel of one hand while the heel of the other hand pushes firmly on top of the posterior surface of the contact hand to regulate the amount of pressure (i.e., force) applied to the soft tissues.
  5. Pressure is applied by the practitioner leaning forward from his or her waist and adjusting with the upper hand how much force is needed to gently stretch the longitudinal paraspinal muscles at 90 degrees to their fiber orientation.
  6. The medial to lateral force is held, without sliding the skin over the underlying muscles, for several seconds or until the tissues soften and increase in compliance; the skin will

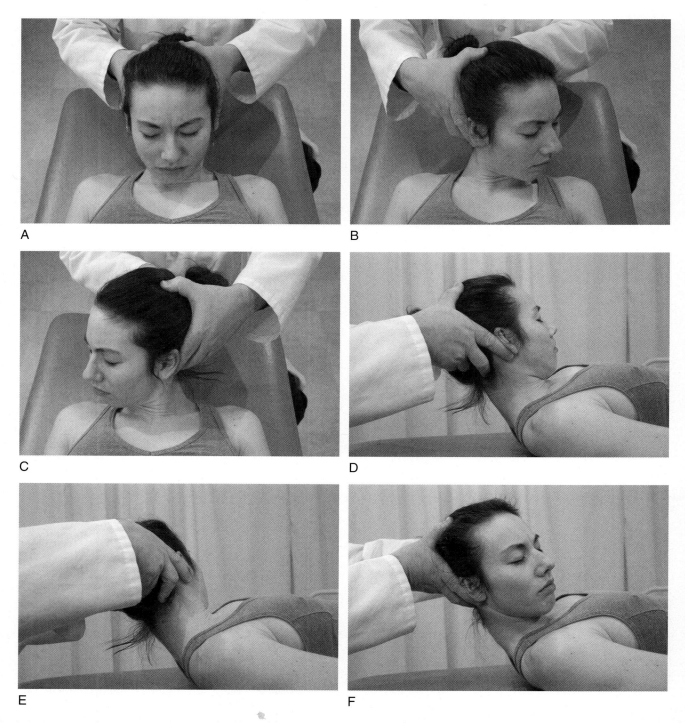

Figure 6.40   A, Flexing the cervical spine before testing atlantoaxial (AA) rotation. **B,** Assessing AA rotation left. **C,** Assessing AA rotation right. **D,** Lateral view: assessing the AA joint with the cervical spine flexed. **E,** Lateral view: assessing AA rotation left. **F,** Lateral view: assessing AA rotation right.

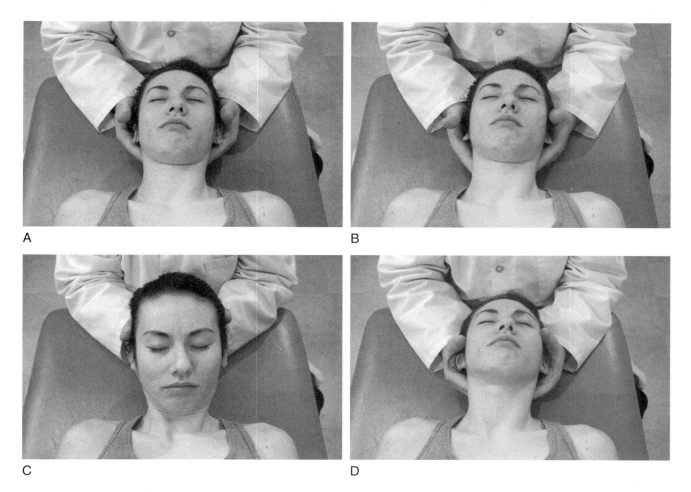

Figure 6.41   A, Palpating cervical pedicles with the cervical spine in the resting or neutral position. **B,** Translate cervical segments to the right to test for restrictive barrier to sidebending left. **C,** Flex the cervical spine and retest lateral translation at the segment that was most resistant to that motion test while in "neutral" position. **D,** Extend the cervical spine and retest lateral translation in the direction that was most resistant in the "neutral" position.

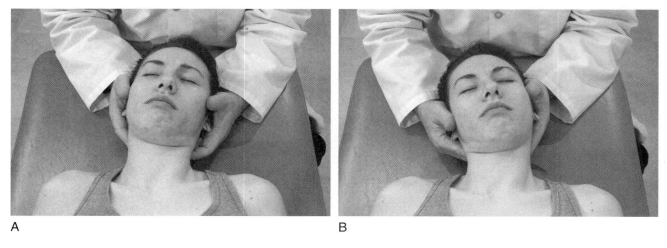

Figure 6.42   A, Testing right lateral translation or left sidebending in the upper cervical spine. **B,** Testing left lateral translation or right sidebending in the upper cervical spine.

Continued

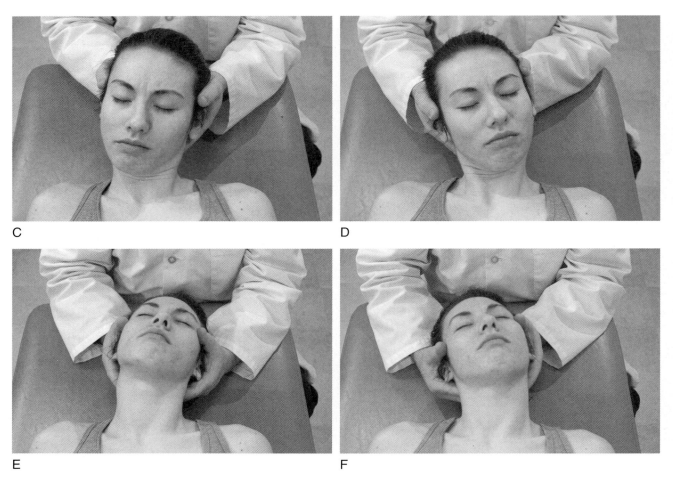

Figure 6.42, cont'd   C, Testing cervical segmental left sidebending in flexion. **D,** Testing cervical segmental right sidebending in flexion. **E,** Testing cervical segmental left sidebending in extension. **F,** Testing cervical segmental right sidebending in extension.

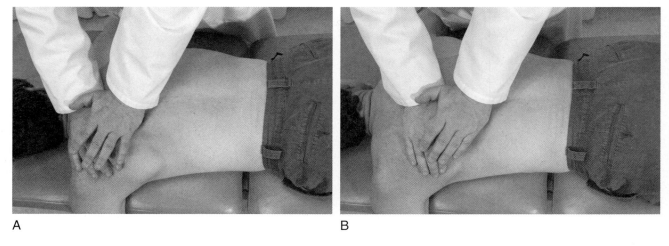

Figure 6.43   A, Prone paraspinal soft tissue lateral stretch. **B,** Prone paraspinal soft tissue lateral stretch at a lower level.

likely turn red and feel warm and boggy due to increased blood flow.

7. The practitioner moves up or down the thoracic levels in a segmental fashion after each lateral stretch maneuver.
8. Steps 4 through 7 are repeated on the other side.

- Reassessment should find softer and more compliant paraspinal muscles.

Upper Thoracic Myofascial Release Treatment

- Diagnosis: any upper thoracic somatic dysfunction that results in restricted neck flexion
- The trapezius myofascial stretch is performed as follows:
  1. The patient is supine on the treatment table (Fig. 6.44).
  2. The practitioner is seated at the head of the table.
  3. The practitioner crosses his or her arms and places the hands firmly on the upper trapezius muscles as they enter the cervical region, which is at the junction of the shoulders and neck.
  4. The patient's occipital region rests on the posterior surface of the practitioner's distal forearm.
  5. The practitioner then lifts the patient's head by using the hand contact area as the fulcrum and elevating his or her arms above the level of the forearms. This can be done most easily by the practitioner moving from a seated to a standing position.
  6. The patient's chin should approximate or touch his or her chest as the neck is taken into full flexion. This maneuver stretches the upper trapezius muscles.
  7. This position is held for several seconds or until increased compliance is observed in neck flexion.
  8. The patient's neck flexion is retested.

Upper Thoracic Articulatory Treatment

- Diagnosis: upper thoracic vertebral or regional motion restriction due to somatic dysfunction
- The head is used as a lever to induce passive motion in the thoracic vertebral levels T1 to T4. The shoulders and trunk are used as the lever for T5 to T12.

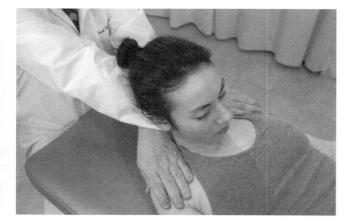

Figure 6.44 Supine trapezius stretch.

- The procedure is performed as follows:
  1. The patient is seated on the treatment table.
  2. The practitioner stands or sits besides the patient on the table.
  3. The restricted thoracic vertebral segments are located, and the restricted motions are identified (e.g., flexion or extension, sidebending right or left, rotation right or left).
  4. The practitioner stabilizes the lower vertebra of the restricted vertebral unit by pinching the spinous process of that vertebra between his or her thumb and index finger and moves the vertebra above it through the restrictive barrier in smooth, gentle, repetitive movements using the head as a lever for T1 to T4 or the shoulders and trunk as the lever for T5 to T12.
  5. After moving through the restrictive barrier, the joint is brought passively back to the resting position, and the restrictive barrier is again engaged and surpassed with the passive movement.
  6. These procedures are repeated several times until improved range of motion occurs.
  7. Passive and active ranges of motion of the affected joints are retested.

Upper Thoracic Muscle Energy Treatment
Type I Somatic Dysfunctions

- Diagnosis: T2 to T4 NS_RR_L
- Restriction: T2 to T4 NS_LR_R
- The procedure is performed as follows:
  1. The patient is seated on a chair or treatment table.
  2. The practitioner stands behind the seated patient on the side of the rotated, or most posterior, transverse process (to the left in this example).
  3. The practitioner's operating hand (left) is placed on the patient's head.
  4. The practitioner monitors the spinous processes of the upper thoracic vertebrae and passively flexes the patient's head until T3 begins to move, but not T4. This localizes the forces at T3 (Fig. 6.45A).
  5. The practitioner's right hand monitors the left transverse process of T3 (i.e., the central and most rotated vertebra of the group) to localize segmental motion.
  6. The practitioner positions the patient's head to engage the motion barrier in all three planes (i.e., neutral, rotation to the right, and sidebending to the left at T3) (see Fig. 6.45B).
  7. The patient is instructed to attempt to return to midline against the practitioner's unyielding counterforce.
  8. This isometric contraction is held for 3 to 5 seconds.
  9. The patient is then instructed to fully relax this effort and neck muscles for 5 seconds.
  10. The practitioner engages the new restrictive barrier, with further rotation to the right and sidebending to the left at T3.
  11. Steps 4 through 7 are repeated three to five times, and a final stretch is given into the restrictive barrier (i.e., rotation to the right and sidebending to the left at T3) after the final repetition.
  12. The patient is retested.

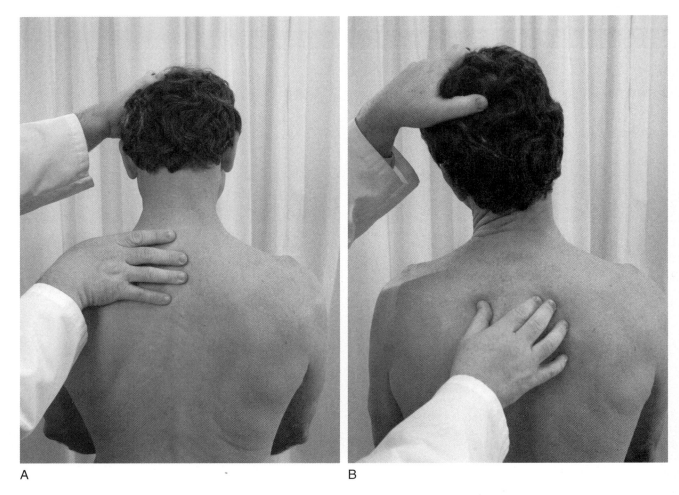

A   B

Figure 6.45   A, The practitioner flexes the patient's head until T3 is engaged to focus forces at T3. **B,** Position for seated muscle energy treatment of T2 to T4 in neutral, sidebent right, and rotated left (NS$_R$R$_L$). The practitioner monitors the posterior transverse process at T3 while engaging the restrictive motion barriers of sidebending left and rotation right with the other hand through contact with the patient's head.

Type II Dysfunctions
- Diagnosis: T3 ER$_L$S$_L$
- Restriction: T3 FR$_R$S$_R$
- The procedure is performed as follows:
  1. The patient is seated on a chair or the treatment table (Fig. 6.46).
  2. The practitioner stands behind the seated patient on the side of the most posterior transverse process (to the left in this example).
  3. The practitioner's operating hand (left) is placed on the patient's head.
  4. The practitioner's right hand monitors the left transverse process of T3 to localize segmental motion.
  5. The practitioner positions the patient's head to engage the barrier in all three planes (i.e., flexion, sidebending to the right, and rotation to the right at T3).
  6. The patient is then instructed to attempt to return to midline against the practitioner's unyielding counterforce.

7. This isometric contraction is held for 3 to 5 seconds.
8. The patient is then instructed to fully relax this effort and neck muscles for 5 seconds.
9. The practitioner engages the new restrictive barrier of further flexion, sidebending to the right, and rotation to the right at T3.
10. Steps 4 through 7 are repeated three to five times, and a final stretch is given into the restrictive barrier (i.e., flexion, sidebending to the right, and rotation to the right at T3) after the final repetition.
11. The patient is retested.

Upper Thoracic Functional Treatment
- Diagnosis: any upper thoracic somatic dysfunction
- Example: T4 has evidence of somatic dysfunction (i.e., ART). It does not matter whether it is flexed or extended because vertebral positioning and motion are not examined or treated in functional technique. What is examined and treated is the

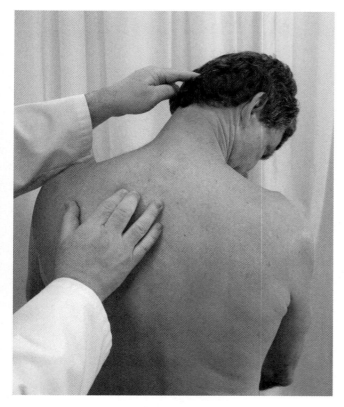

Figure 6.46   Treatment position for seated muscle energy treatment for T3 in extension, rotated left, and sidebent left (ER$_L$S$_L$).

aberrant spinal reflex activity at that level that is hypersensitive and reactive to passive body movements performed in other body regions.

- Typically, the head and neck are used to induce passive motion for functional evaluation and treatment of somatic dysfunction in the upper thoracic spine. The procedure is performed as follows:

  1. The patient is in the seated position.
  2. The practitioner stands beside and faces the patient's back.
  3. The practitioner contacts the patient's forehead with his or her thumb and fifth finger pads of his or her left hand on the lateral angles of the frontal bone. The practitioner instructs the patient to allow his or her head to fall into the practitioner's palm and to relax the neck muscles completely.
  4. The practitioner uses the index and thumb finger pads his or her right hand to monitor the tense tissues overlying the deep segmental paraspinal soft tissues (i.e., rotatores, multifidi, and intertransversarii) on either side of T4 while inducing passive motion by means of the patient's head and neck in one direction at a time.
  5. The practitioner may find, for example, that the paraspinal soft tissues around T4 tighten, or bind, with passive head and neck motion from the midline toward extension, sidebending left, rotation right, translation right and posteriorly, and axial compression and when the patient inhales (Fig. 6.47A).

6. In this example, the paraspinal soft tissues around T4 loosen, or ease, with passive head and neck motion from the midline toward flexion, sidebending right, rotation left, translation left and anteriorly, and axial decompression and when the patient exhales (see Fig. 6.47B).
7. To treat T4 using functional technique, the practitioner passively moves the patient's head and neck from the resting upright midline position toward flexion, sidebending right, rotation left, and translation left and anteriorly and applies axial decompression, in essence stacking the directions of motion that induce ease or compliance in the paraspinal soft tissues around T4.
8. The practitioner instructs the patient to maintain a prolonged natural exhalation (not forced) while fine-tuning the exact directions of motion that produce the most ease of the soft tissues being monitored around T4.
9. The practitioner retests for any presence of ease or bind at T4 during passive head and neck movements.

Anterior Thoracic Counterstrain Treatment
Anterior Thoracic 1 and 2
- Locations: Anterior thoracic 1 (AT1) is found in the midline in the suprasternal notch; anterior thoracic 2 (AT2) is found in the midline in the middle of the manubrium.
- The procedure is performed as follows:
  1. The patient is seated (Fig. 6.48).
  2. The patient's hands are placed on top of the head.
  3. The practitioner stands behind the patient and places his or her arms under the patient's axillae and around the patient's chest, with the practitioner's index finger contacting the tender point (see Fig. 6.48C). An alternate hand position for female patients can be seen in Figure 6.48D.
  4. The patient leans back against the practitioner's chest, inducing marked flexion of the cervical spine.
  5. This position is held for 90 seconds.
  6. The patient is passively, slowly moved back to the resting seated position.
  7. The practitioner retests the tenderness of the point.

Anterior Thoracic 3 and 4
- Location: Anterior thoracic 3 (AT3) is found in the midline of the sternum at the level of the 3rd costal cartilage; anterior thoracic 4 (AT4) is found in the midline of the sternum at the level of the fourth costal cartilage.
- The procedure is performed as follows:
  1. The patient is seated with the arms dangling behind the back (Fig. 6.49).
  2. The practitioner stands behind the patient and grasps the medial side of the patient's forearms bilaterally to add internal rotation and slight posterior traction on the patient's arms.
  3. The patient leans back against the practitioner's chest, creating flexion in the patient's thoracic spine at the desired segmental level.
  4. The practitioner *cannot monitor the counterstrain point with this position.*
  5. This position is held for 90 seconds.
  6. The patient is passively, slowly moved back to resting seated position.
  7. The practitioner retests the tenderness of the point.

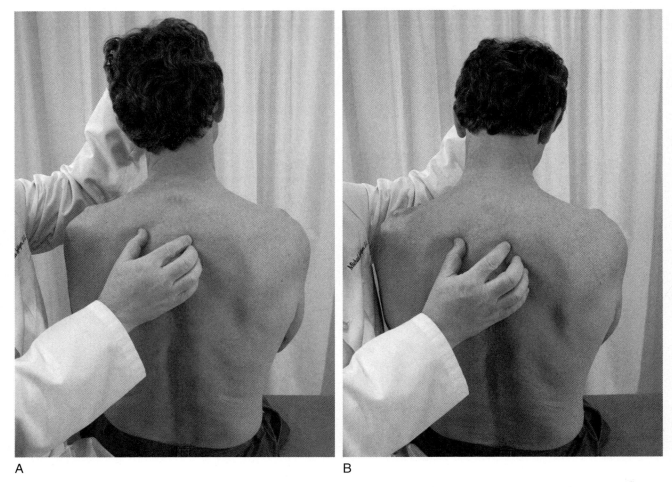

A   B

Figure 6.47   A, The paraspinal soft tissues around T4 tighten, or bind, with passive head and neck motion from the midline toward extension, sidebending left, rotation right, translation right and posteriorly, and axial compression and when the patient inhales. **B,** The paraspinal soft tissues around T4 loosen, or ease, with passive head and neck motion from the midline toward flexion, sidebending right, rotation left, translation left and anteriorly, and axial decompression and when the patient exhales.

Posterior Thoracic Counterstrain Treatment
Posterior Thoracic 1 to 3
- Location: The point of greatest tenderness is located directly on or immediately lateral to the spinous process of the associated vertebra.
- The procedure is performed as follows:
  1. The patient is prone with his or her arms hanging of the sides of the treatment table (Fig. 6.50).
  2. The practitioner stands at the head of the table.
  3. The practitioner uses the pad of the index finger of one hand to palpate and monitor the counterstrain point.
  4. With the other hand the practitioner cups the patient's chin, carries the patient's head into extension, and then adds rotation and sidebending away from the side of the tender point.
  5. This position is held for 90 seconds.
  6. The patient is passively, slowly moved back to the resting position.
  7. The practitioner retests the tenderness of the point.

Posterior Thoracic 4 to 6
- Location: The point of greatest tenderness is located directly on or immediately lateral to the spinous process of the associated vertebra.
- The procedure is performed as follows:
  1. The patient is prone with his or her arms extended off the head of the table (Fig. 6.51).
  2. The practitioner stands at the head of the table.
  3. The practitioner uses the pad of the index finger of one hand to palpate and monitor the counterstrain point.
  4. With the other hand, the practitioner cups the patient's chin, carries the patient's head into extension, and adds rotation and sidebending of the patient's head away from the side of the tender point.
  5. This position is held for 90 seconds.
  6. The patient is passively, slowly moved back to resting position.
  7. The practitioner retests the tenderness of the point.

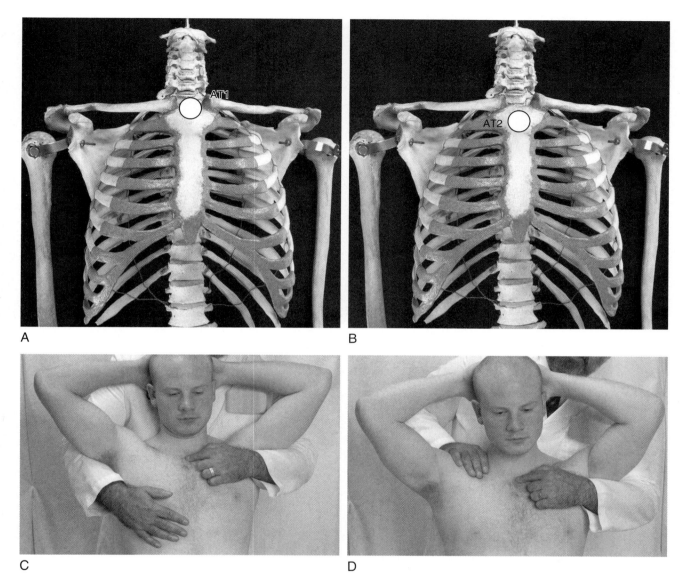

Figure 6.48 **A,** Location of the anterior thoracic 1 (AT1) tender point. **B,** Location of the anterior thoracic 2 (AT2) tender point. **C,** Counterstrain treatment position for AT1. The position for AT2 is similar. **D,** For female patients, the practitioner should place the hand not touching the tender point on the patient's shoulder.

Cervical Spine Treatment Procedures

Cervical Soft Tissue Treatment
Paraspinal Muscle Lateral Stretch
- Diagnosis: any cervical somatic dysfunction
- The procedure is performed as follows:
  1. The patient is supine on the treatment table.
  2. Practitioner stands contralateral to the side of the neck muscles to be stretched or sits at the head of the table.
  3. The practitioner contacts the spinous processes of the patient's cervical spine with his or her finger pads of one hand (Fig. 6.52A).

4. The practitioner flexes his or her distal interphalangeal joints, rolls off of the spinous processes onto the pedicles medial to the paraspinal muscles, and lifts the paraspinal muscles laterally and anteriorly (i.e., toward the ceiling).
5. A counterforce is supplied by the practitioner's other hand with his or her palm across the patient's forehead (see Fig. 6.52B).
6. This force is sustained for several seconds or until the tight muscles begin to soften, which is usually within 5 to 15 seconds.
7. As the neck muscles are stretched (i.e., 90-degree angle to their fibers), the patient's head is rolled toward the side

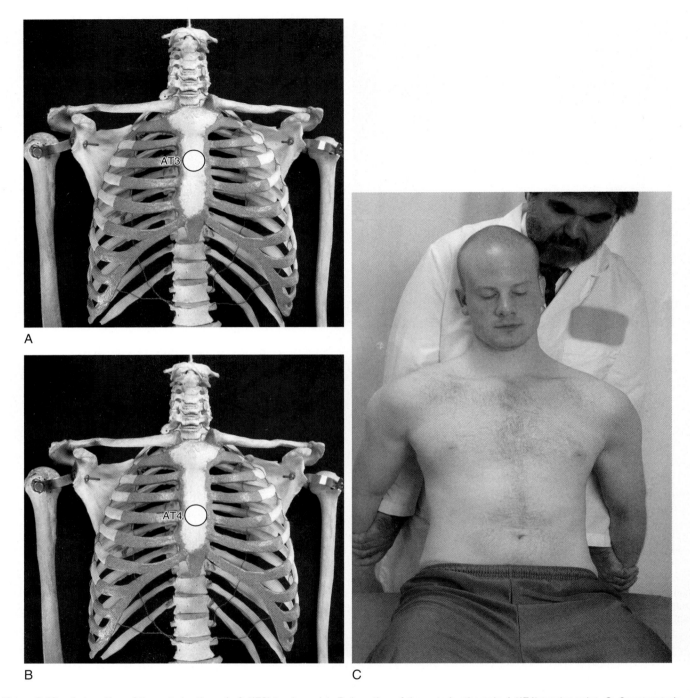

Figure 6.49 **A,** Location of the anterior thoracic 3 (AT3) tender point. **B,** Location of the anterior thoracic 4 (AT4) tender point. **C,** Counterstrain treatment position for AT3 or AT4 tender points.

being stretched. The practitioner's two hands should work together, counterbalancing each other's force so that the patient's head is maintained in the midline, limiting the amount of sidebending or rotation. The counterforce is released, and the patient's head brought back to midline at the same time as the other hand releases the paraspinal muscles and prepares to repeat the stretch.

8. The practitioner continues to passively stretch the tense cervical paraspinal muscles until they are soft and compliant; increased warmth and bogginess occur because of increased blood flow.

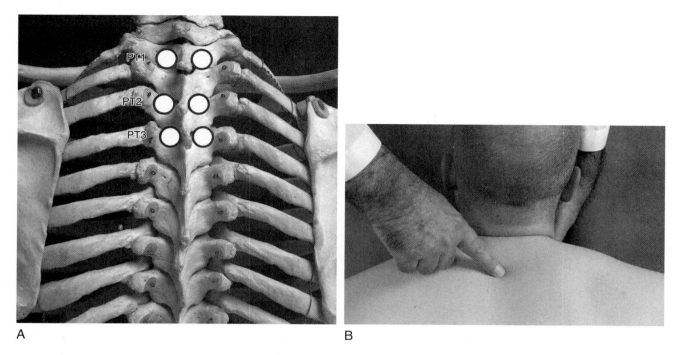

A   B

Figure 6.50   **A,** Location of tender points posterior thoracic 1 (PT1) through PT3. **B,** Counterstrain treatment position for PT1 through PT3. The practitioner extends the patient's upper thoracic spine by gently lifting his or her chin; sidebending and rotation away from the side of the tender point are then added to achieve maximum pain relief at the monitored point.

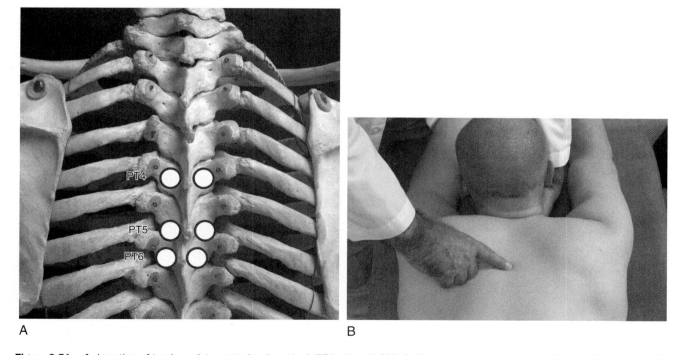

A   B

Figure 6.51   **A,** Location of tender points posterior thoracic 4 (PT4) through PT6. **B,** Counterstrain treatment position for PT4 through PT6.

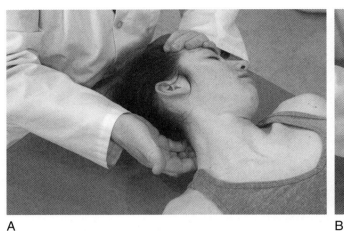
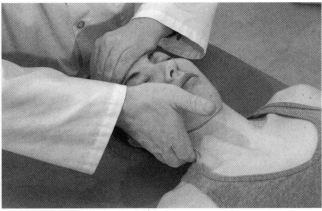

A   B

Figure 6.52   A, Cervical paraspinal muscle lateral stretch hand contact position. The second, third, and fourth fingers are flexed to match the length of the fifth finger so the fingertips are even and broad contact can be made with the patient's paraspinal muscles. **B,** Cervical paraspinal muscle lateral stretch. While passive stretch of the cervical paraspinal muscles is being applied with one hand, a counterforce is applied with the other hand by rolling the patient's head toward the side being treated.

Paraspinal Muscle Axial Stretch

- Diagnosis: any cervical somatic dysfunction
- The procedure is performed as follows:
    1. The patient is supine on the treatment table (Fig. 6.53).
    2. The practitioner sits at the head of the table.
    3. Using the lateral aspect of the distal index fingers, the practitioner contacts the paraspinal muscles overlying the pedicles bilaterally and lifts anteriorly (i.e., toward the ceiling) at each segment successively.
    4. The practitioner should support each index finger by approximating the third to fifth fingers of the same hand flush with it.
    5. These four fingers should be in a C-curve as they contact the paraspinal soft tissue so that the distal phalange of the index fingers contact the tissues at a 90-degree angle.

6. The practitioner holds the stretch at each segment for a few seconds or until the tense tissues soften and become more compliant; increased warmth and bogginess occur because of increased blood flow.

Cervical Myofascial Release Treatment

- Diagnosis: any cervical somatic dysfunction
- The following procedure is most specific for improving cervical sidebending to the left (Fig. 6.54):
    1. Patient is supine.
    2. Practitioner is seated at the head of the table.
    3. The practitioner's left palm contacts the patient's right shoulder over the acromioclavicular joint with thumb contacting the patient's right scapular spine posteriorly and fingers grasping the lateral aspect of the clavicle.

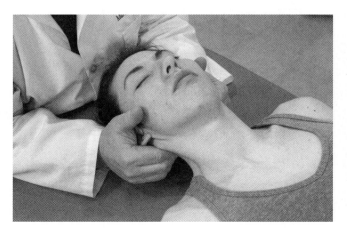

Figure 6.53   Cervical paraspinal soft tissue treatment.

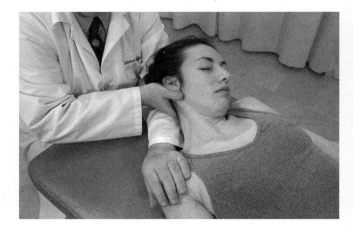

Figure 6.54   Scalene muscles stretch.

4. The practitioner lifts the patient's head with his or her right hand (crossing it over his or her left forearm) by cupping the right occipital region with his or her right palm and fingers, with the thumb positioned along the patient's right mastoid process of the temporal bone.

5. The practitioner passively sidebends the cervical spine to the left, up to the restrictive motion barrier of the tense sternocleidomastoid and scalene muscles and the contiguous fascial tissues. Firm counterforce is maintained on the patient's right shoulder by pressing posteriorly and inferiorly.

6. This stretch is held for several seconds or until there is a sense of release of tension in the tissues as indicated by less resistance to the direct action stretching procedure and ability to move the cervical spine more toward its physiologic and anatomic motion barriers in sidebending left.

7. The patient is retested.

8. The range and quality of motion are reexamined on the opposite side because on relieving restriction in one direction, the opposite side typically is found to have relatively restricted motion compared with the newly released side.

9. Steps 3 through 8 are repeated on the opposite side.

Cervical Articulatory Treatment

- Diagnosis: any cervical vertebral somatic dysfunction
- The procedure is performed as follows:
  1. Patient is supine.
  2. Practitioner is seated at the head of the table.
  3. The restricted cervical vertebral segment is located, and the restricted motions are identified (e.g., flexion or extension, sidebending right or left, rotation right or left).
  4. The practitioner stabilizes the lower vertebra of the restricted vertebral unit with one hand by pinching the spinous process of that vertebra between the thumb and index finger and moves the vertebra above it through the restrictive barrier in smooth, gentle, repetitive movements while using the head as a lever.
  5. The practitioner lifts the patient's head with the other hand by cupping the occiput in his or her palm and localizes movement to the dysfunctional vertebra.
  6. After moving through the restrictive barrier, the joint is brought passively back to resting position, and the restrictive barrier is again engaged and surpassed with the passive movement.
  7. These procedures are repeated several times until an improved range of motion is observed.
  8. Passive and active ranges of motion of the affected joints are retested.

Cervical Muscle Energy Treatment

- There are 10 basic steps to each muscle energy treatment for the cervical spine.
  1. The patient's position is supine.
  2. The practitioner's position is seated at the head of the table.
  3. The practitioner's handhold and contact points on the patient vary according to the dysfunctional joint that needs to be treated.

4. The practitioner motion tests to locate the restrictive barriers in three planes (i.e., flexion and extension, rotation to both sides, and sidebending to both sides).

5. The practitioner instructs the patient to apply an intrinsic, or active, isometric muscle contraction force against the practitioner's equal counterforce using the tight restrictive muscles. This is in the direction of the midline resting position, which is also toward the direction of ease of motion or diagnostic position of the dysfunctional joint. However, no motion occurs because the practitioner is holding the patient's cervical spine and head steady with an equal counterforce.

6. This isometric contraction is held for 5 to 6 seconds.

7. The patient is then directed to fully relax this effort.

8. The practitioner then engages the new restrictive motion barrier in all three planes at the dysfunctional joint. This resets the resting length of the shortened, tight muscles.

9. Steps 5 through 8 are repeated three to five times, with a final stretch of the dysfunctional joint into the restrictive barriers (i.e., flexion or extension, rotation, and sidebending) after the final repetition.

10. The patient is retested.

For each of the treatments listed in the next sections, steps 1, 2, 4, and 6 through 10 are essentially the same. The only differences are the practitioner's hold and contact points on the patient (i.e., step 3) and the practitioner's instructions to the patient (i.e., step 5). These are highlighted.

Occipitoatlantal Joint Treatment for Flexed Somatic Dysfunction

- Diagnosis: OA FR_LS_R
- Restriction: OA ER_RS_L (Fig. 6.55)
- The procedure is performed as follows:
  1. The patient is supine on the treatment table.
  2. The practitioner sits at the head of the table.
  3. *The practitioner cradles the patient's occiput with both hands.*

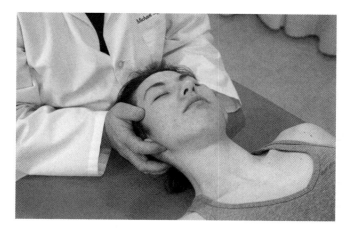

Figure 6.55 Muscle energy treatment position for the occipitoatlantal joint in flexion, rotated left, and sidebent right (OA FR_LS_R).

4. The practitioner engages the motion barriers in all three planes (i.e., extension, right rotation, and left sidebending) at the OA joint.
5. *The patient is instructed to sidebend his or her head toward the right against the practitioner's unyielding and equal counterforce.*
6. This isometric contraction is held for 5 to 6 seconds.
7. The patient is then directed to fully relax this effort.
8. The practitioner engages the new motion barrier in all three planes (i.e., extension, right rotation, and left sidebending) at the OA joint.
9. Steps 5 through 8 are repeated three to five times, with a final stretch of the OA joint into the restrictive barriers (i.e., extension, right rotation, and left sidebending) after the final repetition.
10. The patient is retested.

Occipitoatlantal Joint Treatment for Extended Somatic Dysfunction

- Diagnosis: OA ER_LS_R
- Restriction: OA FR_RS_L (Fig. 6.56)
- The procedure is performed as follows:
    1. The patient is supine on the treatment table.
    2. The practitioner sits at the head of the table.
    3. *The practitioner cradles the patient's occiput with both hands.*
    4. The practitioner engages the motion barriers in all three planes (i.e., flexion, right rotation, and left sidebending) at the OA joint.
    5. *The patient is instructed to sidebend his or her head toward the right against the practitioner's unyielding and equal counterforce.*
    6. This isometric contraction is held for 5 to 6 seconds.
    7. The patient is then directed to fully relax this effort.
    8. The practitioner then engages the new motion barrier in all three planes (i.e., flexion, right rotation, and left sidebending) at the OA joint.
    9. Steps 5 through 8 are repeated three to five times, with a final stretch of the OA joint into the restrictive barriers (i.e., flexion, right rotation, and left sidebending) after the final repetition.
    10. The patient is retested.

Atlantoaxial Joint Treatment

- Diagnosis: AA R_R
- Restriction: AA R_L (Fig. 6.57)
- The procedure is performed as follows:
    1. The patient is supine on the treatment table.
    2. The practitioner sits at the head of the table.
    3. *The practitioner flexes the patient's neck until the shoulders begin to lift off the table to inhibit motion at C2 to C7.*
    4. The practitioner rotates the patient's head to the left side to engage the restrictive barrier.
    5. *The patient is instructed to turn his or her head to the right against the practitioner's unyielding and equal counterforce.*
    6. This isometric contraction is held for 5 to 6 seconds.
    7. The patient is then instructed to fully relax this effort.
    8. The practitioner turns the patient's head further to the left and engages the new restrictive rotational barrier at the AA joint.
    9. Steps 5 through 8 are repeated three to five times, with a final stretch into the restrictive barrier (rotation) after the final repetition.
    10. The patient is retested.

Typical Cervical Joints (C2 to C7): Treatment for Flexed Somatic Dysfunction

- Diagnosis: C4 FS_RR_R
- Restriction: C4 ES_LR_L
- The procedure is performed as follows:
    1. The patient is supine on the treatment table (Fig. 6.58).
    2. The practitioner sits at the head of the table.
    3. *The practitioner cradles the patient's occiput with the palms of both hands, while the pads of the index or middle fingers contact the articular pillars of the restricted segment.*
    4. The practitioner engages the motion barriers in all three planes (i.e., extension, left sidebending, and left rotation) of the restricted segment.
    5. *The practitioner instructs the patient to sidebend his or her head toward the right against the practitioner's unyielding and equal counterforce.*

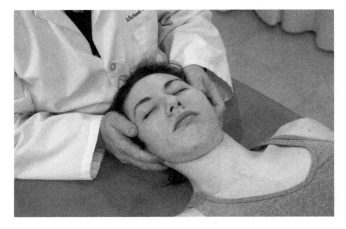

Figure 6.56 Muscle energy treatment position for the occipitoatlantal joint in extension, rotated left, and sidebent right (OA ER_LS_R).

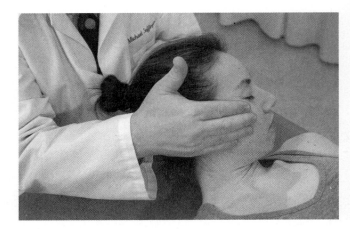

Figure 6.57 Muscle energy treatment position for the atlantoaxial joint rotated right (AA R_R).

6. This isometric contraction is held for 5 to 6 seconds.
7. The patient is then instructed to fully relax this effort.
8. The practitioner engages the new motion barrier in all three planes (i.e., extension, left sidebending, and left rotation) at the involved vertebral segment.
9. Steps 5 through 8 are repeated three to five times, with a final stretch into the restrictive barrier after the final repetition.
10. The patient is retested.

Typical Cervical Joints: Treatment for Extended Somatic Dysfunction

- Diagnosis: C4 ES_RR_R (i.e., representative case for C2 to C7 joints)
- Restriction: C4 FS_LR_L
- The procedure is performed as follows:
    1. The patient is supine on the treatment table (Fig. 6.59).
    2. The practitioner sits at the head of the table.
    3. *The practitioner cradles the patient's occiput with the palms of both hands, while the pads of the index or middle fingers contact the articular pillars of the restricted segment.*
    4. The practitioner engages the motion barriers in all three planes (i.e., flexion, left sidebending, and left rotation) of the restricted segment.
    5. *The practitioner instructs the patient to sidebend his or her head toward the right against the practitioner's unyielding and equal counterforce.*
    6. This isometric contraction is held for 5 to 6 seconds.
    7. The patient is then instructed to fully relax this effort.
    8. The practitioner engages the new motion barrier in all three planes (i.e., flexion, left sidebending, and left rotation) at the involved vertebral segment.
    9. Steps 5 through 8 are repeated three to five times, with a final stretch into the restrictive barrier after the final repetition.
    10. The patient is retested.

Cervical Functional Treatment

- Diagnosis: any cervical vertebral somatic dysfunction

- Example: C5 has evidence of somatic dysfunction (i.e., ART). It does not matter whether it is flexed or extended because vertebral positioning and motion are not examined or treated in functional technique. What is examined and treated is the aberrant spinal reflex activity at that level that is hypersensitive and reactive to passive body movements performed in other body regions.
- The procedure is performed as follows:
    1. The patient is in the supine position on a plinth or treatment table.
    2. The practitioner sits at the head of the table.
    3. The practitioner uses the index finger and thumb pads of one hand to monitor the tense tissues overlying the deep segmental paraspinal soft tissues (i.e., rotatores, multifidi) on either side of C5 (Fig. 6.60) while inducing slight passive motions by means of the patient's head in one direction at a time (e.g., flexion, extension, sidebending left then right, rotation left then right), mostly moving the OA and AA joints.
    4. The practitioner may find, for example, that the paraspinal soft tissues around C5 tighten, or bind, with passive head motion from the midline toward extension, sidebending left, rotation left, translation right and posteriorly, and axial compression and when the patient inhales (Fig. 6.61).
    6. In this example, the paraspinal soft tissues around C5 will loosen, or ease, with passive head motion from the midline toward flexion, sidebending right, rotation left, translation left and anteriorly, and axial decompression and when the patient exhales.
    7. To treat C5 using functional technique, the practitioner passively moves the patient's head from the resting midline position toward flexion, sidebending right, rotation right, and translation left and anteriorly and applies axial decompression, in essence stacking the directions of motion that induce ease or compliance in the paraspinal soft tissues around C5 (Fig. 6.62).
    5. The practitioner instructs the patient to maintain a prolonged natural exhalation (not forced) while fine-tuning

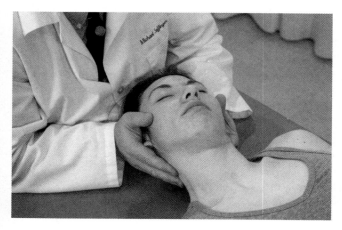

Figure 6.58 Muscle energy treatment position for the fourth cervical vertebra in flexion, sidebent right, and rotated right (C4 FS_RR_R).

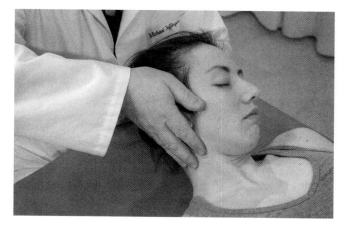

Figure 6.59 Muscle energy treatment position for the fourth cervical vertebra in extension, sidebent right, and rotated right (C4 ES_RR_R).

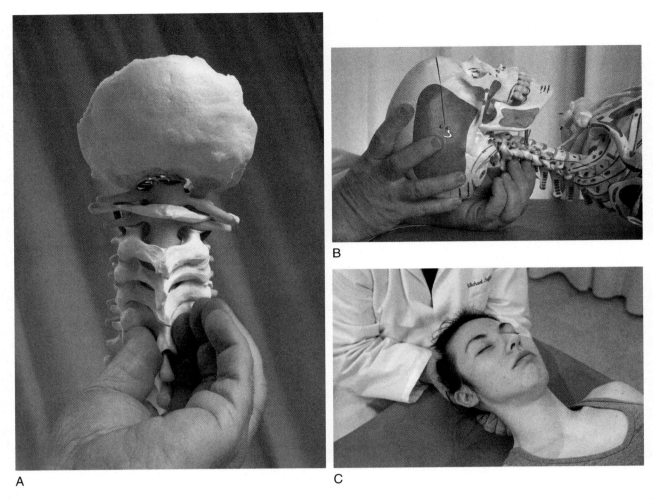

A

B

C

Figure 6.60 **A,** "Monitoring hand" position for functional treatment of the cervical spine. **B** and **C,** Hand positions for functional treatment of the cervical spine.

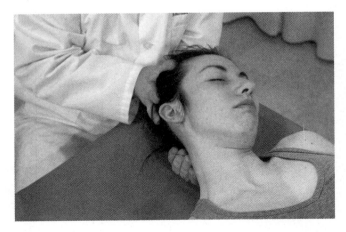

Figure 6.61 The practitioner may find that the paraspinal soft tissues around C5 tighten, or bind, with passive head motion from the midline toward extension, sidebending left, rotation left, translation right and posteriorly, and axial compression and when the patient inhales.

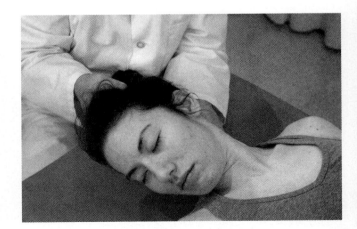

Figure 6.62 Functional treatment for the somatic findings in Figure 6.61 entails passively moving the patient's head from the resting midline position toward flexion, sidebending right, rotation right, and translation left and anteriorly while applying axial decompression, in essence stacking the directions of motion that induce ease, or compliance, in the paraspinal soft tissues around C5. The patient is instructed to inhale during these motions to facilitate the treatment.

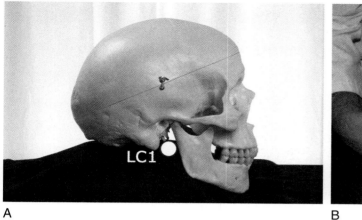
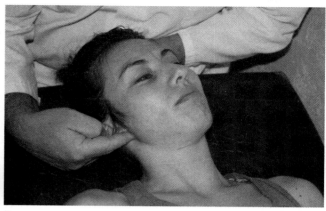

A   B

Figure 6.63   **A,** Location of counterstrain tender point lateral cervical 1 (LC1). **B,** Counterstrain treatment position for LC1.

the exact directions of motion that produce the most ease of the soft tissues being monitored around C5.

6. The practitioner retests for any presence of ease or bind at C5 during passive head movements.

Cervical Counterstrain Treatment
Lateral Cervical 1
- Location: The lateral cervical 1 (LC1) point is found at the tip of the transverse process of C1, located by pressing medially in the area between mastoid process and mandible, just below the occiput.
- The procedure is performed as follows:
  1. The patient is supine (Fig. 6.63).
  2. The practitioner is seated at the head of the table.
  3. The practitioner sidebends the patient's head toward the tender point.
  4. This position is held for 90 seconds.

5. The patient is passively, slowly moved back to the resting position.
6. The practitioner retests the tenderness of the point.

Anterior Cervical 1
- Location: The anterior cervical 1 (AC1) point is found on the posterior edge of the ascending ramus of the mandible at the level of the ear lobe.
- The procedure is performed as follows:
  1. The patient is supine (Fig. 6.64).
  2. The practitioner is seated at the head of the table.
  3. The practitioner rotates the patient's head away from the tender point, up to 90 degrees.
  4. This position is held for 90 seconds.
  5. The patient is passively, slowly moved back to the resting position.
  6. The practitioner retests the tenderness of the point.

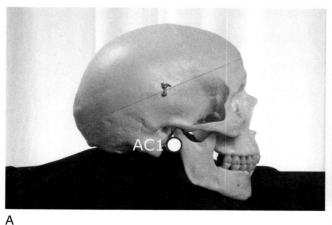
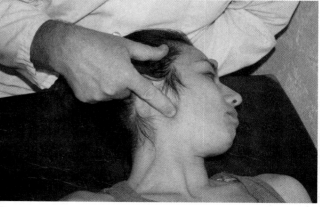

A   B

Figure 6.64   **A,** Location of counterstrain tender point anterior cervical 1 (AC1). **B,** Counterstrain treatment position for AC1.

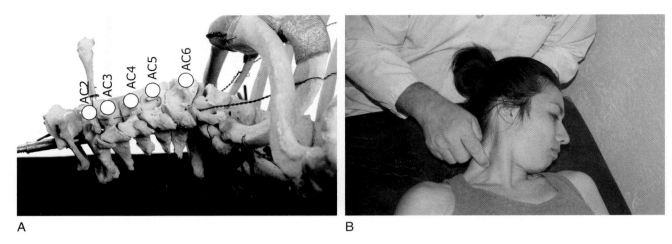

Figure 6.65 **A,** Location of counterstrain tender points anterior cervical 2 (AC2) through AC6. **B,** Counterstrain treatment position for AC2 through AC6 is demonstrated for AC4.

Anterior Cervical 2 to 6

- Location: Anterior cervical 2 to 6 (AC2 to AC6) points are found on the anterior surface of the tips of the transverse processes of the corresponding vertebrae.
- The procedure is performed as follows:
  1. The patient is supine (Fig. 6.65).
  2. The practitioner is seated at the head of the table.
  3. The practitioner flexes the patient's neck and head to the level of the affected vertebra.
  4. The practitioner then sidebends and rotates the patient's head away from the side of the counterstrain point.
  5. This position is held for 90 seconds.
  6. The patient is passively, slowly moved back to the resting position.
  7. The practitioner retests the tenderness of the point.

Anterior Cervical 7

- Location: The anterior cervical 7 (AC7) point is found about 3 cm lateral to the medial end of the clavicle on the superior surface, at the clavicular attachment of the sternocleidomastoid muscle.
- The procedure is performed as follows:
  1. The patient is supine (Fig. 6.66).
  2. The practitioner is seated at the head of the table.
  3. The practitioner markedly flexes the patient's cervical spine.
  4. The practitioner then sidebends the patient's head toward and rotates it away from the side of the counterstrain point.
  5. This position is held for 90 seconds.
  6. The patient is passively, slowly moved back to the resting position.
  7. The practitioner retests the tenderness of the point.

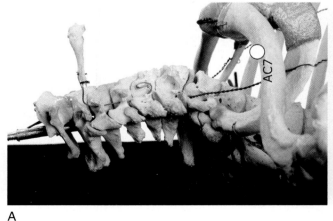
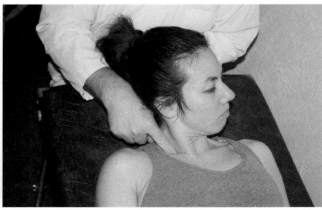

Figure 6.66 **A,** Location of counterstrain tender point anterior cervical 7 (AC7). **B,** Counterstrain treatment position for AC7.

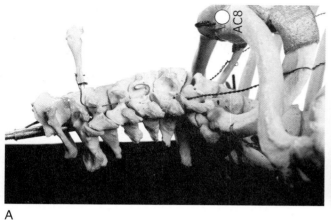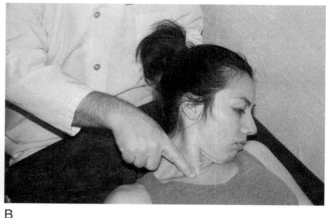

A

B

Figure 6.67 **A,** Location of counterstrain tender point anterior cervical 8 (AC8). **B,** Counterstrain treatment position for AC8.

Anterior Cervical 8

- Location: The anterior cervical 8 (AC8) point is found on the medial end of the clavicle in the suprasternal notch.
- The procedure is performed as follows:
  1. The patient is supine (Fig. 6.67).
  2. The practitioner is seated at the head of the table.
  3. The practitioner flexes the patient's head and neck to the level of the affected vertebra.
  4. The practitioner then sidebends and rotates the patient's head away from the side of the counterstrain point.
  5. This position is held for 90 seconds.
  6. The patient is passively, slowly moved back to resting position.
  7. The practitioner retests the tenderness of the point.

Inion

- Location: The inion (IC1) is found 2 cm below the external occipital protuberance, medial to the muscle mass.
- The procedure is performed as follows:
  1. The patient is supine (Fig. 6.68).
  2. The practitioner is seated at the head of the table.
  3. The practitioner markedly flexes the patient's head on his or her neck.
  4. This position is held for 90 seconds.
  5. The patient is passively, slowly moved back to the resting position.
  6. The practitioner retests the tenderness of the point.

Posterior Cervical 1

- Location: The posterior cervical 1 (PC1) point is found 2 cm lateral to the suboccipital muscle mass, on the occiput at the occipitocervical junction.
- The procedure is performed as follows:
  1. The patient is supine (Fig. 6.69).
  2. The practitioner is seated at the head of the table.
  3. The practitioner induces extension of the patient's neck at C1 to C2.
  4. The practitioner then adds *slight* sidebending and rotation away from the counterstrain point.

5. This position is held for 90 seconds.
6. The patient is passively, slowly moved back to the resting position.
7. The practitioner retests the tenderness of the point.

Posterior Cervical 2

- Location: The posterior cervical 2 (PC2) point is found on the superior surface of the spinous process of C2 or in the muscle mass lateral to the spinous process of C2.
- The procedure is performed as follows:
  1. The patient is supine (Fig. 6.70).
  2. The practitioner is seated at the head of the table.
  3. The practitioner induces slight extension in the patient's neck.
  4. The practitioner then sidebends and rotates the patient's head away from the counterstrain point.
  5. This position is held for 90 seconds.
  6. The patient is passively, slowly moved back to the resting position.
  7. The practitioner retests the tenderness of the point.

Posterior Cervical 3

- Location: The posterior cervical 3 (PC3) point is found on the inferior portion of the spinous process of C2.
- The procedure is performed as follows:
  1. The patient is supine (Fig. 6.71).
  2. The practitioner is seated at the head of the table.
  3. The practitioner induces approximately 45 degrees of flexion into the patient's neck.
  4. The practitioner then sidebends and rotates the patient's head away from the counterstrain point.
  5. This position is held for 90 seconds.
  6. The patient is passively, slowly moved back to the resting position.
  7. The practitioner retests the tenderness of the point.

Posterior Cervical 4 to 8

- Location: The posterior cervical 4 (PC4) point is found on the spinous process of C3, PC5 on the spinous process of C4,

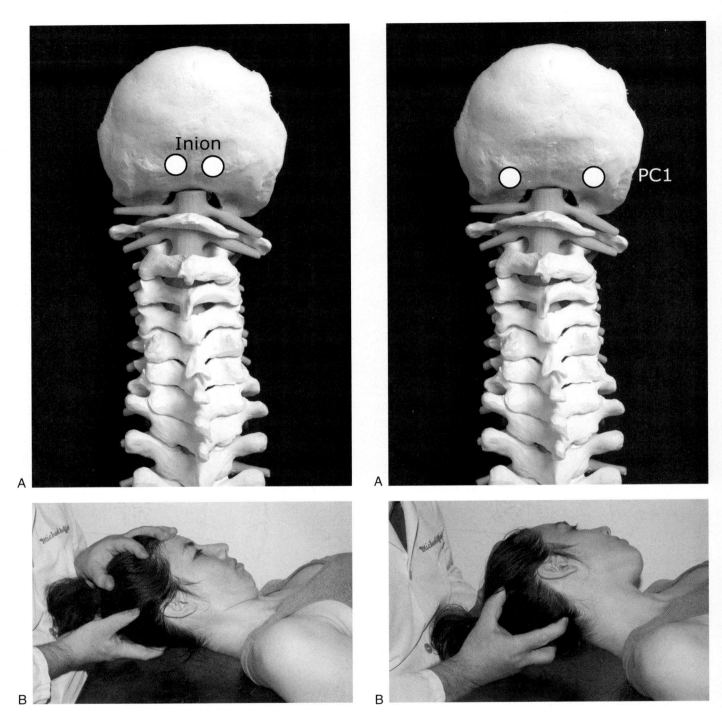

Figure 6.68   A, Location of counterstrain tender point inion (IC1). **B,** Counterstrain treatment position for IC1.

Figure 6.69   A, Location of counterstrain tender point posterior cervical 1 (PC1). **B,** Counterstrain treatment position of PC1.

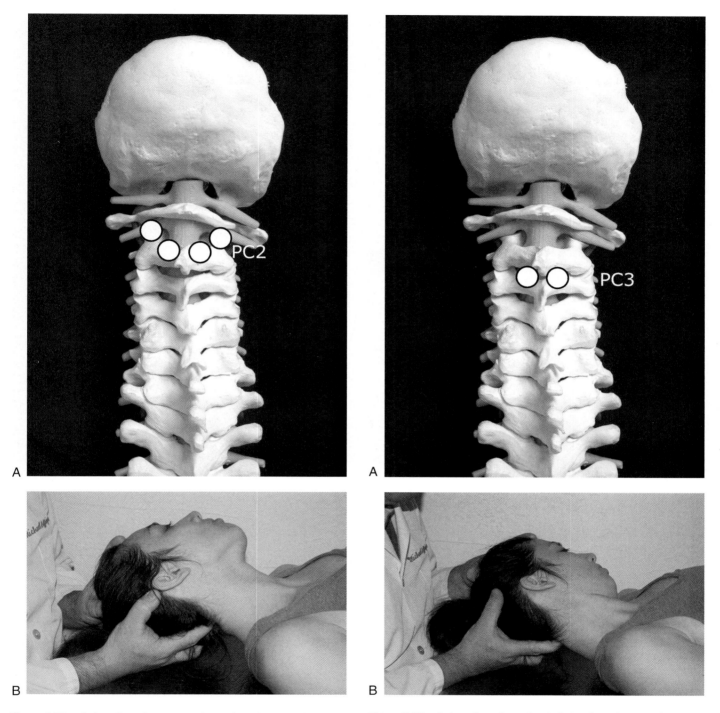

Figure 6.70 **A,** Location of counterstrain tender point posterior cervical 2 (PC2). **B,** Counterstrain treatment position of PC2.

Figure 6.71 **A,** Location of counterstrain tender point posterior cervical 3 (PC3). **B,** Counterstrain treatment position for PC3.

PC6 on the spinous process of C5, PC7 on the spinous process of C6, and PC8 on the spinous process of C7.

- The procedure is performed as follows:
  1. The patient is supine (Fig. 6.72).
  2. The practitioner is seated at the head of the table.
  3. The practitioner brings the patient toward himself or herself, so that the patient's head is over the edge of the table, extended, and supported in the practitioner's hands.
  4. The practitioner then sidebends and rotates the patient's head away from the counterstrain point.
  5. This position is held for 90 seconds.
  6. The patient is passively, slowly moved back to the resting position.
  7. The practitioner retests the tenderness of the point.

ADJUNCT TREATMENTS

- Analgesic or corticosteroid injections, bracing, posture and ergonomic instruction, physical modalities to ease pain, and exercise to restore motion and strength can be beneficial.
- Interventions that promote activity and mobilization, such as exercise,[55] physical therapy,[56] analgesics, and nonsteroidal anti-inflammatory drugs (NSAIDs), are effective for the short term, but the prolonged use of soft collars, rest, and inactivity probably prolongs disability.
- Most of the commonly used adjunctive therapies have not been rigorously tested and therefore remain unproven (see Table 6.14).
- Cold compresses, typically used as often as 20 minutes per hour in more severe cases, and heat and massage may not be scientifically proven, but they are sufficiently anecdotally acknowledged as safe pain relievers to justify their use.[57]

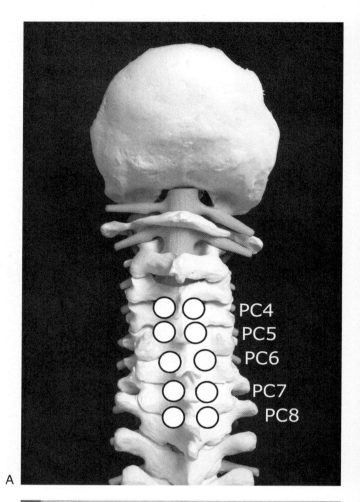

A

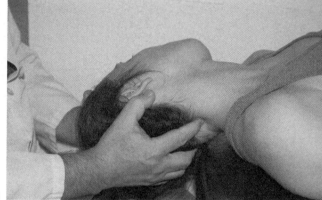

B

Figure 6.72 **A,** Location of counterstrain tender points posterior cervical 4 (PC4) through PC8. **B,** Counterstrain treatment position for PC4 through PC8.

Table 6.14   Commonly used adjunct treatments*

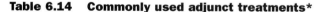

Acupuncture

Cervical pillows

Epidural or intrathecal injections

Heat

Ice

Laser

Massage

Muscle relaxants

Postural training

Psychosocial interventions

Short-wave diathermy

Spray and stretch

Transcutaneous nerve stimulation

Ultrasound

*Adjunct treatments have not been rigorously tested for effectiveness.

- A home program, consisting of ischemic pressure and sustained stretching, can be effective in reducing trigger point sensitivity and pain intensity in individuals with neck and upper back pain.[58]
- Returning to work depends on the severity of the pain, chronicity of the pain, work environment, automobile usage, home environment, and psychosocial and economic factors.
- A surgical consultation is warranted if there is refractory radiculopathy or progressive neurologic deficit.

Education

- Patients should be instructed on the cause, nature, and prognosis based on the current epidemiologic understanding of the condition.
- Patients should be encouraged to avoid activities that exacerbate the condition, such as prolonged neck flexion, arm and shoulder activities, and poor postural mechanics.
- Comorbid conditions should be addressed and managed.
- Coping skills and counseling may be needed if the condition is prolonged and unresolved.

Exercises

Neck Exercises to Improve Range of Motion

The following neck exercises can be done sitting comfortably in a chair (Fig. 6.73).

Neck Flexion Stretch

- The exercise is performed as follows:
  1. Slowly bring your chin toward your chest (Fig. 6.74).
  2. Return to the normal resting position (i.e., head upright and looking straight ahead).
  3. Repeat five times.
  4. For additional stretch, put pressure on the back of your head with one hand (Fig. 6.75).

Neck Extension Stretch

- The exercise is performed as follows:
  1. Slowly extend your neck, looking up toward the ceiling as far as is comfortable (Fig. 6.76).
  2. Return to the normal resting position.
  3. Repeat five times.

Neck Sidebending (Lateral Flexion) Stretch

- The exercise is performed as follows:
  1. Slowly tilt your head to one side such that your ear approaches the shoulder on the same side while keeping your face straight forward.

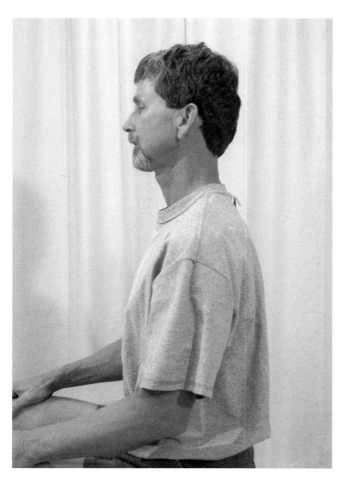

Figure 6.73   Starting or rest position for neck exercises.

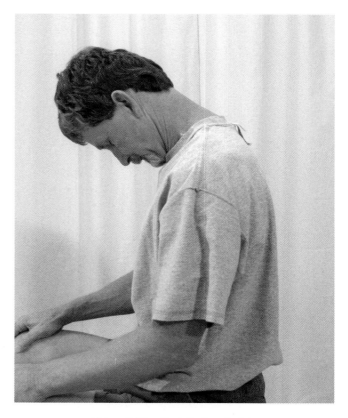

Figure 6.74   Neck flexion stretch.

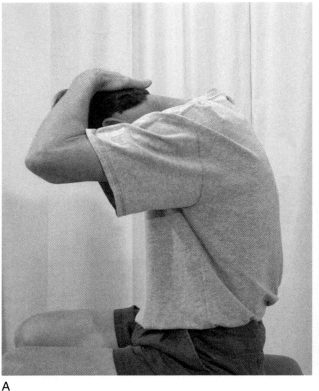
A

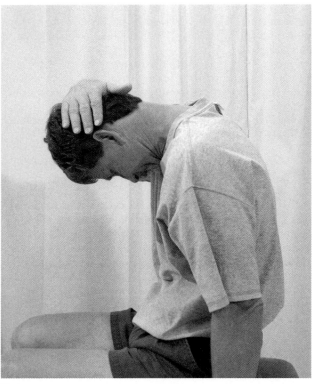
B

Figure 6.75   **A,** Passive neck flexion stretch. **B,** Reverse angle view of a passive neck flexion stretch.

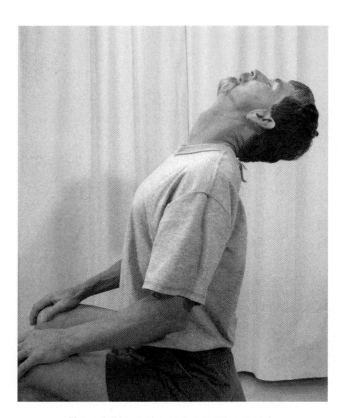

Figure 6.76   Active neck extension stretch.

2. Return to normal resting position (Fig. 6.77).
3. Repeat five times.
4. Repeat steps 1 through 3 to the other side.
5. You can increase the stretch by reaching over to the other side of your head and gently pulling the head toward the shoulder (Fig. 6.78).

Neck Rotation Stretch
- The exercise is performed as follows:
    1. Slowly turn your head in one direction as if to look over your shoulder (Fig. 6.79).
    2. Return to the normal resting position.
    3. Repeat five times.
    4. Repeat steps 1 and 2 to the other side.

Neck Exercises to Improve Muscle Tone
The following exercises can be done in the seated position.

Isometric Contraction for Anterior Neck Muscles
- The exercise is performed as follows:
    1. Place the palm of one of your hands in the center of your forehead, and press forward with your head just enough to contract the anterior neck muscles but not enough to overcome the force of your palm pushing against the forehead (Fig. 6.80). There should be muscle tightening in the front part of your neck but no movement.

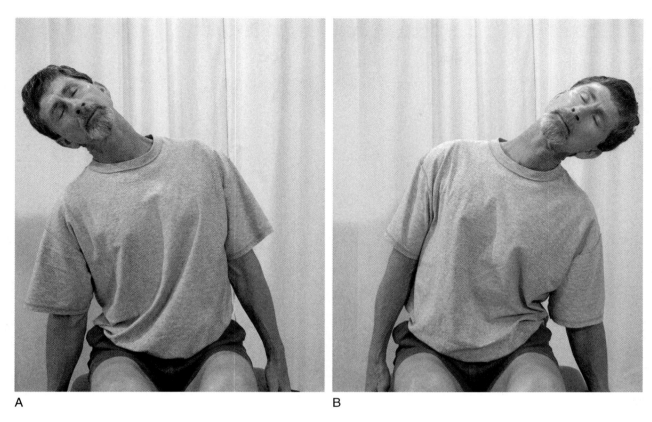

A

B

Figure 6.77   **A,** Active neck right sidebending stretch. **B,** Active neck left sidebending stretch.

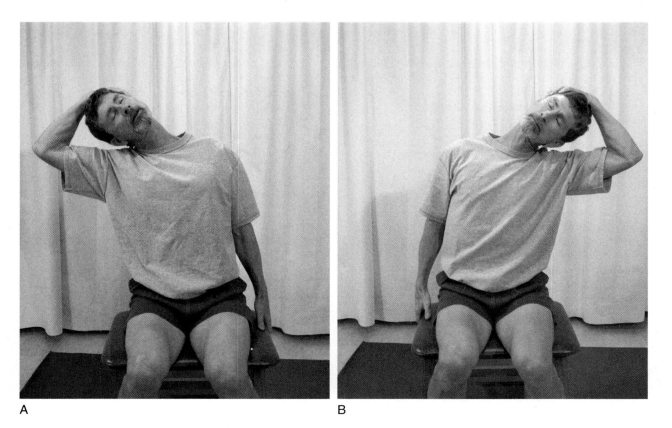

A

B

Figure 6.78   **A,** Passive neck right sidebending stretch. **B,** Passive neck left sidebending stretch.

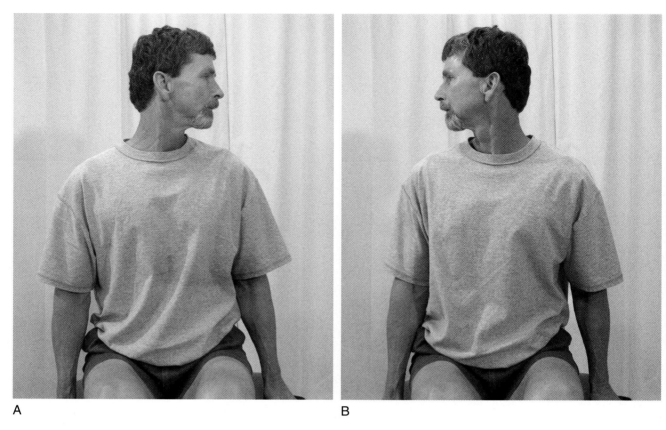

A   B

Figure 6.79   **A,** Active neck left rotation stretch. **B,** Active neck right rotation stretch.

2. Maintain that contraction without moving for 5 seconds, relax the muscles completely, and stop pressing on your forehead with your palm.

3. After a few seconds of rest, repeat steps 1 and 2.

4. Repeat steps 1 through 3 five times.

Isometric Contraction of Posterior Neck Muscles
• The exercise is performed as follows:

1. Place the palm of one of your hands in the middle of the back of your head, and push your head backwards toward your hand with just enough force to tighten the posterior neck muscles but not enough to overcome the resistance of the hand pressing against the back side of your head (Fig. 6.81). There should be no movement of your head away from its resting midline position.

2. Maintain that contraction without moving for 5 seconds, relax the muscles completely, and stop pressing on the back of your head with your hand.

3. After a few seconds of rest, repeat steps 1 and 2.

4. Repeat steps 1 through 3 five times.

Isometric Contraction of Lateral Neck Muscles
• The exercise is performed as follows:

1. Place the palm of your right hand just above your right ear on your head, and tilt your head toward it with just enough

force to tighten the lateral neck muscles but not enough to overcome the resistance of the palm that is pressing against the side of your head (Fig. 6.82). There should be no movement of your head away from its resting midline position.

2. Maintain that contraction without moving for 5 seconds, relax the muscles completely, and stop pressing on the side of your head with your palm.

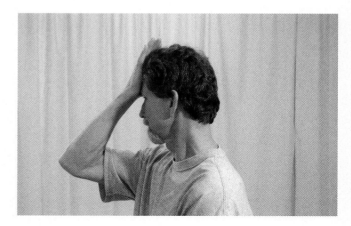

Figure 6.80   Isometric contraction for anterior neck muscles.

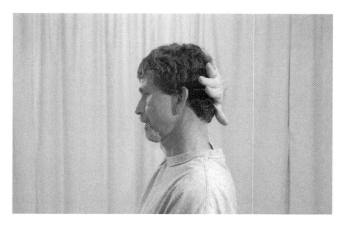

Figure 6.81 Isometric contraction for posterior neck muscles.

3. After a few seconds of rest, repeat steps 1 and 2.
4. Repeat steps 1 through 3 five times.
5. Repeat steps 1 through 4 on the opposite side.

Lateral Neck and Anterior Chest Muscle Stretches

The following neck exercises can be done in the seated position on a plinth or treatment table.

Scalene and Anterior Neck Muscle Stretches
- The exercise is performed as follows:
  1. Sit on a plinth, massage table, or treatment table (Fig. 6.83).
  2. Reach behind you with one hand, and grab the side of the table as shown in Figure 6.83A.
  3. Tilt your head away from the side that is grabbing the table, and look upward to extend the neck and stretch the scalene muscles.
  4. Hold the position for 5 seconds.
  5. Release the table, relax the muscles, and return to the resting seated position.

6. Repeat three times.
7. Repeat steps 1 through 6 on the other side (see Fig. 6.83B).
8. Reach behind you with both hands, grab the side of the table (see Fig. 6.83C), tilt your head straight backward, and look upward to stretch the anterior neck and chest muscles.
9. Repeat steps 4 through 6 on the opposite side.

Suboccipital Neck Muscle Stretch
The following technique is done lying down on your back (supine) on the floor or a plinth, massage table or treatment table.

Posterior Occipital Muscle Stretch
- The exercise is performed as follows:
  1. Place a 2- to 3-inch-thick book under your occiput (Fig. 6.84).
  2. Tuck your chin toward your chest.
  3. Hold this position for 5 seconds.
  4. Relax.
  5. Repeat steps 3 through 5 five times.

CONTROVERSIES

There has been concern expressed regarding the use of high-velocity, low-amplitude (HVLA) manipulative procedures in the treatment of upper cervical somatic dysfunction. There have been reports of vertebral artery dissection and stroke. However, no direct causal relationship can be established because the natural incidence of this catastrophic event occurs at a higher rate than has been reported with the use of cervical HVLA.[59,60] Although these techniques are not presented in this textbook, it is important to understand the controversy associated with HVLA of the upper cervical spine and to be aware of the reports in the literature and the policies of organized professional medical societies. For example, the AAO (March 2003) and the AOA (August 2004) developed position papers on osteopathic manipulation of the cervical spine. They included a concise review of

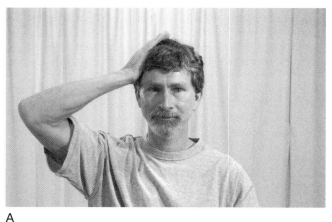

A

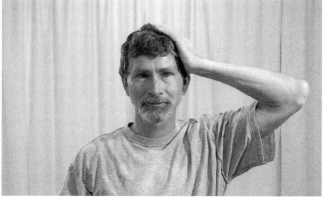

B

Figure 6.82 **A,** Isometric contraction for right lateral neck muscles. **B,** Isometric contraction for left lateral neck muscles.

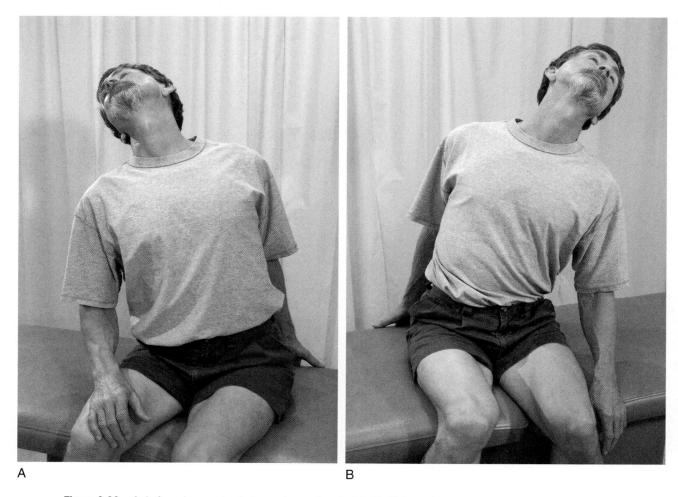

A   B

Figure 6.83   **A,** Left scalene and anterior neck muscles stretch. **B,** Right scalene and anterior neck muscles stretch.

the literature and strong statements of support for osteopathic manipulation of the cervical spine, including HVLA manipulative procedures.

There have been no complications from any of the manipulative procedures performed in any of the clinical trials of spinal manipulation (>100 in the past 25 years). However, because of the controversy surrounding the HVLA manual procedures for the cervical spine and the belief that these procedures should be learned under the direct supervision of licensed and trained professionals, we decided not to include HVLA manual procedures in this textbook. Moreover, a randomized clinical trial demonstrated that mobilization of the cervical spine yields clinical outcomes comparable to those from HVLA procedures.[61] This study provides support for the concept that it is not necessary to use the HVLA procedures, which carry a small risk and substantial social stigmatism, to facilitate rehabilitation of a cervical somatic dysfunction. The procedures presented in this textbook have not caused injury and are safe for most patients of all age groups. The most common reasons for complications arising from a manipulative procedure are practitioner related rather than procedure related: misdiagnosis, lack of skill, or lack of consultation with a skilled manipulator.

Realizing that data alone do not make clinical decisions and that expert opinion is still needed to help guide us, the RAND corporation put together a panel of experts consisting of an orthopedic spine surgeon, a neurosurgeon, two neurologists, one primary care practitioner, and four chiropractors in the Los Angeles area.[62] (There were no osteopathic practitioners or physical therapists on the panel). The panelists were asked to independently review the literature on spinal manipulative therapy and to rate the level of appropriateness of this treatment for a patient presenting with the complaint of neck pain in a variety of clinical scenarios. They determined that patients likely to benefit from a trial of spinal manipulative treatment (SMT, such as HVLA) for a complaint of neck pain include the following:
• Acute neck pain (< 3 weeks' duration)
  1. No radiculopathy
      Painful or limited range of motion
      Pain anatomically consistent with musculotendinous distribution

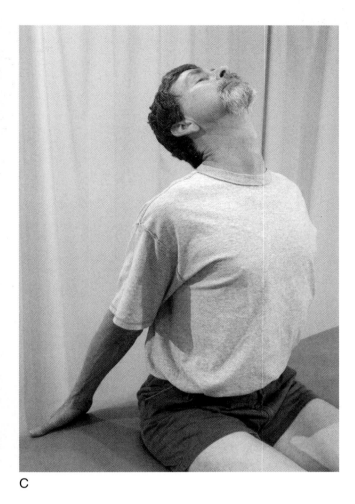

C

Figure 6.83, cont'd   C, Anterior neck and chest muscles stretch.

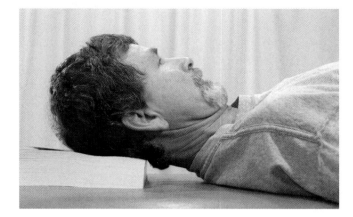

Figure 6.84   Suboccipital muscles stretch.

Nontraumatic or minimally traumatic origin
Absence of clinical risk factors or radiographic contraindications
No prior SMT or favorable response to prior SMT
  2. Possible radiculopathy
No radiographic contraindications
Advanced imaging study shows no herniated disc, spinal foramina osteophytosis, or spinal stenosis
Prior favorable response to SMT
If no prior SMT, add nontraumatic or minimally traumatic origin
- Subacute or chronic neck pain (>3 weeks' duration)
  1. No radiculopathy
Painful or limited range of motion
Pain anatomically consistent with musculotendinous distribution
Nontraumatic or minimally traumatic origin
No radiographic contraindications
No prior SMT or favorable response to prior SMT
  2. Possible radiculopathy
No radiographic contraindications

Advanced imaging study shows no herniated disc, spinal foramina osteophytosis, or spinal stenosis
Prior favorable response to SMT
Nontraumatic or minimally traumatic origin
No prior SMT or favorable response to prior SMT
- Generalized neck pain
  1. Morning stiffness
  2. No clinical suspicion of connective tissue disease
  3. Radiographs showing less than advanced degeneration of the cervical spine
  4. Nonmanipulative care for this condition not helpful

The following clinical factors associated with indications that the panel rated as inappropriate for cervical spine manipulation (i.e., HVLA) included:
- Presence of a clinically substantial traumatic origin for neck pain in the absence of cervical radiographs
- The presence of clinical risk factors in the absence of cervical radiographs
- The presence of radiographic contraindications
- The presence of clinically significant cervical disc herniation
- Spinal foramina osteophytosis
- Spinal canal stenosis (>50%)

Whereas the neurosurgical literature insists that chiropractic cervical manipulation (i.e., HVLA) is inappropriate in the face of cervical radiculopathy,[9] the National Guidelines Clearinghouse states that chiropractic (i.e., HVLA) manipulation of the cervical spine is contraindicated only in patients with a risk for stroke (i.e., cerebral vascular accident).

OPPORTUNITIES FOR RESEARCH

- On physical examination, patients with palpable passive cervical motion asymmetries in the absence of neck pain complaints have abnormal muscle firing patterns, decreased strength, and endurance as demonstrated by electromyography.[63]
- In a 7-year prospective longitudinal study, patients with hypertension were found to have a chronic pattern of somatic

dysfunction (diagnosed by palpatory findings of paraspinal muscle tension, decreased range of motion, and skin or soft tissue texture abnormalities) in the neck and upper back at C6, T2, and T6.[64]

- These findings suggest the possibility that the physical examination can detect abnormal muscle function in the cervical spine that may predate the onset of pain.
- Unfortunately, the subjects in these studies were not followed with pain questionnaires over time.
- The added benefit of exercise needs to be further explored. Factorial design would help determine the active treatment agents within a treatment mix. Phase II trials would help identify the most effective treatment characteristics and dosages. Greater attention to methodologic quality is needed.[50,51]

REFERENCES

1. Côté P, Cassidy JD, Carroll LJ, et al: The annual incidence and course of neck pain in the general population: A population-based cohort study. Pain 112:267-273, 2004.
2. Hartvigsen J, Christensen K, Frederiksen H: Back and neck pain exhibit many common features in old age: A population-based study of 4,486 Danish twins 70-102 years of age. Spine 29:576-580, 2004.
3. Walker-Bone K, Reading I, Coggon D, et al: The anatomical pattern and determinants of pain in the neck and upper limbs: An epidemiologic study. Pain 109:45-51, 2004.
4. Ståhl M, Mikkelsson M, Kautiainen H, et al: Neck pain in adolescence: A 4-year follow-up of pain-free preadolescents. Pain 110:427-431, 2004.
5. Chapline JF, Ferguson SA, Lillis RP, et al: Neck pain and head restraint position relative to the driver's head in rear-end collisions. Accid Anal Prev 32:287-297, 2000.
6. Hill J, Lewis M, Papageorgiou AC, et al: Predicting persistent neck pain: A 1-year follow-up of a population cohort. Spine 29:1648-1654, 2004.
7. Vogt MT, Simonsick EM, Harris TB, et al: Neck and shoulder pain in 70- to 79-year-old men and women: Findings from the Health, Aging and Body Composition Study. Spine J 3:435-441, 2003.
8. Bot SD, van der Waal JM, Terwee CB, et al: Incidence and prevalence of complaints of the neck and upper extremity in general practice. Ann Rheum Dis 64:118-123, 2005.
9. Narayan P, Haid RW: Treatment of degenerative cervical disc disease. Neurol Clin 19:217-229, 2001.
10. Bilkey WJ: Manual medicine approach to the cervical spine and whiplash injury. Phys Med Rehabil Clin North Am 7:749-759, 1996.
11. Sleszynski SL, Glonek T: Outpatient osteopathic SOAP note form: Preliminary results in osteopathic outcomes-based research. J Am Osteopath Assoc 105:181-205, 2005.
12. Côté P, Cassidy JD, Carroll L: Is a lifetime history of neck injury in a traffic collision associated with prevalent neck pain, headache and depressive symptomatology? Accid Anal Prev 32:151-159, 2000.
13. Côté P, Cassidy JD, Carroll L: The factors associated with neck pain and its related disability in the Saskatchewan population. Spine 25:1109-1117, 2000.
14. Bunketorp L, Stener-Victorin E, Carlsson J: Neck pain and disability following motor vehicle accidents: A cohort study. Eur Spine J 14:84-89, 2005.
15. Borghouts JA, Koes BW, Vondeling H, et al: Cost-of-illness of neck pain in The Netherlands in 1996. Pain 80:629-636, 1999.
16. United States National Health Survey, 1999-2000: Ambulatory Care Visits to Practitioner Offices, Hospital Outpatient Departments, and Emergency Departments. Washington, DC, U.S. Government Printing Office, September 2004.
17. Borghouts JA, Koes BW, Bouter LM: The clinical course and prognostic factors of non-specific neck pain: A systematic review. Pain 77:1-13, 1998.
18. Siivola SM, Levoska S, Latvala K, et al: Predictive factors for neck and shoulder pain: A longitudinal study in young adults. Spine 29:1662-1669, 2004.
19. Grooten WJ, Wiktorin C, Norrman L, et al: Seeking care for neck/shoulder pain: A prospective study of work-related risk factors in a healthy population. J Occup Environ Med 46:138-146, 2004.
20. Borg K, Hensing G, Alexanderson K: Risk factors for disability pension over 11 years in a cohort of young persons initially sick-listed with low back, neck, or shoulder diagnoses. Scand J Public Health 32:272-278, 2004.
21. Andersen JH, Kaergaard A, Mikkelsen S, et al: Risk factors in the onset of neck/shoulder pain in a prospective study of workers in industrial and service companies. Occup Environ Med 60:649-654, 2003.
22. Ciancaglini R, Testa M, Radaelli G: Association of neck pain with symptoms of temporomandibular dysfunction in the general adult population. Scand J Rehabil Med 31:17-22, 1999.
23. Bleasdale-Barr KM, Mathias CJ: Neck and other muscle pains in autonomic failure: Their association with orthostatic hypotension. J R Soc Med 91:355-359, 1998.
24. Zapletal J, Hekster RE, Straver JS, et al: Relationship between atlanto-odontoid osteoarthritis and idiopathic suboccipital neck pain. Neuroradiology 38:62-65, 1996.
25. Larsson R, Oberg PA, Larsson SE: Changes of trapezius muscle blood flow and electromyography in chronic neck pain due to trapezius myalgia. Pain 79:45-50, 1999.
26. Hoving JL, Koes BW, De Vet HC, et al: Manual therapy, physical therapy or continued care by the general practitioner for patients with neck pain: Short-term results from a pragmatic randomized trial. Ann Intern Med 136:713-722, 2002.
27. Ariëns GA, van Mechelen W, Bongers PM, et al: Physical risk factors for neck pain. Scand J Work Environ Health 26:7-19, 2000.
28. Ariëns GA, van Mechelen W, Bongers PM, et al: Psychosocial risk factors for neck pain: A systematic review. Am J Ind Med 39:180-193, 2001.
29. Ariëns GA, Bongers PM, Douwes M, et al: Are neck flexion, neck rotation, and sitting at work risk factors for neck pain? Results of a prospective cohort study. Occup Environ Med 58:200-207, 2001.
30. Krause N, Ragland DR, Greiner BA, et al: Physical workload and ergonomic factors associated with prevalence of back and neck pain in urban transit operators. Spine 22:2117-2127, 1997.
31. Lauren H, Luoto S, Alaranta H, et al: Arm motion speed and risk of neck pain: A preliminary communication. Spine 22:2094-2099, 1997.
32. Guez M, Hildingsson C, Stegmayr B, et al: Chronic neck pain of traumatic and non-traumatic origin: A population-based study. Acta Orthop Scand 74:576-579, 2003.
33. Murphy S, Buckle P, Stubbs D: Classroom posture and self-reported back and neck pain in schoolchildren. Appl Ergon 35:113-120, 2004.
34. Viikari-Juntura E, Martikainen R, Luukkonen R, et al: Longitudinal study on work related and individual risk factors affecting radiating neck pain. Occup Environ Med 58:345-352, 2001.
35. Friedman MH, Nelson AJ Jr: Head and neck pain review: Traditional and new perspectives. J Orthop Sports Phys Ther 24:268-278, 1996.
36. Lord SM, Barnsley L, Wallis BJ, et al: Chronic cervical zygapophysial joint pain after whiplash: A placebo-controlled prevalence study. Spine 21:1737-1745, 1996.
37. Speldewinde GC, Bashford GM, Davidson IR: Diagnostic cervical zygapophyseal joint blocks for chronic cervical pain. Med J Aust 174:174-176, 2001.
38. Norlander S, Gustavsson BA, Lindell J, et al: Reduced mobility in the cervico-thoracic motion segment—A risk factor for musculoskeletal neck-shoulder pain: A two-year prospective follow-up study. Scand J Rehabil Med 29:167-174, 1997.
39. Norlander S, Aste-Norlander U, Nordgren B, et al: Mobility in the cervico-thoracic motion segment: An indicative factor of musculo-skeletal neck-shoulder pain. Scand J Rehabil Med 28:183-192, 1996.
40. Norlander S, Nordgren B: Clinical symptoms related to musculoskeletal neck-shoulder pain and mobility in the cervico-thoracic spine. Scand J Rehabil Med 30:243-251, 1998.
41. Cleland JA, Childs JD, McRae M, et al: Immediate effects of thoracic manipulation in patients with neck pain: A randomized clinical trial. Man Ther 10:127-135, 2005.
42. Chong CL, Ooi SB: Neck pain after minor neck trauma—Is it always neck sprain? Eur J Emerg Med 7:147-149, 2000.
43. McPartland JM, Brodeur RR, Hallgren RC: Chronic neck pain, standing balance, and suboccipital muscle atrophy—A pilot study. J Manipulative Physiol Ther 20:24-29, 1997.
44. Hagen KB, Harms-Ringdahl K, Enger NO, et al: Relationship between subjective neck disorders and cervical spine mobility and motion-related pain in male machine operators. Spine 22:1501-1507, 1997.
45. Dyrehag LE, Widerstrom-Noga EG, Carlsson SG, et al: Relations between self-rated musculoskeletal symptoms and signs and psychological distress in chronic neck and shoulder pain. Scand J Rehabil Med 30:235-242, 1998.
46. Seffinger MA, Najm WI, Mishra SI, et al: Reliability of spinal palpation for diagnosis of neck or back pain: A systematic review of the literature. Spine 29:413-425, 2004.
47. Hurwitz EL, Aker PD, Adams AH, et al: Manipulation and mobilization of the cervical spine: A systematic review of the literature. Spine 21:1746-1760, 1996.
48. Gross AR, Aker PD, Quartly C: Musculoskeletal medicine: Manual therapy in the treatment of neck pain. Rheum Dis Clin North Am 22:579-98, 1996.
49. Fiechtner JJ, Brodeur RR: Manual and manipulation techniques for rheumatic disease. Rheum Dis Clin North Am 26:83-96, 2000.
50. Gross AR, Hoving JL, Haines TA, et al: Cervical overview group. A Cochrane review of manipulation and mobilization for mechanical neck disorders. Spine 29:1541-1548, 2004.
51. Gross AR, Hoving JL, Haines TA, et al: Cervical overview group: Manipulation and mobilisation for mechanical neck disorders. Cochrane Database Syst Rev (2):CD004249, 2004.

52. McMorland G, Suter E: Chiropractic management of mechanical neck and low-back pain: A retrospective, outcome-based analysis. J Manipulative Physiol Ther 23: 307-311, 2000.

53. Work Loss Data Institute: Disorders of the Neck and Upper Back. Corpus Christi, TX, Work Loss Data Institute, 2003.

54. Korthals-de Bos IBC, Hoving JL, van Tulder MW, et al: Cost effectiveness of physiotherapy, manual therapy, and general practitioner care for neck pain: Economic evaluation alongside a randomised controlled trial. BMJ 326:911-914, 2003.

55. Waling K, Sundelin G, Ahlgren C, et al: Perceived pain before and after three exercise programs—A controlled clinical trial of women with work-related trapezius myalgia. Pain 85:201-207, 2000.

56. Giebel GD, Edelmann M, Huser R: Sprain of the cervical spine: Early functional vs. immobilization treatment. Zentralbl Chir 122:517-521, 1997.

57. Swezey RL: Musculoskeletal medicine: Chronic neck pain. Rheum Dis Clin North Am 22:411-437, 1996.

58. Hanten WP, Olson SL, Butts NL, et al: Effectiveness of a home program of ischemic pressure followed by sustained stretch for treatment of myofascial trigger points. Phys Ther 80:997-1003, 2000.

59. Haldeman S, Kohlbeck FJ, McGregor M: Risk factors and precipitating neck movements causing vertebrobasilar artery dissection after cervical trauma and spinal manipulation. Spine 24:785-794, 1999.

60. Haldeman S, Kohlbeck FJ, McGregor M: Stroke, cerebral artery dissection, and cervical spine manipulative therapy. J Neurol 249:1098-1104, 2002.

61. Hurwitz EL, Morgenstern H, Harber P, et al: A randomized trial of chiropractic manipulation and mobilization for patients with neck pain: Clinical outcomes from the UCLA neck-pain study. Am J Public Health 92:1634-1641, 2002.

62. Shekelle PG, Coulter I: Cervical spine manipulation: Summary report of a systematic review of the literature and a multidisciplinary expert panel. J Spinal Disord 10: 223-228, 1997.

63. Vorro J, Johnston WL: Clinical biomechanic correlates of cervical dysfunction. Part 4. Altered regional motor behavior. J Am Osteopath Assoc 98:317-323, 1998.

64. Kelso AF, Johnston WL: The status of a C6-T2-T6 (CT) pattern of segmental somatic dysfunction in research subjects after 3-7 years. J Am Osteopath Assoc 89:1356, 1989.

SUGGESTED READING

Barton PM, Hayes KC: Neck flexor muscle strength, efficiency, and relaxation times in normal subjects and subjects with unilateral neck pain and headache. Arch Phys Med Rehabil 77:680-687, 1996.

Berglund A, Alfredsson L, Cassidy JD, et al: The association between exposure to a rear-end collision and future neck or shoulder pain: A cohort study. J Clin Epidemiol 53: 1089-1094, 2000.

Bogduk N, Mercer S: Biomechanics of the cervical spine. I. Normal kinematics. Clin Biomech (Bristol, Avon) 15:633-648, 2000.

Bronfort G: Spinal manipulation: Current state of research and its indications. Neurol Clin North Am 17:91-111, 1999.

Coulter ID: The Appropriateness of Manipulation and Mobilization of the Cervical Spine. Santa Monica, CA, RAND, 1996.

Dvořák J, Dvořák V: Diagnostics. In Gilliar WG, Greenman PE (trans, eds): Manual Medicine. New York, Geog Thieme, 1984.

Feise RJ, Menke JM: Functional rating index: A new valid and reliable instrument to measure the magnitude of clinical change in spinal conditions. Spine 26:78-87, 2001.

Fjellner A, Bexander C, Faleij R, et al: Interexaminer reliability in physical examination of the cervical spine. J Manipulative Physiol Ther 22:511-516, 1999.

Giles LG, Singer KP: Clinical Anatomy and Management of Cervical Spine Pain. Boston, Butterworth-Heinemann, 1997.

Goldstein M (ed): The Research Status of Spinal Manipulative Therapy. NINCDS monograph no. 15, DHEW (NIH) publication no. 76-998. Bethesda, MD, U.S. Department of Health, Education and Welfare, 1975

Greenman PE: Principles of Manual Medicine, 3rd ed. Philadelphia, Lippincott Williams & Wilkins, 2003.

Hagberg M, Harms-Ringdahl K, Nisell R, et al: Rehabilitation of neck-shoulder pain in women industrial workers: A randomized trial comparing isometric shoulder endurance training with isometric shoulder strength training. Arch Phys Med Rehabil 81:1051-1058, 2000.

Hagino C, Boscariol J, Dover L, et al: Before/after study to determine the effectiveness of the align-right cylindrical cervical pillow in reducing chronic neck pain severity. J Manipulative Physiol Ther 21:89-93, 1998.

Hallgren RC, Greenman PE, Rechtien JJ: Atrophy of suboccipital muscles in patients with chronic pain: A pilot study. J Am Osteopath Assoc 94:1032-1038, 1994.

Hoving JL, Gross AR, Gasner D, et al: A critical appraisal of review articles on the effectiveness of conservative treatment for neck pain. Spine 26:196-205, 2001.

Iwata JL, Rados JJ, Glonek T, et al: Comparing psychotic and affective disorders by musculoskeletal structural examination. J Am Osteopath Assoc 97:715-721, 1997.

Jordan A, Bendix T, Nielsen H, et al: Intensive training, physiotherapy, or manipulation for patients with chronic neck pain. A prospective, single-blinded, randomized clinical trial. Spine 23:311-319, 1998.

Jordan A, Manniche C, Mosdal C, et al: The Copenhagen Neck Functional Disability Scale: A study of reliability and validity. J Manipulative Physiol Ther 21:520-527, 1998.

Karjalainen K, Malmivaara A, van Tulder M, et al: Multidisciplinary biopsychosocial rehabilitation for neck and shoulder pain among working age adults: A systematic review within the framework of the Cochrane collaboration back review group. Spine 26:174-181, 2001.

Kemppainen P, Hamalainen O, Kononen M: Different effects of physical exercise on cold pain sensitivity in fighter pilots with and without the history of acute in-flight neck pain attacks. Med Sci Sports Exerc 30:577-582, 1998.

Kolbinson DA, Epstein JB, Burgess JA, et al: Temporomandibular disorders, headaches, and neck pain after motor vehicle accidents: A pilot investigation of persistence and litigation effects. J Prosthet Dent 77:46-53, 1997.

Kuchera ML, DiGiovanna EL, Greenman PE: Efficacy and complications. In Ward RC (ed): Foundations for Osteopathic Medicine, 2nd ed. Philadelphia, Lippincott Williams & Wilkins, 2003, pp 1143-1152.

Larsson R, Cai H, Zhang Q, et al: Visualization of chronic neck-shoulder pain: Impaired microcirculation in the upper trapezius muscle in chronic cervico-brachial pain. Occup Med (Lond) 48:189-194, 1998.

Leboeuf-Yde C, Hennius B, Rudberg E, et al: Side effects of chiropractic treatment: A prospective study. J Manipulative Physiol Ther 20:511-515, 1997.

Linton SJ: A review of psychological risk factors in back and neck pain. Spine 25: 1148-1156, 2000.

Lord SM, Barnsley L, Wallis BJ, et al: Chronic cervical zygapophysial joint pain after whiplash. A placebo-controlled prevalence study. Spine 21:1737-1745, 1996.

Madeleine P, Lundager B, Voigt M, et al: Shoulder muscle co-ordination during chronic and acute experimental neck-shoulder pain. An occupational pain study. Eur J Appl Physiol Occup Physiol 79:127-140, 1999.

Maigne JY, Chatellier G: Assessment of sexual activity in patients with back pain compared with patients with neck pain. Clin Orthop 385:82-87, 2001.

Mercado AC, Carroll LJ, Cassidy JD, et al: Coping with neck and low back pain in the general population. Health Psychol 19:333-338, 2000.

Mikkelsson M, Sourander A, Salminen JJ, et al: Widespread pain and neck pain in school-children: A prospective one-year follow-up study. Acta Paediatr 88:1119-1124, 1999.

Mitchell FL Jr, Mitchell PKG: The Muscle Energy Manual, vol 1. Cervical Spine. East Lansing, MI, MET Press, 1995.

Nachemson AL, Jonsson E (eds): Neck and Back Pain: The Scientific Evidence of Causes, Diagnosis, and Treatment. Philadelphia, Lippincott Williams & Wilkins, 2000.

Nadler S, Cooke P: Myofascial pain in whiplash injuries: Diagnosis and treatment. Spine 12:357-376, 1998.

Nebe J, Keidel M, Ludecke C, et al: Pain quantification after whiplash trauma using computer-interactive pressure-pain measurement. Nervenarzt 69:924-928, 1998.

Olson SL, O'Connor DP, Birmingham G, et al: Tender point sensitivity, range of motion, and perceived disability in subjects with neck pain. J Orthop Sports Phys Ther 30:13-20, 2000.

Powell FC, Hanigan WC, Olivero WC: A risk/benefit analysis of spinal manipulation therapy for relief of lumbar or cervical pain. Neurosurgery 33:73-79, 1993.

Purdy WR, Frank JJ, Oliver B: Suboccipital dermatomyotomic stimulation and digital blood flow. J Am Osteopath Assoc 96:285-289, commentary 279, 1996.

Schrader H, Obelieniene D, Bovim G, et al: Natural evolution of late whiplash syndrome outside the medicolegal context. Lancet 347:1207-1211, 1996.

Sheather-Reid RB, Cohen ML: Psychophysical evidence for a neuropathic component of chronic neck pain. Pain 75:341-347, 1998.

Skargren EI, Oberg BE: Predictive factors for 1-year outcome of low back and neck pain in patients treated in primary care: Comparison between the treatment strategies chiropractic and physiotherapy. Pain 77:201-207, 1998.

Smedmark V, Wallin M, Arvidsson I: Inter-examiner reliability in assessing passive intervertebral motion of the cervical spine. Man Ther 5:97-101, 2000.

Sobel JB, Sollenberger P, Robinson R, et al: Cervical non-organic signs: A new clinical tool to assess abnormal illness behavior in neck pain patients: A pilot study. Arch Phys Med Rehabil 81:170-175, 2000.

Sturzenegger M, Radanov BP, Di Stefano G: The effect of accident mechanisms and initial findings on the long-term course of whiplash injury. J Neurol 242:443-449, 1995.

Taimela S, Takala EP, Asklof T, et al: Active treatment of chronic neck pain: A prospective randomized intervention. Spine 25:1021-1027, 2000.

Tinazzi M, Fiaschi A, Rosso T, et al: Neuroplastic changes related to pain occur at multiple levels of the human somatosensory system: A somatosensory-evoked potentials study in patients with cervical radicular pain. J Neurosci 20:9277-9283, 2000.

Toomingas A: Characteristics of pain drawings in the neck-shoulder region among the working population. Int Arch Occup Environ Health 72:98-106, 1999.

van Tulder MW, Goossens ME, Hoving JL: Nonsurgical treatment of chronic neck pain. In Nachemson AL, Jonsson E (eds): Neck and Back Pain: The Scientific Evidence of

Causes, Diagnosis and Treatment. Philadelphia, Lippincott Williams & Wilkins, 2000, pp 339-354.

Vasseljen O, Holte KA, Westgaard RH: Shoulder and neck complaints in customer relations: Individual risk factors and perceived exposures at work. Ergonomics 44:355-372, 2001.

Vernon HT, Aker P, Burns S, et al: Pressure pain threshold evaluation of the effect of spinal manipulation in the treatment of chronic neck pain: A pilot study. J Manip Physiol Ther 13:13-16, 1990.

Visscher CM, Lobbezoo F, de Boer W, et al: Clinical tests in distinguishing between persons with or without craniomandibular or cervical spinal pain complaints. Eur J Oral Sci 108:475-483, 2000.

Walko EJ, Janouschek C: Effects of osteopathic manipulative treatment in patients with cervicothoracic pain: Pilot study using thermography. J Am Osteopath Assoc 94:135-141, 1994.

Westgaard RH: Muscle activity as a releasing factor for pain in the shoulder and neck. Cephalalgia 19:1-8, 1999.

Appendix 6.1
Osteopathic Manipulative Treatment of the Cervical Spine

The American Osteopathic Association (AOA) position paper on osteopathic manipulative treatment of the cervical spine was passed by the AOA House of Delegates on July 2004 and is reprinted here with their permission.

BACKGROUND AND STATEMENT OF ISSUE

There has been increasing concern about the safety of cervical spine manipulation. Specifically, this concern has centered on devastating negative outcomes such as stroke. This paper presents the evidence behind the benefit of cervical spine manipulation, explores the potential harm, and makes a recommendation about its use.

BENEFIT

Spinal manipulation has been reviewed in a meta-analysis published as early as 1992, showing a clear benefit for low back pain.[1] There is less available information in the literature about manipulation in regard to neck pain and headache, but the evidence does show benefit.[2-6] There have been at least 12 randomized, controlled trials of manipulative treatment of neck pain. Some of the benefits shown include relief of acute neck pain: reduction in neck pain as measured by validated instruments in subacute and chronic neck pain compared with muscle relaxants or usual medical care. There is also short-term relief from tension-type headaches.[7] Manipulation relieves cervicogenic headache and is comparable to commonly used first-line prophylactic prescription medications for tension-type headache and migraine.[8] Meta-analysis of five randomized, controlled trials showed that there was a statistically significant reduction in neck pain using a visual analogue scale.[9]

HARM

Since 1925, there have been approximately 275 cases of adverse events reported with cervical spine manipulation.[10-13] It has been suggested by some that there is an under-reporting of adverse events.[10] A conservative estimate of the number of cervical spine manipulations per year is approximately 33 million and may be as high as 193 million in the United States and Canada.[14,15] The estimated risk of adverse outcome after cervical spine manipulation ranges from 1 in 400,000 to 1 in 3.85 million manipulations.[16-19] The estimated risk of major impairment after cervical spine manipulation is 6.39 per 10 million manipulations.[20] Most of the reported cases of adverse outcome have involved "thrust" or "high-velocity/low-amplitude" types of manipulative treatment.[11] Many of the reported cases do not distinguish the type of manipulative treatment provided. However, the risk of a vertebrobasilar accident (VBA) occurring spontaneously is nearly twice the risk of a VBA resulting from cervical spine manipulation.[7] This includes cases of ischemic stroke and vertebral artery dissection.

A concern has been raised by a recent report that VBA following cervical spine manipulation is unpredictable.[10] This report is biased because all of the cases were involved in litigation. The nature of litigation can lead to inaccurate reporting by the patient or provider. However, it did conclude that VBA after cervical spine manipulation is "idiosyncratic and rare." Further review of this data showed that 25% of the cases presented with sudden onset of new and unusual headache and neck pain often associated with other neurologic symptoms that might have represented a dissection in progress.[21] In direct contrast to this concern about unpredictability, another report states that cervical spine manipulation may worsen preexisting cervical disc herniation or even cause cervical disc herniation. This report describes complications such as radiculopathy, myelopathy, and vertebral artery compression by a lateral cervical disc herniation.[12] The authors concluded that the incidence of these types of complications could be lessened by rigorous adherence to published exclusion criteria for cervical spine manipulation.[12]

The current literature does not clearly distinguish the type of provider (i.e., MD, DO, DC, or PT) or manipulative treatment (manipulation versus mobilization) provided in cases associated with VBA. This information may help to understand the mechanism of injury leading to VBA, because there are differences in education and practice among the various professions that use this type of treatment.

COMPARISON OF ALTERNATIVE TREATMENTS

Nonsteroidal anti-inflammatory drugs (NSAIDs) are the most commonly prescribed medications for neck pain. Approximately 13 million Americans use NSAIDs regularly.[32] Eighty-one percent of gastrointestinal (GI) bleeds related to NSAID use occur without prior symptoms.[32] Research in the United Kingdom has shown NSAIDs will cause 12,000 emergency admissions and

2500 deaths per year due to GI tract complications.[22] The annual cost of GI tract complications in the United States is estimated at $3.9 billion, with up to 103,000 hospitalizations and at least 16,500 deaths per year.[23,24,32] This makes GI toxicity from NSAIDs the 15th most common cause of death in the United States.[32]

Epidural steroid injection is a popular treatment for neck pain. Common risks include subdural injection, intrathecal injection and intravascular injection.[35] Subdural injection occurs in about 1% of procedures.[35] Intrathecal injection occurs in about 0.6% to 10.9% of procedures.[35] Intravascular injection is the most significant risk and occurs in about 2% of procedures and about 8% of procedures in pregnant patients.[35] Cervical epidural abscess is rare, but has been reported in the literature.[36]

PROVOCATIVE TESTS

Provocative tests such as the DeKline test have been studied in animals and humans. This test and others like it were found to be unreliable for demonstrating reproducibility of ischemia or risk of injuring the vertebral artery.[25-30]

RISK FACTORS

VBA accounts for 1.3 in 1000 cases of stroke, making this a rare event. Approximately 5% of patients with VBA die as a result, whereas 75% have a good functional recovery.[33] The most common risk factors for VBA are migraine, hypertension, oral contraceptive use, and smoking.[31] Elevated homocysteine levels, which have been implicated in cardiovascular disease, may be a risk factor for VBA.[34] A study done in 1999 reviewing 367 cases of VBA reported from 1966 to 1993 showed 115 cases related to cervical spine manipulation; 167 were spontaneous, 58 from trivial trauma, and 37 from major trauma.[31] Complications from cervical spine manipulation most often occur in patients who have had prior manipulation uneventfully and without obvious risk factors for VBA.[7] "Most vertebrobasilar artery dissections occur in the absence of cervical manipulation, either spontaneously or after trivial trauma or common daily movements of the neck, such as backing out of the driveway, painting the ceiling, playing tennis, sneezing, or engaging in yoga exercises."[10] In some cases, manipulation may not be the primary insult causing the dissection, but an aggravating factor or coincidental event.[21]

It has been proposed that thrust techniques that use a combination of hyperextension, rotation, and traction of the upper cervical spine will place the patient at greatest risk of injuring the vertebral artery. In a retrospective review of 64 medical legal cases, information on the type of manipulation was available in 39 (61%) of the cases; 51% involved rotation, with the remaining 49% representing a variety of positions, including lateral flexion, traction, and isolated cases of nonforce or neutral position thrusts. Only 15% reported any form of extension.[21]

CONCLUSIONS

Osteopathic manipulative treatment of the cervical spine, including but not limited to high-velocity/low-amplitude treatment, is effective for neck pain and is safe, especially in comparison to other common treatments. Because of the very small risk of adverse outcomes, trainees should be provided with sufficient information so they are advised of the potential risks. There is a need for research to distinguish the risk of VBA associated with manipulation done by provider type and to determine the nature of the relationship between different types of manipulative treatment and VBA.

It is the position of the American Osteopathic Association that all modalities of osteopathic manipulative treatment of the cervical spine, including high velocity/low amplitude, should continue to be taught at all levels of education and that osteopathic practitioners should continue to offer this form of treatment to their patients.

REFERENCES

1. Shekelle P, Adams A, Chassin MR, et al: Spinal manipulation for low-back pain. Ann Intern Med 117:590-598, 1992.
2. Koes BW, Bouter LM, et al: The effectiveness of manual therapy, physiotherapy, and treatment by the general practitioner for nonspecific back and neck complaints, a randomized clinical trial. Spine 17:28-35, 1992.
3. Koes B, Bouter L, et al: Randomised clinical trial of manipulative therapy and physiotherapy for persistent back and neck complaints: Results of one year follow-up. BMJ 304:601-605, 1992.
4. Koes BW, Bouter LM, van Marmeren H, et al: A randomized clinical trial of manual therapy and physiotherapy for persistent neck and back complaints: Sub-group analysis and relationship between outcome measures. J Manipulative Physiol Ther 16:211-219, 1993.
5. Cassidy JD, Lopes AA, Yong-Hing K: The immediate effect of manipulation versus mobilization on pain and range of motion in the cervical spine: A randomized controlled trial. J Manipulative Physiol Ther 15:570-575, 1992.
6. Jensen OK, Nielsen FF, Vosmar L: An open study comparing manual therapy with the use of cold packs in the treatment of posttraumatic headache. Cephalgia 10:241-250, 1990.
7. Hurwitz EL, Aker PD, Adams AH, et al: Manipulation and Mobilization of the Cervical Spine. A systematic review of the literature. Spine 21:1746-1756, 1996.
8. Bronfort G, Assendelft WJ, Evans R, et al: Efficacy of spinal manipulation for chronic headache: A systematic review. J Manipulative Physiol Ther 27:457-466, 2001.
9. Gross AR, Aker PD, Goldsmith CH, et al: Conservative management of mechanical neck disorders: A systematic overview and meta-analysis. Online J Curr Clin Trials, doc no. 200-201, 1996.
10. Haldeman S, Kohlbeck FJ, McGregor M: Unpredictabilty of cerebrovascular ischemia associated with cervical spine manipulation: A review of 64 cases after cervical spine manipulation therapy. Spine 27:49-55, 2002.
11. Assendelft WJJ, Bouter LM, Knipschild PG: Complications of spinal manipulation: A comprehensive review of the literature. J Fam Pract 42:475-480, 1996.
12. Malone DG, Baldwin NG, Tomecek FJ, et al: Complications of cervical spine manipulation therapy: 5-year retrospective study in a single-group practice. Neurosurg Focus 13:1, 2002.
13. Vick DA, McKay C, Zengerle CR: The safety of manipulative treatment: Review of the literature from 1925 to 1993. J Am Osteopath Assoc 96:113-115, 1996.
14. Haldeman S, Carey P, Townsend M, et al: Arterial dissection following cervical manipulation. The chiropractic experience. CMAJ 165:905-906, 2001.
15. Hurwitz EL, Coulter ID, Adams AH, et al: Use of chiropractic services from 1985 through 1991 in the United States and Canada. Am J Public Health 88:771-776, 1998.
16. Jenson et al: Complications of cervical manipulation. Gen Forensic Sci 32:1089-1094, 1987.
17. Koss RW: Quality assurance monitoring of osteopathic manipulative treatment. J Am Osteopath Assoc 90:427-433, 1990.
18. Dvorak J, Orelli F: How dangerous is manipulation to the cervical spine? Case report and results of a survey. Man Med 2:1-4, 1985.
19. Carey P: A report on the occurrence of cerebral vascular accidents in chiropractic practice. J Can Chiropract Assoc 37:104-106, 1993.
20. Coulter ID, Hurwitz EL, Adams AH, et al: The Appropriateness of Manipulation and Mobilization of the Cervical Spine. Santa Monica, CA, Rand, 1996.
21. Haldeman S, Kohlbeck FJ, McGregor M: Stroke, cerebral artery dissection, and cervical spine manipulative therapy. J Neurol 249:1098-1104, 2002.

22. Blower AI, Brooks A, Fenn CG, et al: Emergency admissions for upper gastrointestinal disease and their relation to NSAIDs use. Aliment Pharmacol Ther 11:283-291, 1997.

23. Fries JF, Miller SR, Spitz PW, et al: Toward an epidemiology of gastropathy associated with nonsteroidal anti-inflammatory drug use. Gastroenterology 96:647-655, 1989.

24. Bloom BS: Direct medical costs of disease and gastrointestinal side effects during treatment for arthritis. Am J Med 84:20-24, 1988.

25. Licht PB, Christensen HW, Svendensen P, et al: Vertebral artery flow and cervical manipulation: An experimental study. J Manipulative Physiol Ther 22:431-435, 1999.

26. Cote P, Kreitz BG, Cassidy JD, et al: The validity of extension-rotation tests as a clinical screening procedure before neck manipulation: A secondary analysis. J Manipulative Physiol Ther 19:159-164, 1996.

27. Refshauge KM: Rotation: A valid premanipulative dizziness test? Does it predict safe manipulation? J Manipulative Physiol Ther 17:15-19, 1994.

28. Stevens A: A functional Doppler sonography of the vertebral artery and some considerations about manual techniques. J Man Med 6:102-105, 1991.

29. Theil H, Wallace K, Donat J, et al: Effect of various head and neck positions on vertebral artery blood flow. Clin Biomech 9:105-110, 1994.

30. Weingart JR, Bischoff HP: Doppler sonography of the vertebral artery with regard to head positions appropriate to manual medicine. J Man Med 6:62-65, 1992.

31. Haldeman S, Kohlbeck FJ, McGregor M: Risk factors and precipitating neck movements causing vertebrobasilar artery dissection after cervical trauma and spinal manipulation. Spine 24:785-794, 1999.

32. Wolfe M, Lichtenstein D, Singh G: Gastrointestinal toxicity of nonsteroidal antiinflam-matory drugs. N Engl J Med 340:1888-1899, 1999.

33. Schievink W: Spontaneous dissection of the carotid and vertebral arteries. N Engl J Med 344:898-906, 2001.

34. Rosner A: Spontaneous cervical artery dissections and implications for homocys-teine. J Manipulative Physiol Ther 27:124-132, 2004.

35. Mulroy M, Norris M, Spencer L: Safety steps for epidural injection of local anesthetics: Review of the literature and recommendations. Anesth Analg 85:1346-1356, 1997.

36. Huang RC: Cervical epidural abscess after epidural steroid injection. Spine 29:E7-E9, 2004.

CHAPTER 7

Cervicogenic Headache

DEFINITION

- Pain referred to the head region, typically unilaterally, from cervical musculoskeletal dysfunction.
- It is characterized by the presence of cervical somatic dysfunction as exhibited by muscle spasm, decreased range of motion and pain on digital provocation, worse with movement and better with rest.
- It can be associated with cervical muscles' tendonitis, trigger points, or tender points in the cervical or head region, or cervical joint inflammation.
- Pain is alleviated by successful treatment of the somatic dysfunction, and there is a lack of systemic or local head region pathology to account for the pain.
- The Cervicogenic Headache International Study Group diagnostic criteria for cervicogenic headache (CHA) are listed in Table 7.1.[1]
- The International Headache Society diagnostic criteria for CHA are listed in Table 7.2.[2]

EPIDEMIOLOGY

Age

- All ages are affected.
- The mean age is 42.9 years.[3]

Gender

- CHA is four times more common in female than male patients.[3,4]

Prevalence

- CHA accounts for 14% to 18% of all chronic and recurrent headaches.[5,6]
- CHA is a common symptom after neck trauma; 54% to 66% of patients with whiplash-associated disorder complain of headache.[7]

- On average, 54.8% (range, 36.2% to 80%) of patients seen by pain specialists have CHA or CHA in combination with other types of headache.[3]
- The prevalence of CHA in the general population is estimated to be 0.4% to 2.5%.[3]

Natural Clinical Course

- CHAs often lack a regular pattern.
- Quality of life is affected, particularly loss of physical functioning.[8]
- CHAs are often recurrent and episodic, lasting hours to days per episode.
- Most de novo CHAs occurring after whiplash resolve within a year.[9,10] However, previous car accidents and preexisting headache and neck pain may lead to chronic CHA after whiplash injury.[10]

Effects on Society

- From a U.S. survey totaling 13,343 respondents, 9.4% reported missing work more than rarely because of headache, 31% reported that their work level was reduced more than rarely by headache, and 9.2% reported that their work level was reduced more than 50% by headaches during work.[11]
- In accounting for actual lost workdays and reduced effectiveness at work, individuals lost the equivalent of 4.2 days per year because of headache.
- Subjects with migraine headache were much more likely (57%) to report actual lost workdays because of headache, whereas tension-type and other headache types accounted for a large proportion (64%) of decreased work effectiveness because of headache.
- Headache type, headache severity, and education level were each independent predictors of workplace impact of headache.
- In a 2001-2002 random sample telephone survey of 28,902 American workers, 13% of the total workforce experienced a loss in productive time during a 2-week period due to a common pain condition.[12]
- Headache was the most common (5.4%) pain condition resulting in lost productive time, accounting for a mean loss of 3.5 hours in productive time per week.

Table 7.1 Diagnostic criteria for cervicogenic headache from the Cervicogenic Headache International Study Group

Criteria	Method
Symptoms and signs of neck involvement	Precipitation of head pain usually similar to one occurring
	By neck movement or sustained awkward head positioning
	By external pressure over the upper cervical or occipital region on the symptomatic side
	Restriction of the range of motion in the neck
	Ipsilateral neck, shoulder, or arm pain of a rather vague nonradicular nature, or occasionally arm pain of a radicular nature
Confirmatory evidence	Obtained by diagnostic anesthetic blockades
Unilaterality of the head pain	Head pain without side shift

From Sjaastad O, Fredriksen TA, Pfaffenrath V: Cervicogenic headache: Diagnostic criteria. Headache 38:442-445, 1998.

- Among active workers, lost productive time from common pain conditions (e.g., headache, back pain, arthritis) costs an estimated $61.2 billion per year, with $20 billion due to headache.
- The majority (76.6%) of the lost productive time was not caused by absence from work but was explained by reduced performance while at work.

Table 7.2 Diagnostic criteria for cervicogenic headache from the International Headache Society

Criteria	Diagnostic Method
A. Pain	Referred from a source in the neck and perceived in one or more regions of the head and face, fulfilling criteria C and D
B. Clinical, laboratory, and imaging evidence	A disorder or lesion within the cervical spine or soft tissues of the neck known to be or generally accepted as a valid cause of headache
C. Evidence that the pain can be attributed to a neck disorder or lesion based on at least one of the following conditions	Demonstration of clinical signs that implicate a source of pain in the neck Abolition of headache after diagnostic block of a cervical structure or its nerve supply by use of a placebo or other adequate controls
D. Resolution after treatment	Pain that resolves within 3 months after successful treatment of the causative disorder or lesion

From International Headache Society: The international classification of headache disorders, 2nd edition. Cephalalgia 24(Suppl 7):114-116, 2004.

Risk Factors

- Head or neck traumatic injuries, especially whiplash, often predispose a patient to CHA symptoms.
- Sustained neck postures or movements typically precipitate the symptoms, but patients often have difficulty in recognizing aggravating factors.
- Significant compensatory cervical somatic dysfunctions, resulting from primary thoracic, lumbar, pelvic, shoulder, or costal cage somatic dysfunctions, are common.
- Stress may be a provocative factor, because it is common for many headache types.

FUNCTIONAL ANATOMY

Functional anatomy is covered in the section on the neck region in Chapter 6.

Muscles

- The suboccipital muscles adjust the level of the occiput and temporal bones to the horizon to ensure the visual and vestibular systems function optimally (Fig. 7.1A).
- The oblique capitis superior muscle connects the transverse process of the atlas to the occiput, inserting between the superior and inferior nuchal lines. It sidebends the head toward the same side as the unilaterally contracting muscle.
- The oblique capitis inferior muscle originates at the spine of the axis and inserts on the transverse processes of the atlas. Unilateral contraction rotates the atlas and head around the odontoid process of C2 such that the face turns toward the side of the contraction.
- The trapezius is the most superficial of the posterior muscles. It connects the thoracic spine, shoulders, neck, and head and functions primarily as an elevator and adductor of the upper extremity.
- Deep to the trapezius, the semispinalis, splenius capitis, and longissimus capitis muscles connect the thoracic spine to the head and neck and function in concert to extend the head and neck when acting bilaterally. Splenius capitis and longissimus capitis muscles sidebend and rotate the head and neck to the same side when acting unilaterally. However, unilateral contraction of the semispinalis capitis muscle rotates the head and face to the opposite side of the contracting muscle.
- The sternocleidomastoid muscle is also superficial, originates on the manubrium of the sternum and the medial one third of the clavicle, and inserts on the mastoid process of the temporal bone and lateral aspects of the superior nuchal line. Bilateral action facilitates head and neck flexion. Unilateral contraction sidebends the head and neck toward the same side and rotates them to the opposite side of the contracting muscle.
- The rotatores and multifidi muscles are responsible for segmental motion in the cervical region, just as they are in other spinal regions (see Chapter 6, Fig. 6.19). The multifidi traverse one to three spinal levels, and the rotatores connect successive vertebrae. Because their origins are inferior and lateral to their insertions, unilateral contraction of these muscles rotates the

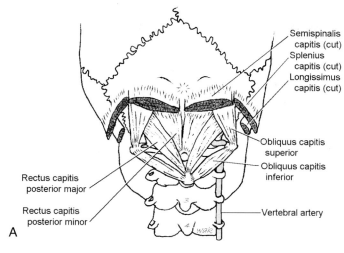

Attachments of:

Figure 7.1 **A,** Suboccipital muscles. Notice the rectus capitis posterior minor (RCPm) in relation to the other muscles. **B,** The myodural bridge. The rectus capitis posterior minor muscle attaches to the cervical spinal dura. (**A,** With permission from Simons DG, Travell JG, Simons LS: Myofascial Pain and Dysfunction, Vol. I: Upper Half of the Body, Second Edition, Baltimore, Williams and Wilkins, 1999:474.

body of the superior vertebra of the unit toward the side opposite of the contracting muscle (i.e., contraction of a left rotatores or multifidus rotates the superior vertebra of the unit toward the right).

- The intertransversarii muscles connect the cervical vertebrae by their transverse processes. Bilateral contraction facilitates

head and neck extension, and unilateral contraction sidebends the superior vertebra of the unit toward the side of the contracting muscle.

- The rectus capitis posterior major and rectus capitis posterior minor are the most medial of the suboccipital muscles. The origin of the minor is the posterior tubercle of the atlas and that of the major is the spine of the axis, where it joins the origins of the oblique capitis inferior, semispinalis, multifidi, and interspinales muscles. Both recti muscles insert onto the occiput between the foramen magnum and the inferior nuchal line. Bilateral contraction facilitates head extension (i.e., counternutation), and unilateral contraction, like the inferior obliques, facilitates sidebending and rotation to the same side.

The Myodural Bridge

- The rectus capitis posterior minor muscle fascia and tendon, along with the perivascular sheaths in that region, form the posterior atlanto-occipital membrane and fuse with the spinal dura between C1 to C2 and C2 to C3, creating a *myodural bridge*, strengthening the dura, and preventing dural enfolding during extension of the craniocervical junction.[13,14] (see Fig. 7.1B)
- The cervical spinal dura is innervated by sensory nerves that are stretch responsive, such that strain or prolonged contraction of the posterior suboccipital muscles can be considered as a potential mechanism for eliciting pain felt in the posterior occipital region and emanating from the stretched spinal or intracranial dura.

Nerves

Central Nervous System
- The tectospinal tract coordinates eye and neck movements.
- Vestibular function (i.e., balance and equilibrium) is linked to neck motion.
- Neck motion is linked with shoulder and upper back motion.

Cranial (Parasympathetic) Nerves
- Cervical somatic dysfunction refers pain to the head and face through the trigeminal nerve (cranial nerve [CN] V).[15]
- The trigeminal nerve (CN V) innervates cranial and facial structures, including the cerebral blood vessels (i.e., the trigeminovascular system) and dura mater, sending its sensory information to the pons in the midbrain en route to the thalamus and somatosensory cortex. The trigeminal nerve also has tracts that descend into the spine. The upper cervical spinal cord contains the trigeminal nucleus caudalis (TNC).
- The TNC descends as low as C4,[15] and it is contiguous with the spinal gray matter in the substantia gelatinosa in lamina II of the dorsal horn.
- C1 to C3 spinal nerves innervate the zygapophyseal joints, uncovertebral joints, intervertebral discs, cervical muscles and ligaments, the vertebral artery, the cervical spinal dura, the posterior scalp, and even the lower layer of the tentorium cerebelli. The afferents from these structures converge with the TNC within the spinal cord.[15]
- Because sensory nerve fibers from the upper cervical region (C1 to C3) converge with the TNC, pain signals from the neck can be referred to the same receptive field in the thalamus as that of the head and face, giving the patient the sensation that the pain is emanating from the head or face although it is coming from the cervical spine.[15]

- Lower cervical (C5 to C7) nociceptive stimuli can refer pain to the head and face through the TNC because afferent nociceptive information can ascend one to three levels before entering the dorsal horn and interacting with interneurons that connect with the TNC.[15]
- Nociceptive input originating from cervical structures can be perceived as head pain in the regions innervated by the trigeminal nerve, such as the temporal, frontal, and orbital regions.[15,16]
- The superior and inferior vagal ganglia lie superior and inferior to the jugular foramina, respectively. The vagus nerve (CN X) is a mixed nerve with motor, sensory, and parasympathetic components. Of interest to the topic of CHAs is that nociceptive or inflammatory stimuli from the larynx and pharynx, as well as the thoracic and abdominal viscera, are transmitted by the vagus and converge with upper cervical afferents.[17] The increased afferent activity converging in the upper cervical region is thought to increase the efferent discharge of cervical spinal motor neurons, accounting for the palpable increase in myofascial tissue tension in the upper cervical spine (i.e., viscerosomatic reflex).
- Primary sensory axons from the superior vagal ganglia terminate in the TNC and convey general sensation from the external auditory meatus, external surface of the tympanic membrane, and skin of the ear to the trigeminal receptive field in the thalamus.
- The spinal accessory nerve (CN XI), which sends motor efferents to the trapezius and sternocleidomastoid muscles, also has some sensory afferents that may converge with the TNC[15,16] (Fig. 7.2).

Sympathetic Nerves
- Sympathetic nerve fibers are dense in the basal region of the occipital dura mater and alongside, as well as independent from blood vessels.[18]
- The superior cervical ganglia lie anterior to the articular pillars of C2. They have postganglionic fibers that innervate the vasculature and mucous membranes of the head region, including the middle ear, the lacrimal glands, and pupils of the eyes. Their preganglionic cell bodies emanate from the spinal cord at levels T1 to T4.

Peripheral Nerves
- The greater and lesser occipital nerves originate from C1 to C3; the medial branches of C2 and C3 dorsal rami form the greater occipital nerve and the third occipital nerve. They greater and lesser occipital nerves innervate the posterior scalp. Occipital neuralgia arises from entrapment or trauma to these nerves, the upper cervical zygapophyseal joints or the C2 spinal root.[16]
- The suboccipital (C1) nerve innervates the occipitoatlantal (OA) joint and can refer pain from somatic dysfunction to the occipital region.[16]
- The AA joint and C2 to C3 are innervated by the C2 spinal nerve. C2 neuralgia causes a deep or dull pain that usually radiates from the occipital to parietal, temporal, frontal, and periorbital regions. A paroxysmal sharp or shock like pain is often superimposed over the constant pain. Ipsilateral eye lacrimation and conjunctival injection are common associated signs.[16]

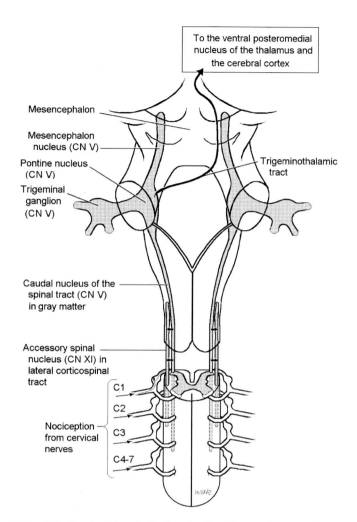

To the ventral posteromedial nucleus of the thalamus and the cerebral cortex

Mesencephalon

Mesencephalon nucleus (CN V)

Pontine nucleus (CN V)

Trigeminal ganglion (CN V)

Trigeminothalamic tract

Caudal nucleus of the spinal tract (CN V) in gray matter

Accessory spinal nucleus (CN XI) in lateral corticospinal tract

C1

C2

Nociception from cervical nerves

C3

C4-7

Figure 7.2 Cervical-trigeminal referred pain pathways. Afferent pain impulses from cervical structures enter the spinal cord through spinal nerves and cranial nerve XI, and they converge in the trigeminal nucleus caudalis (TNC). The nociceptive information ascends to the pons and then to the contralateral ventral trigeminothalamic tract, although some information ascends ipsilaterally. The sensory information is then processed in the ventral posteromedial nucleus of the thalamus en route to the sensory cortex in the postcentral gyrus, where it is perceived as coming from the trigeminal sensory receptive field of the face and head.

- The third occipital nerve (i.e., dorsal ramus of C3) innervates the C2 to C3 joints. Somatic dysfunction of these joints, which often occurs in relation to whiplash injuries, transmits referred pain to the frontotemporal and periorbital regions.[16]

PATHOPHYSIOLOGY

- The cause of CHA is cervical spine somatic dysfunction, and alleviation of this musculoskeletal dysfunction alleviates the headache.
- In general, CHA is often related to somatic dysfunction of the OA and atlantoaxial (AA) joints, and neck pain most often related to C2 to C7 somatic dysfunction. Fifty percent of whiplash patients with chronic neck pain and dominant headache symptoms have C2 to C3 zygapophyseal joint pain that is abolished with nerve blocks.[19,20] Nerve blocks of the greater occipital nerve and lower cervical segments have also abolished headache symptoms, indicating that sensitization of these structures is also involved in the genesis of CHA.[21,22]

- Cervical somatic dysfunction can involve the trigeminal and spinal accessory cranial nerves, which innervate structures in the cervical and head regions. The TNC in the upper cervical spinal cord is thought to interact with upper cervical peripheral afferents and spinal accessory nerves (CN XI) to account for the bidirectional referral of painful sensations between the neck and the trigeminal receptive sensory fields of the face and head.[16]

- Upper cervical and occipital muscle spasm may induce tension transmitted through the myodural connective tissue and elicit head pain.

- The C1 to C2 facet produces pain in the posterior auricular area in the distribution of the greater occipital nerve.

- Organic disease from structures innervated by the vagus nerve can cause sensitization of upper cervical spinal segments and may predispose the patient to upper cervical somatic dysfunction, leading to CHA.[23]

- Cervicogenic pain has also been abolished with cervical myofascial trigger point and botulinum toxin injections, indicating that peripheral sensitization in the soft tissues plays a role in CHA genesis.

- Increased levels of proinflammatory cytokines and nitric oxide are higher in patients with CHA compared with patients with migraine headaches, and they likely promote hyperalgesia (i.e., peripheral sensitization).[24] However, the lack of calcitonin gene–related peptide in symptomatic CHA patients indicates that the trigeminovascular system is not activated by this condition as it is in migraineurs.[25]

DIFFERENTIAL DIAGNOSIS

- The differential diagnosis of CHA includes hemicrania continua, occipital neuralgia, migraine, and tension-type headache, but the main diagnostic challenge is distinguishing CHA from migraine without aura and tension-type headache (Table 7.3).

- Red flag causes of headache and their distinguishing characteristics are listed in Table 7.4.

- In patients with acute or chronic headache, if there are no signs of serious pathology that require emergent treatment, findings of cervical somatic dysfunction indicate treatment of the cervical spine with manual medicine. An algorithm for headache evaluation is presented in Figure 7.3.

- Other causes of head pain that come from cervical pathology include the following:

1. Arteriovenous malformation
2. Cervical spondylosis
3. Greater occipital nerve compression or inflammation
4. Herniated cervical disc
5. Rheumatoid arthritis

Table 7.3   Characteristics of similar headache types

Feature	Cervicogenic Headache	Cluster	Hemicrania Continua	Migraine without Aura	Tension-Type Headache
Associated symptoms	Usually absent or similar to migraine but milder, decreased neck movement, neck pain with movement	Ipsilateral autonomic symptoms, such as tearing, rhinorrhea, ptosis, miosis	Autonomic symptoms may occur, can have tender points in the cervical paraspinal tissues	Nausea, vomiting, phonophobia, photophobia, visual scotoma	Occasionally decreased appetite, photophobia or phonophobia
Associated triggers	Neck movement, digital pressure over C1-3 facets	Alcohol, headaches occur at predictable times of day	None typical	Various chemicals, foods, stress	Stress, jaw clenching, temporomandibular joint syndrome
Character of pain	Moderate, not excruciating or throbbing	Severe, constant	Moderately severe, waxing and waning	Excruciating, throbbing or pulsating	Bilateral, not throbbing, moderate, bandlike head pressure
Duration	Intermittent or constant with attacks	15 to 180 min, several per day	Constant with attacks	4 to 72 hr	Days to weeks
Gender	F > M	M > F	F > M	F > M	F > M
Laterality	Unilateral without side shift	Unilateral without side shift	Unilateral without side shift	Unilateral with side shift	Bilateral
Location	Occipital to frontoparietal and orbital	Orbital, temporal	Frontal, temporal, orbital, hemicranial	Frontal, orbital, temporal, hemicranial	Frontal, occipital, circumferential
Treatment	Cervical manipulation; local anesthetic blockade is diagnostic	Oxygen, medications such as ergot, triptans	Medications such as indomethacin	Sleep, medications such as ergot, triptans, β-blockers, or calcium channel blockers	Cervical and cranial manipulation sometimes effective, analgesics, cognitive behavioral therapy

6. Trauma
7. Tumors
8. Vasculitis
9. Vertebral artery dissection

HISTORY

Intensity

- Moderate to severe, deep, nonthrobbing, and nonlancinating pain

Precipitating Factors

- Neck movement and sustained head positioning can precipitate head pain.
- Whiplash and head or neck injury can occur before the onset of symptoms.
- Patients often report difficulties in identifying factors that precipitate, aggravate, or ease their headaches.

Location

- Headache is posterior, lateral, at the vertex, behind the orbit, or in the frontal region.
- Unilateral head or face pain without side shift; the pain occasionally may be bilateral.[1]

Radiation

- Ipsilateral head, neck, shoulder, and nonradicular or, occasionally, radicular arm pain[1]
- Scalp paresthesias or dysesthesia

Characteristics

- CHAs may be constant or fluctuating, dull, or aching, or they may be viselike in character.
- Episodes have various durations.
- There is often a lack of response to medication that is successful for other headache forms.

Table 7.4   Red flag differential diagnosis for headache

Condition	Characteristics and Tests
Arteriovenous malformations	Symptoms: headache, visual disturbances, lapses of consciousness Signs: seizures, extremity weakness Tests: angiogram, MRI
Cerebral aneurysm	Symptoms: explosive headache Signs: nuchal rigidity, neurologic deficits Tests: bloody CSF from spinal tap, angiogram
Chiari malformation	Symptoms: loss of coordination, imbalance, exertional headache Signs: ataxia and varying degrees of upper motor neuron signs Tests: angiogram, MRI
Glaucoma	Symptoms: general headache, disturbed vision Signs: dilated pupil, increased ocular pressure Tests: tonometry
Meningitis	Symptoms: headache, nausea, vomiting, photophobia Signs: nuchal rigidity, fever, may have Kernig's sign or Brudzinski's sign from meningeal irritation Tests: brain CT, spinal tap for CSF analysis
Posterior fossa tumors	Symptoms: vertigo, nausea, exertional headache Signs: ataxia, dysarthria, papilledema Tests: brain MRI
Pseudotumor cerebri	Symptoms: headache Signs: young, obese female and papilledema Tests: brain CT scan; markedly elevated opening pressures on lumbar puncture
Subdural hemorrhage (SDH), subarachnoid hemorrhage (SAH), or epidural hemorrhage	Symptoms: headache, nausea, vomiting. For SAH, patient often states it is "the worst headache my life"; with SDH, there is often a history of head trauma; epidural hemorrhage may manifest with head trauma, followed by a period of lucidity with gradually worsening arousal. Signs: nuchal rigidity, Kernig's sign, Brudzinski's sign, Battle's sign (i.e., ecchymosis behind the ear), hemotympanum may suggest occult skull fracture Tests: brain CT, MRI
Vasculitis (giant cell or temporal arteritis)	Symptoms: age > 50 years, throbbing headache, jaw claudication, blurred vision Signs: tortuous, nodular, tender temporal artery, papilledema, end-stage blindness Tests: ESR, temporal artery muscle biopsy
Vertebral artery dissection	Symptoms: headache, nausea, severe local pain Signs: dysarthria, ataxia, tender artery Tests: neck and brain angiogram, MRI

CSF, cerebrospinal fluid; CT, computed tomography; ESR, erythrocyte sedimentation rate; MRI, magnetic resonance imaging

Associated Symptoms

- CHAs may be associated with occasional nausea, phonophobia, photophobia, dizziness, ipsilateral "blurred vision," difficulties swallowing, or ipsilateral periorbital edema.
- A Valsalva maneuver, cough, or sneeze may trigger the pain.

PHYSICAL FINDINGS

- Physical examination of the cervical spine in patients with headache has been demonstrated to have acceptable interexaminer reliability between experienced neurologists.[26]
- Kappa reliability scores were greater than 0.4 (i.e., acceptable reliability range) for restriction of cervical rotation, pain induced by motion, and digital pain provocation of tender points, but digital pressure for zygapophyseal joint pain was not reliable.
- Acceptable levels of intraexaminer and interexaminer reliability (kappa > 0.4) of active and passive segmental mobility and pain provocation tests for the upper cervical spine in patients with CHA has been demonstrated by physical therapists.[27]
- Restriction of motion of the AA (C1 to C2) joint using the passive flexion-rotation test is the most common finding in patients with CHA.[28]
- The practitioner should look for asymmetric neck and head position in relation to the shoulders.
- Head pain is reproduced by external digital pressure over the upper cervical (OA, C2 to C4) or occipital region (especially over the greater occipital nerve) on the symptomatic side. The applied digital pressure is up to 4 kg, or until the examiner's finger nail bed is one-fourth to one-half blanched by the pressure.
- Restriction of active and passive neck range of motion, especially in the upper three cervical joints, is common.
- There is neck muscle stiffness but not nuchal rigidity.

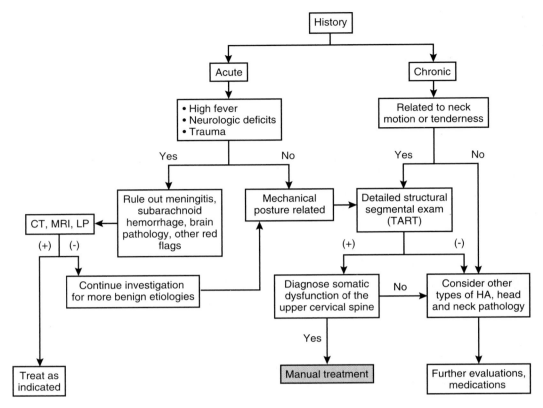

Figure 7.3 Algorithm for acute or chronic headache (HA) presentation. CT, computed tomography; LP, lumbar puncture; MRI, magnetic resonance imaging; TART, asymmetry of musculoskeletal structural landmarks, altered quantity or quality of active or passive neck motion, tissue texture abnormalities, including tenderness and temperature variations.

- Digital provocations of suboccipital, cervical, or shoulder muscle trigger points refer pain to the ipsilateral head region.
- There are poor activation levels and endurance capacity of the deep and postural supporting neck and shoulder girdle muscles.[29]

LABORATORY AND RADIOGRAPHIC FINDINGS

- Blood test results for systemic pathology are negative.
- Neck and head radiographs, magnetic resonance imaging (MRI),[30] and computed tomography (CT) myelograms are negative.
- Cervical disc bulging is not specific.

MANUAL MEDICINE

Best Evidence

- Manual therapists suspect that cervical mobilization and manipulation procedures decrease the afferent stimulus into the spinal cord from cervical joint receptors by relaxing the paraspinal muscles and releasing strain on the connective tissues and joints.

- Manual treatment and physical conditioning exercises for moderate to severe pain of any duration are effective for patients of all ages and both genders[31-34] (grade A evidence) (Table 7.5).
- Ongoing exercise and physical conditioning programs are beneficial for long-term prevention and control of symptoms.[35]

Risks

- Chapter 6 addresses the risks associated with upper cervical rotatory high-velocity, low-amplitude (HVLA) manipulation.

Table 7.5   Evidence-based practice recommendation

Evidence Level*	Recommendation	Studies
A	Manual treatment and physical conditioning exercises are effective for cervicogenic headache.	Nilsson et al, 1997[31] Jull et al, 2002[32] Bronfort et al, 2004[34]

*Evidence levels: A, randomized, controlled trials, meta-analyses, and systematic reviews; B, case-control or cohort studies, retrospective studies, and certain uncontrolled studies; C, consensus statements, expert guidelines, usual practice, and opinion.

- There have been no reported complications associated with cervical mobilization procedures, as described in this textbook, for treating somatic dysfunction related to CHA.
- The practitioner should be aware that patients with congenital anomalies, such as those with Down syndrome, may have deformities of the upper cervical spine that can alter the biomechanics in that region.
- Caution is warranted in treating patients with rheumatoid arthritis because there may be laxity of the alar (odontoid) ligament and hypermobility of the AA joint (C1 to C2).

Benefits

- Decreased pain frequency, intensity, and duration[31] (grade A evidence)
- Improved functionality in activities of daily living and at work
- Decreased reliance on analgesic and other medications that can have side effects and complications

Practice Recommendations

- Most professionals agree that CHA should be treated with a combination of manual treatment, exercise, locally injected and oral medications, stress-reduction counseling, and education.
- Surgery is reserved for refractory conditions.

DIAGNOSTIC PROCEDURES

- The ICD-9 diagnostic code for cervical somatic dysfunction is 739.1.
- Although other codes are used, they are not specific as indicators for manual treatment.
- Physical evaluation procedures for CHA are the same as for upper back and neck pain (see Chapter 6). A general screening examination of the musculoskeletal system (see Chapter 3) is followed by a regional examination and by a segmental examination of the cervical spine. Consult the appropriate chapters for the diagnostic examinations for cervical somatic dysfunction.
- Asymmetry of musculoskeletal structural landmarks; altered quantity or quality of active or passive neck motion; and tissue texture abnormalities, including tenderness and temperature variations (ART), lead the practitioner to consider mechanical neck disorder or a cervical somatic dysfunction diagnosis.
- Observing for pharyngeal and tonsil inflammation, glandular hypertrophy or tenderness, and lymphadenopathy can alert the practitioner to internal organic problems that can be an underlying cause of the somatic findings through viscerosomatic reflexes. Thoracic or abdominal visceral diseases may also cause palpable soft tissue abnormalities in the upper cervical spine.
- Cervical somatic dysfunction can be primary, or it can result from somatic dysfunction in the thoracic, low back, and shoulder regions.

- Physician practitioners typically also auscultate the carotid arteries with a stethoscope, listening in particular for any bruits that indicate a compromised vascular lumen (i.e., from cholesterol buildup or an aneurysm). A neurologic examination shows deficits in the case of cervical peripheral nerve impingement with radiculopathy or spinal cord impingement from a herniated cervical disc.
- Identification of cervical somatic dysfunction can provide the indication for manual treatment of the cervical spine.
- Confirmation of the diagnosis is achieved by alleviation of head pain on resolution of the somatic dysfunction or after local anesthetic blockade (injection) of a related zygapophyseal joint, cervical nerve, or its medial branch.

TREATMENT PROCEDURES

- Treatment procedures for CHA are the same as those for neck pain. These include soft tissue, articulatory, myofascial release, muscle energy, functional, and counterstrain procedures. Chapter 6 addresses cervical somatic dysfunction treatment procedures.
- Several techniques lend themselves to treating upper cervical somatic dysfunction in addition to those described in Chapter 6:
  1. Direct myofascial release of the suboccipital soft tissues
  2. Indirect myofascial release of the upper cervical paraspinal tissues
  3. Isometric muscle energy using patient eye movements as an activating force. (This technique uses the tectospinal tract, which coordinates eye movement with neck movements. For example, looking to the right contracts the suboccipital muscles in preparation for a strong contraction and turning of the head to the right.)
  4. Isometric muscle energy activation for the treatment of OA somatic dysfunction using one primary direction of motion
  5. Functional treatment of the OA joint with the patient supine and the patient's head off the table in the practitioner's hands

Myofascial Release

Myofascial Release: Suboccipital Release
- Diagnosis: suboccipital myofascial tension
- The procedure is performed as follows:
  1. The patient is supine (Fig. 7.4).
  2. The practitioner sits at the head of the treatment table.
  3. The occiput should be held bilaterally just inferior to the condyles, with the practitioner's palms against the occiput and thumbs just superior to the ears.
  4. The practitioner contacts the suboccipital fascia with the finger pads and applies slight traction in a superior direction. The practitioner moves his or her hands in a clockwise and counterclockwise direction and observes the direction of ease of movement.
  5. The practitioner holds the fascia in the position of ease.

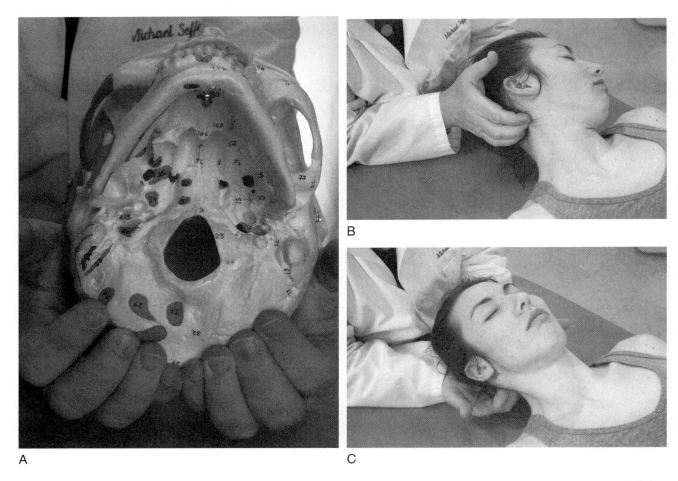

Figure 7.4 **A,** Inferior view of a skull model shows the hand position for suboccipital myofascial release. **B,** Hand position for suboccipital myofascial release. **C,** Suboccipital myofascial release.

6. The practitioner allows the fascia to unwind until the tissues are relaxed and the unwinding stops.
7. The practitioner then retests the motion of the fascia.

Myofascial Release: Occiptioatlantal Indirect Release

- Diagnosis: suboccipital myofascial tension
- The procedure is performed as follows:
  1. The patient is supine.
  2. The practitioner sits at the head of the table (Fig. 7.5).
  3. The practitioner contacts the posterior tubercle of the atlas, just below the occiput, with one hand and places the opposite hand on the vertex of the patient's head.
  4. The practitioner assesses the fascial motion at the OA joint by gliding the hand on the posterior tubercle of the atlas in the following directions: superior-inferior, clockwise-counterclockwise, and laterally in both directions.
  5. The practitioner stacks the fascia into the positions of ease of the three directions.
  6. The practitioner allows the fascia to unwind until the tissues are relaxed and the unwinding stops.

7. The practitioner retests the motion of the fascia in all planes.

Myofascial Release: C2 to C3 Indirect Release

- Diagnosis: upper cervical myofascial tension
- The procedure is performed as follows:
  1. The patient is supine (see Fig. 7.5).
  2. The practitioner is seated at the head of the table.
  3. The practitioner contacts the posterior aspects of the transverse processes of C2 with the thumb and index finger (or thumb and middle finger) of one hand and places the opposite hand on the vertex of the patient's head.
  4. The practitioner observes the ease of motion in flexion or extension, sidebending, left and right rotation, and compression or distraction when applicable.
  5. The practitioner stacks the cervical fascia into the direction of ease for each of the motions tested.
  6. The practitioner allows the fascia to unwind until the tissues are relaxed and the unwinding stops.
  7. The practitioner slowly returns the tissues to the neutral position and retests the fascia in all planes of motion.

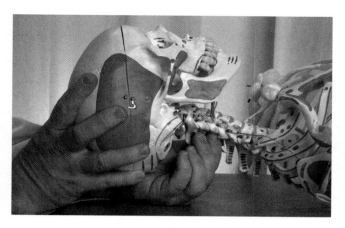

Figure 7.5 Handhold for upper cervical indirect myofascial release is shown on a skeletal model.

Cervical Muscle Energy Techniques: Using Eye Movements

Occipitoatlantal Joint

- Diagnosis: OA FR$_R$S$_L$ (i.e., E, extended; F, flexed; N, neutral, R, rotated; S, sidebent; subscripted L and R, left and right sides)
- Restriction: OA ER$_L$S$_R$
- The procedure is performed as follows:
  1. The patient is supine on the treatment table (Fig. 7.6).
  2. The practitioner sits at the head of the table.
  3. The practitioner cradles the patient's occiput with both hands and places his or her thumbs on the patient's zygomas (i.e., lateral bones of the orbit and cheek) bilaterally.
  4. The practitioner engages the motion barriers in all three planes (i.e., extension, left rotation, and right sidebending) at the OA joint.
  5. The patient is instructed to look toward the right (i.e., back toward the midline) without moving the head, meeting the practitioner's counterforce supplied by his or her thumb on the patient's zygoma.
  6. This eye position is held for 5 to 6 seconds.
  7. The patient is then directed to fully relax this effort.
  8. The practitioner then engages the new motion barrier in all three planes (i.e., extension, left rotation, and right sidebending) at the OA joint.
  9. Steps 5 through 8 are repeated three to five times.
  10. The practitioner retests.

Occipitoatlantal Joint

- Diagnosis: OA ER$_L$S$_R$
- Restriction: OA FR$_R$S$_L$
- The procedure is performed as follows:
  1. The patient is supine on the treatment table.
  2. The practitioner sits at the head of the table.
  3. The practitioner cradles the patient's occiput with both hands and thumbs on the patient's zygomas (lateral orbit/cheek bones).
  4. The practitioner engages the motion barriers in all three planes (flexion, right rotation, left side bending) at the OA joint.

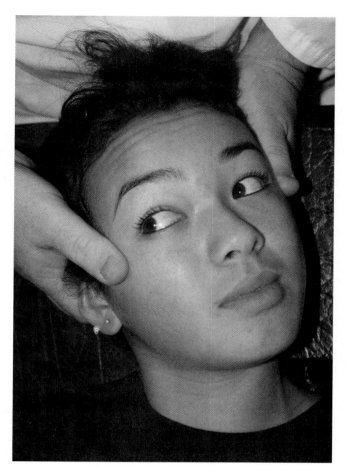

Figure 7.6 Isometric muscle energy for the occipitoatlantal joint flexed, rotated right, and sidebent left using eye movements as the activating force. The patient is instructed to look toward the right (i.e., back toward the midline) after the practitioner localizes at the restrictive barriers in extension, rotation left, and sidebending right. Notice that the practitioner's right thumb on the patient's zygoma provides the resistive counterforce. The practitioner's index and middle fingertips (not visible behind the patient's ears) can monitor the isometric contraction of the head rotator muscles at the base of the occiput.

  5. The patient is instructed to look toward the left (back toward midline) without moving his/her head.
  6. This eye position is held for 5-6 seconds.
  7. The patient is then directed to fully relax this effort.
  8. The practitioner then engages the new motion barrier in all three planes (flexion, right rotation, left side bending) at the OA joint.
  9. Steps 5 through 8 are repeated three to five times.
  10. The practitioner retests.

Atlantoaxial Joint

- Diagnosis: AA R$_R$
- Restriction: AA R$_L$
- The procedure is performed as follows:
  1. The patient is supine on the treatment table (Fig. 7.7).
  2. The practitioner sits at the head of the table.

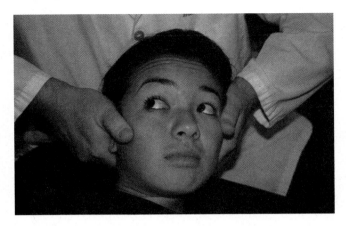

Figure 7.7 Isometric muscle energy for the atlantoaxial (AA) joint rotated right using eye movements as the activating force. The patient is instructed to look to the right (i.e., back toward the midline) after the practitioner localizes at the left rotation restrictive barrier. Notice that the patient's cervical spine is flexed to isolate the activating force at the AA joint.

3. The practitioner flexes the patient's neck until the shoulders begin to lift off the table to inhibit motion at C2 to C7.
4. The practitioner then rotates the patient's head toward the left side to engage the restrictive barrier.
5. The patient is instructed to look toward the right (i.e., back toward the midline) without moving his to her head.
6. This eye position is held for 5 to 6 seconds.
7. The patient is then instructed to fully relax this effort.
8. The practitioner then rotates the patient's head further to the left to engage the new restrictive rotational barrier at the AA joint.
9. Steps 5 through 8 are repeated three to five times.
10. The practitioner retests.

• Muscle energy treatments of the OA can also be performed with a focus on one primary plane of motion, such as flexion or extension, because nodding and looking upward are primary motions of the OA and the most common motions to be restricted. Sidebending and rotation are less prominent at the OA (Figs. 7.8 and 7.9).

Functional Technique for Occipitoatlantal Somatic Dysfunction

• Diagnosis: OA somatic dysfunction (any positional diagnosis)
• The procedure is performed as follows:
   1. The patient is supine (Figs. 7.10 and 7.11).
   2. The practitioner is seated at the head of table.
   3. The practitioner monitors the paraspinal tissues between the occiput and atlas (see Fig. 7.10).
   4. The practitioner observes the relative ease and bind between paired motions (e.g., flexion and extension). With the functional technique, it is the *response of the tissues at the initiation of motion in a particular direction* that determines ease versus bind, not the end range of motion.
   5. The practitioner rests his or her elbows on his or her knees to get better control, moving the knees up, down, and side to side and raising or lowering the forearms to create flexion, extension, sidebending, and rotation at the OA while the fingertips monitor the response of the soft tissues around the OA (see Fig. 7.11).
   6. The practitioner observes the relative directions of ease or bind while introducing the following motions at the OA junction:
      Flexion is induced by lifting the heels, which indirectly flexes the patient's OA joint (see Fig. 7.11A), and then lowering the heels and the forearms to allow extension at the patient's OA joint (see Fig. 7.11B). These maneuvers

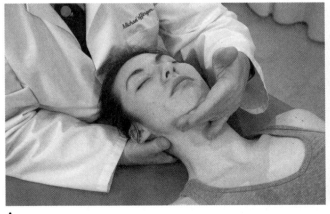

A

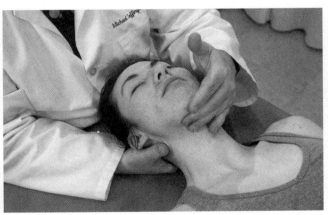

B

Figure 7.8 **A,** Treating a flexed (nutated) occipitoatlantal (OA) joint with an isometric muscle energy technique in one plane. The patient is instructed to gently bring her chin toward her chest as the practitioner provides an equal and unyielding counterforce with two fingers placed underneath her chin. **B,** Final stretch after treating a flexed OA joint with an isometric muscle energy technique in one plane.

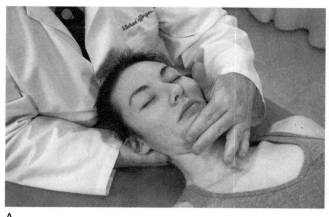
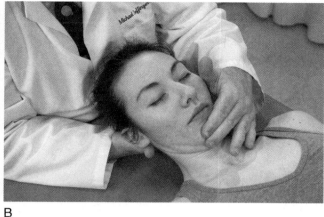

A   B

Figure 7.9 **A,** Treating an extended (counternutated) occipitoatlantal (OA) joint with an isometric muscle energy technique in one plane. The patient is instructed to gently tilt her head upward against the equal and unyielding counterforce provided by the practitioner with two fingers on the anterior surface of her chin. **B,** Final stretch after treating an extended OA joint with an isometric muscle energy technique in one plane.

do not interfere with the sensing fingers assessing compliance versus resistance to the initiation of the passive motions.

Rotating the hips to move one knee more anteriorly than the other induces sidebending (see Fig. 7.11C and D).

Rotation is accomplished by lifting one heel or letting only one forearm at a time drop lower than the other (see Fig. 7.11E).

Compression and distraction are induced sequentially by gently leaning forward toward and then away from the patient (see Fig. 7.11F).

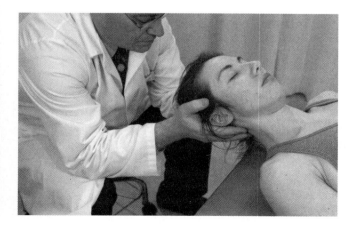

Figure 7.10 Functional technique for an occipitoatlantal (OA) joint somatic dysfunction with the patient supine and the head off the table and in the practitioner's hands. The practitioner monitors the patient's suboccipital tissues with his finger pads while directing passive motion with his foot, leg, and arm motions. Notice that his elbows are resting on his knees.

The patient is then instructed to inhale and exhale while the practitioner monitors the soft tissue response at the OA joint.

7. Treatment is accomplished by combining (stacking) all the directions of ease and then adding the respiratory motion that facilitates more compliance.

8. The practitioner retests the various motions to ensure resolution of any resistance to the initiation of passive motion in any direction.

• After a direction of motion is discovered to elicit compliance of the soft tissues around the OA joint, there is no need to move into the opposite direction that causes resistance while testing the other directions of motion. By the time the last plane of motion is tested, all the directions eliciting ease have been stacked (i.e., combined); the patient need only breath in and then out while the practitioner fine-tunes the directions of motion that elicit a sense of ease in the soft tissues being monitored, and the treatment will be complete. Sometimes, it is necessary to have the patient hold his or her breath in the phase of respiration that induces more ease as the practitioner fine-tunes the various motions until complete relaxation is palpable at the OA joint.

ADJUNCT TREATMENTS

• Only a few adjunct treatments have been studied in randomized, controlled trials (RCTs).[16]
• Adjunct treatments include the following:
  1. Occipital traction to relax suboccipital muscles and inhibit greater occipital nerve
  2. Anesthetic blockade of the greater and lesser occipital nerves
  3. Anesthetic blockade in conjunction with exercises and mobilization
  4. Analgesic medication

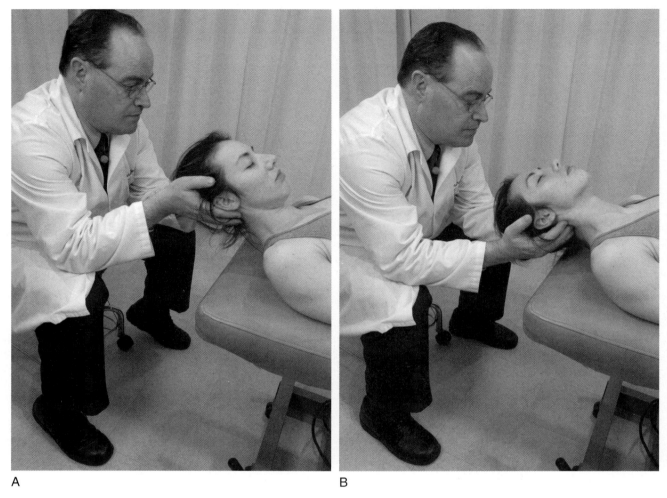

A   B

Figure 7.11   A, The practitioner induces passive flexion while monitoring the tissue response around the patient's suboccipital region. Notice that the practitioner has elbows on his knees and is raising his heels. **B,** The practitioner induces passive extension while monitoring the tissue response around the patient's suboccipital region. Notice that the practitioner is lowering his forearms.

5. Antiepileptic medication for neuropathic pain
6. Antidepressants to modulate pain and improve sleep
7. Muscle relaxants
8. Botulinum toxin type A injection into pericranial and cervical muscles
9. Narcotics for short-term relief while awaiting the effects of other therapies
10. Trigger point injections
11. Radiofrequency neurolysis for refractory cases
12. Beneficial psychological counseling, biofeedback, relaxation meditations, and cognitive-behavioral therapies[36]
13. Cervical epidural steroids in patients with multilevel disc or spine degeneration
14. Surgical relief of nerve entrapments
15. Surgical transection of the greater occipital nerve
16. Surgical implantation of occipital or cervical spinal nerve stimulators
17. Surgical neurectomy, dorsal rhizotomy, or microvascular decompression of nerve roots or peripheral nerves, which are considered as last resorts unless well-defined pathology is discovered by radiographic procedures during evaluation

EDUCATION

• Posture and ergonomics of entire spine, especially the cervical spine, are essential.
• Patients are reassured about the nondisease nature of the pathophysiology.

EXERCISES

• Physical conditioning and neck stretches and strengthening exercises for treatment and prevention are essential.[34]
• Improving tone and strength of deep neck flexors and extensors is desirable.[29]
• Exercises for the cervical spine are helpful (see Chapter 6).

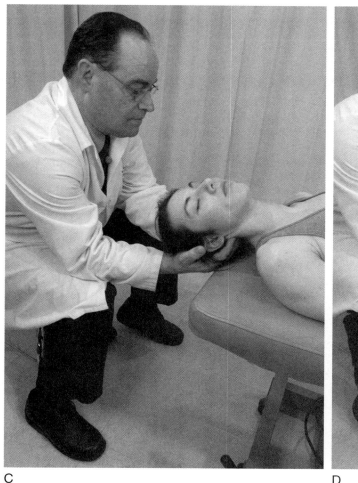
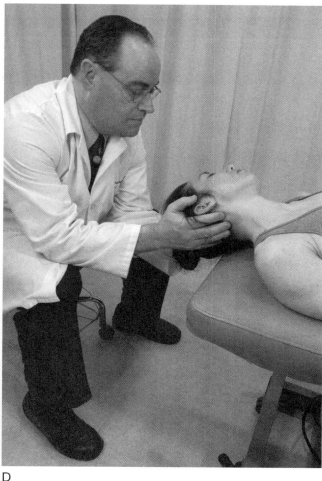

C   D

Figure 7.11, cont'd   C, The practitioner induces passive sidebending right at the patient's occipitoatlantal (OA) joint by rotating his hip to the right, which moves his right knee to a more anterior position. His fingertips are monitoring the tissue response around the patient's suboccipital region. **D,** The practitioner induces passive sidebending left by rotating his hips to the left while monitoring the tissue response around the patient's suboccipital region.

Continued

CONTROVERSIES

- It is unclear to what extent the observed treatment effects can be explained by manipulation or by nonspecific factors (e.g., personal attention, patient expectation) or whether manipulation produces long-term effects.[37]
- It is unclear whether the cervical somatic dysfunction found in patients with CHA is primary or results from the headache symptoms.
- Upper cervical manipulation using forceful adjustments, such as thrusting or HVLA, is controversial (see Chapter 6).

OPPORTUNITIES FOR RESEARCH

- Better controlled RCTs should be designed to compare behavioral factors and relaxation measures that are known to help decrease headache symptoms and the effects specifically attributable to cervical manipulation.

- The results on headache intensity, frequency, and duration should be obtained with the same methods that have been employed by other clinical trials assessing headache therapies.[38]
- The long-term effects of cervical manipulation should be determined.
- The methodology of the RCTs on spinal manipulation for CHA can be improved by adhering to the following guidelines[37]:
  1. Clearly define the experimental and control conditions, the setting, and outcome measures.
  2. Use randomization of subjects and power calculations to determine sample size.
  3. If possible, use sham-controlled or patient-blinded and evaluator-blinded protocols.
  4. Use test statistics that are predefined and relate to intergroup comparisons rather than differences before and after manipulation.
  5. Use a multidisciplinary team of researchers and clinicians who use manual therapies to treat patients with CHA.

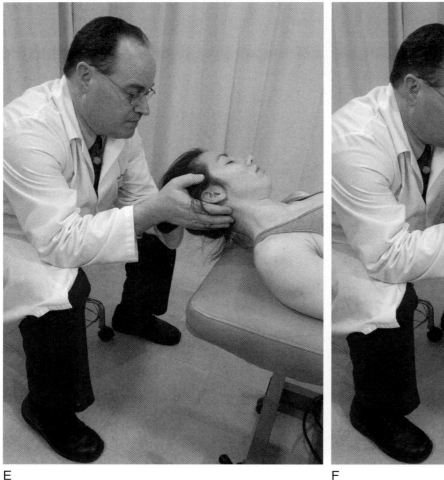
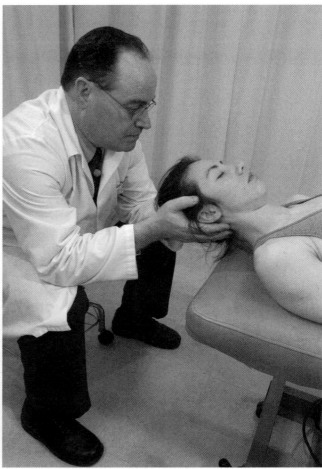

E   F

Figure 7.11, cont'd   **E,** The practitioner induces passive rotation left (i.e., the practitioner can raise the right heel or lower the left forearm) while monitoring the tissue response around the patient's suboccipital region. Passive rotation right is accomplished by raising the left heel or lowering right forearm, or both. **F,** The practitioner induces passive axial compression and distraction of the OA joint while assessing the response of the patient's suboccipital region with his finger pads.

REFERENCES

1. Sjaastad O, Fredriksen TA, Pfaffenrath V: Cervicogenic headache: Diagnostic criteria. Headache 38:442-445, 1998.
2. International Headache Society: The international classification of headache disorders (2nd edition). Cephalalgia 24(Suppl 7):114-116, 2004.
3. Haldeman S, Dagenais S: Cervicogenic headaches: A critical review. Spine J 1:31-46, 2001.
4. Pöllmann W, Keidel M, Pfaffenrath V: Headache and the cervical spine: A critical review. Cephalalgia 17:801-816, 1997.
5. Pfaffenrath V, Kaube H: Diagnostics of cervicogenic headache. Funct Neurol 5:159-164, 1990.
6. Nilsson N: The prevalence of cervicogenic headache in a random population sample of 20-59 year olds. Spine 20:1884-1888, 1995.
7. Skovron ML: Epidemiology of whiplash. In Gunzbrug R and Szpalski M (eds): Whiplash Injuries: Current Concepts in Prevention, Diagnosis, and Treatment of the Cervical Whiplash Syndrome. Philadelphia, Lippincott-Raven, 1998.
8. van Suijlekom HA, Lame I, Stomp-van den Berg SG, et al: Quality of life of patients with cervicogenic headache: A comparison with control subjects and patients with migraine or tension-type headache. Headache 43:1034-1041, 2003.
9. Drottning M, Staff PH, Sjaastad O: Cervicogenic headache after whiplash injury. Cephalalgia 17:288-289, 1997.
10. Drottning M, Staff PH, Sjaastad O: Cervicogenic headache (CEH) after whiplash injury. Cephalalgia 22:165-171, 2002.
11. Schwartz BS, Stewart WF, Lipton RB: Lost workdays and decreased work effectiveness associated with headache in the workplace. J Occup Environ Med 39:320-327, 1997.
12. Stewart WF, Ricci JA, Chee E, et al: Lost productive time and cost due to common pain conditions in the U.S. workforce. JAMA 290:2443-2454, 2003.
13. Hack GD, Koritzer RT, Robinson WL, et al: Anatomic relation between the rectus capitis posterior minor muscle and the dura mater. Spine 20:2484-2486, 1995.
14. Nash L, Nicholson H, Lee ASJ, et al: Configuration of the connective tissue in the posterior atlantooccipital interspace. Spine 30:1359-1366, 2005.
15. Biondi DM: Cervicogenic headache: Mechanisms, evaluation, and treatment strategies. J Am Osteopath Assoc 100(Suppl):S7-S14, 2000.
16. Biondi DM: Cervicogenic headache: A review of diagnostic and treatment strategies. J Am Osteopath Assoc 105(Suppl):S16-S22, 2005.
17. Foreman RD: Integration of viscerosomatic sensory input at the spinal level. Prog Brain Res 122:209-221, 2000.
18. Artico M, Cavallotti C: Catecholaminergic and acetylcholine esterase containing nerves of cranial and spinal dura mater in humans and rodents. Microsc Res Tech 53:212-220, 2001.
19. Lord SM, Barnsley L, Wallis BJ: Third occipital nerve headache: A prevalence study. J Neurol Neurosurg Psychiatry 57:1187-1190, 1994.
20. Lord SM, Barnsley L, Wallis BJ: Chronic cervical zygapophysial joint pain after whiplash. A placebo-controlled prevalence study. Spine 21:1737-1744, 1996.

21. Bovim G, Berg R, Dale LG: Cervicogenic headache: Anesthetic blockades of cervical nerves (C2-C5) and facet joint (C2/C3). Pain 49:315-320, 1992.

22. Bovim G, Sand T: Cervicogenic headache, migraine without aura and tension-type headache. Diagnostic blockade of greater occipital and supra-orbital nerves. Pain 51:43-48, 1992.

23. Kuchera ML: Osteopathic principles and practice/osteopathic manipulative treatment considerations in cephalgia. J Am Osteopath Assoc 98:S14-S19, 1998.

24. Martelletti P, van Suijlekom HA: Cervicogenic headache: Practical approaches to therapy. CNS Drugs 18:793-805, 2004.

25. Frese A, Schilgen M, Edvinsson L, et al: Calcitonin gene-related peptide in cervicogenic headache. Cephalalgia 25:700-703, 2005.

26. van Suijlekom HA, de Vet HC, van den Berg SG, et al: Interobserver reliability in physical examination of the cervical spine in patients with headache. Headache 40:581-586, 2000.

27. Hanten WP, Olson SL, Ludwig GM: Reliability of manual mobility testing of the upper cervical spine in subjects with cervicogenic headache. J Man Manipul Ther 10:76-82, 2002.

28. Hall T, Robinson K: The flexion-rotation test and active cervical mobility—A comparative measurement study in cervicogenic headache. Man Ther 9:197-202, 2004.

29. Jull G: Management of cervical headache. Man Ther 2:182-190, 1997.

30. Coskun O, Ucler S, Karakurum B, et al: Magnetic resonance imaging of patients with cervicogenic headache. Cephalalgia 23:842-845, 2003.

31. Nilsson N, Christensen HW, Hartvigsen J: The effect of spinal manipulation in the treatment of cervicogenic headache. J Manipulative Physiol Ther 20:326-330, 1997.

32. Jull GA, Trott P, Potter H, et al: A randomized controlled trial of exercise and manipulative therapy for cervicogenic headache. Spine 27:1835-1843, 2002.

33. Jull GA, Stanton WR: Predictors of responsiveness to physiotherapy management of cervicogenic headache. Cephalalgia 25:101-108, 2005.

34. Bronfort G, Nilsson N, Haas M, et al: Non-invasive physical treatments for chronic/recurrent headache. Cochrane Database Syst Rev (3):CD001878, 2004; doi: 10.1002/14651858.CD001878.pub2.

35. Biondi DM: Physical treatments for headache: A structured review. Headache 45:738-746, 2005.

36. Jerome J: Pain management. In Ward RC (ed): Foundations for Osteopathic Medicine. Philadelphia, Lippincott Williams & Wilkins, 2003.

37. Astin JA, Ernst E: The effectiveness of spinal manipulation for the treatment of headache disorders: A systematic review of randomized clinical trials. Cephalalgia 22:617-623, 2002.

38. Fernández-de-las-Peñas C, Alonso-Blanco C, Cuadrado ML, et al: Spinal manipulative therapy in the management of cervicogenic headache. Headache 45:1260-1263, 2005.

CHAPTER 8

Temporomandibular Joint Dysfunction

DEFINITION

- There is no universal agreement on a definition.[1]
- Dysfunction of the temporomandibular joint (TMJ) refers to a number of clinical problems that involve the muscles of mastication or the TMJ, and its associated structures, or both.
- TMJ dysfunction usually is manifested by phenomena such as joint sounds, limitation of jaw movement, muscle tenderness, joint tenderness, and pain, especially in the preauricular region.
- Associated complaints include headache, earache, and orofacial pain, as well as hypertrophy of the muscles of mastication and abnormal occlusion.
- Other complaints include tinnitus, ear fullness, and perceived hearing loss.

EPIDEMIOLOGY

Age

- TMJ dysfunction usually occurs in adults.
- Most patients are between 20 and 50 years old.

Gender

- Men and women are affected.
- TMJ dysfunction is more common in women between the ages of puberty and menopause.

Prevalence

- Reliable data are lacking.[1]
- Cross-sectional studies of nonpatient populations show the following:
  1. Approximately 75% have at least one sign of TMJ dysfunction.
  2. Approximately 33% have at least one symptom.

Natural Clinical Course

- TMJ dysfunction commonly begins as popping or clicking sounds on opening or closing the jaw.
- Internal derangement of the TMJ disc occurs. The disc may be intermittently displaced or permanently dislocated.
- Initial signs and symptoms progress to episodes of intermittent locking of jaw.
- The disorder can lead to a chronic, "closed lock" position of jaw and to chronic pain.
- Ligamentous laxity and damage may occur.
- Joint may become remodeled, and degenerative joint disease may appear.
- There is a high rate of comorbidity between TMJ dysfunction and certain other medical problems, such as mitral valve prolapse, hypermobile joints, and fibromyalgia.[2-4]

Effect on Society

- No reliable data are available for the societal effects of TMJ dysfunction.

Risk Factors

- Several risk factors for the development of TMJ dysfunction have been identified.
- The most common risk factors are shown in Table 8.1.

PATHOPHYSIOLOGY

- Causes of TMJ dysfunction include the following:
  1. Malocclusion
  2. Bruxism
  3. Trauma
  4. Inflammation
  5. Degenerative joint diseases
  6. Somatic dysfunctions of the head, neck, and upper back regions (somatic dysfunction of the lower thoracic, lumbar,

Table 8.1   Risk factors

Grinding or clinching teeth
Tension of the muscles of mastication
Stress
Poorly aligned teeth
Poorly fitting dentures
Osteoarthritis or rheumatoid arthritis

pelvic, and lower extremity regions may also be implicated in TMJ dysfunction)

7. Congenital anomalies of the mandible or temporomandibular joint
8. Psychological stress

- Other postulated causes, such as hormonal imbalances and nutritional deficiencies, remain controversial.[6]

DIFFERENTIAL DIAGNOSIS

- Neuralgia of the trigeminal or facial nerves
- Tumors
- Inflammatory disorders
- Infection[6,7]

HISTORY

- Headache
- Dull, aching unilateral preauricular pain that radiates to the temple, back of the head, and along the mandible
- Tenderness of the muscles of mastication
- Clicking or popping sounds when opening the mouth
- Inability to open the jaw completely
- Aching back, shoulders, or neck
- Pain brought on by yawning
- History of bruxism
- History of trauma to the head, neck, or upper back regions[1]

PHYSICAL FINDINGS

- Malocclusion
- Crepitus in the TMJ
- Popping or clicking of the TMJ on opening or closing the jaw
- Deviation of the mandible on opening or closing the jaw
- Limitation of jaw opening
- Pain and hypertonicity of the muscles of mastication and the muscles of the neck and upper back
- Palpable findings of somatic dysfunction of the head, neck, or upper back areas[1,6]

LABORATORY AND RADIOGRAPHIC FINDINGS

- Plain radiographs provide limited information regarding the TMJ. They are limited to providing a screening assessment for gross bony abnormalities, such as developmental abnormalities; damage as a result of trauma; or arthritic diseases.[7]
- Arthrography is useful for diagnosing soft tissue abnormalities and TMJ disc displacement or dislocation.
- Computed tomography (CT) scanning is useful for analyzing bone structure and density, and CT is particularly applicable in cases of trauma or degenerative diseases of bone.
- Magnetic resonance imaging (MRI) is superior for imaging TMJ soft tissues, and MRI can be particularly helpful in assessing the TMJ disc position. Its major advantages over arthrography are its noninvasive nature and the fact that MRI requires no ionizing radiation.
- Laboratory tests typically are not useful for a TMJ dysfunction diagnosis, unless a specific cause, such as inflammatory disease or infection, is suspected.[8]

MANUAL MEDICINE

Best Evidence

- Reviews of the literature on the use of manual treatments for TMJ dysfunction have been mixed. The RAND group[9] reported that current information neither supports nor refutes the use of cervical spine manipulation in the treatment of TMJ problems.
- Certain manipulative techniques for manual reduction of TMJ disc displacement have been effective.[10]
- Chiropractic and physical therapy approaches have been reported as beneficial in the treatment of TMJ dysfunction.[11-13]
- Other researchers[2,14,15] have demonstrated through case reports that various forms of manual treatment show a tendency to be effective in the treatment of TMJ dysfunction.
- Much research needs to be done before a clear picture of the effectiveness of manual treatment for TMJ dysfunction is established.

Risks

- Little has been written regarding the risks of using manual treatments for TMJ dysfunction. However, the literature on complications from spinal manipulation procedures has shown that it is a highly safe method of treatment for a wide variety of conditions.[16-18]
- With neck pain being a common complaint in patients with TMJ dysfunction, the risks associated with manipulation of the cervical spine are of interest to the practitioner. The cervical region is most commonly associated with complications of manual treatment.
- The most frequent of all complications reported is vertebral artery injury. Investigation shows that this complication is thought to arise from high-velocity, low-amplitude (HVLA) manipulation applied with the neck in a position of extreme rotation and extension. Other common reasons given for these complications include an inadequately trained practitioner and an erroneous or incomplete diagnosis.
- There have been no reports of complications from any of the non-HVLA manipulative techniques. Experts advise that the

best way to avoid complications from manual treatment is to have a precise diagnosis of somatic dysfunction; to rule out other causes by a complete history, physical examination, and appropriate diagnostic studies; and to take appropriate precautions.

Benefits

- Manipulative treatment for somatic dysfunction associated with TMJ dysfunction can result in an earlier return to more normal functional status, less need for medication and other adjunctive treatments, and avoidance of unnecessary invasive procedures.[2,14]
- Several outcome findings have been reported for TMJ dysfunction manipulation:
  1. Pain reduction or alleviation
  2. Less medication usage
  3. Reduced or eliminated need for other therapies
  4. Increased patient satisfaction

Practice Recommendations

- No official guidelines for the diagnosis and treatment of TMJ dysfunction have been developed.

FUNCTIONAL ANATOMY

- Each temporomandibular joint consists of the articulation between the articular fossa of the temporal bone and the condyle of the mandible (Fig. 8.1). The articular disc divides the joint into upper and lower parts. A fibrous capsule surrounds the joint and is attached above to the articular tubercle of the temporal bone and the squamotympanic fissure and below to the neck of the mandible itself. A synovial membrane lines the fibrous capsule.

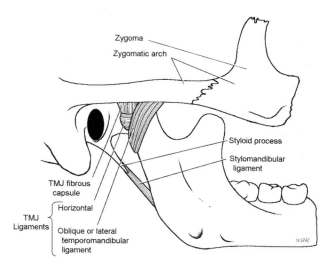

Figure 8.2   The temporomandibular joint (TMJ) ligament.

- Closely related to the fibrous capsule is the lateral temporomandibular ligament, which is attached above to the zygomatic process of the temporal bone and below to the lateral surface and posterior border of the neck of the mandible (Fig. 8.2).
- The sphenomandibular ligament is a flat, thin band stretching from the spine of the sphenoid to the lingula of the mandible. The stylomandibular ligament runs from the tip of the styloid process of the temporal bone to the angle and posterior border of the ramus of the mandible (Fig. 8.3).

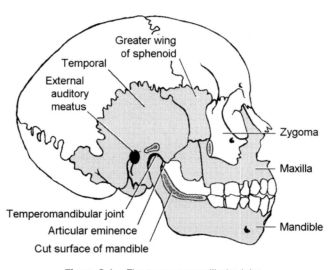

Figure 8.1   The temporomandibular joint.

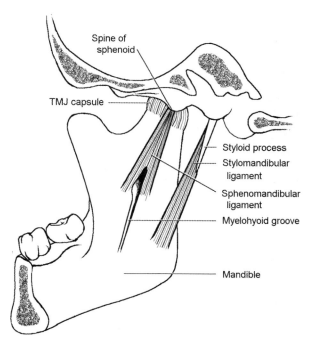

Figure 8.3   The sphenomandibular and stylomandibular ligaments. TMJ, temporomandibular joint.

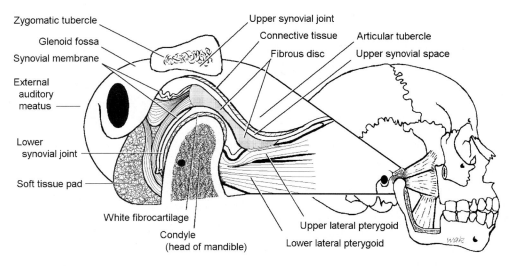

Figure 8.4 The temporomandibular joint showing the fibrous disc and the lateral pterygoid muscle.

- The articular disc is a somewhat oval body of fibrous tissue, which is convex on its upper surface to accommodate itself to the shape of the articular fossa and concave on its inferior surface to conform to the head of the mandible. The disc divides the joint into upper and lower compartments. The circumference of the disc is connected to the fibrous capsule, and the front portion of the disc is connected to the lateral pterygoid muscle. There are fibrous bands attaching from the disc to the medial and lateral aspects of the mandibular head (Fig. 8.4).
- The innervation of the TMJ is derived from the mandibular nerve, specifically the auriculotemporal and masseteric branches. The arterial blood supply is from the superficial temporal and maxillary arteries.
- Each condyle of the mandible articulates with the ipsilateral temporal bone.
- The gross physiologic motion of the TMJ is as follows:
  1. In depressing the mandible, the condyles of the mandible translate forward and rotate about a horizontal axis.
  2. The muscular action involved includes contraction of the lateral pterygoid muscles and some assistance from the mylohyoid, geniohyoid, and digastric muscles.
  3. Approximating the mandible to the maxillae involves reversal of the condylar motion previously described and the action of the temporal, masseter, and medial pterygoid muscles. All of these muscles assist in maintaining the mandible in a nonocclusal resting position (Fig. 8.5).

MANUAL DIAGNOSTIC PROCEDURES

- The procedure to assess range and quality of motion of the TMJ is performed as follows:
  1. Observe the patient while he or she is speaking, and notice any deviation of the mandible from the midline.

2. Observe whether the patient can fit three fingerbreadths between his or her front teeth (i.e., incisors) after opening the mouth as wide as possible.
3. Have the patient open his or her jaw as far as comfortably possible. Observe whether there is any restriction of jaw opening (Fig. 8.6). The range of motion for jaw opening can also be measured with a ruler or tongue blade. The normal range of motion for jaw opening is 40 to 50 mm.
4. Have the patient move his or her jaw from side to side, and observe whether there is any restriction in lateral movement of the TMJ (Fig. 8.7). The normal range of motion for lateral jaw movement is 8 mm to each side.
5. Have the patient protrude and retrude his or her jaw, and observe any restrictions of these motions. The normal range of motion for protrusion is 6 to 8 mm and, for retrusion, 3 mm (Fig. 8.8).
6. To assess the quality of motion, observe whether the jaw opening and closing motion is smooth and comfortable or there is observable limitation of movement, jerkiness of motion, or patient discomfort.

- Palpation of the TMJ is performed as follows:
  1. The patient is seated on the examination table.
  2. The practitioner stands facing the patient.
  3. The practitioner places the pads of his or her index fingers into the patient's external auditory canals, with the palmar surfaces pressing lightly anteriorly to contact the head of the mandible as it articulates with the temporomandibular fossa.
  4. The patient is instructed to slowly open and close his or her mouth.
  5. The practitioner observes or palpates to determine the following:
     Which side of the jaw moves first on opening?
     Which side returns first on closing?

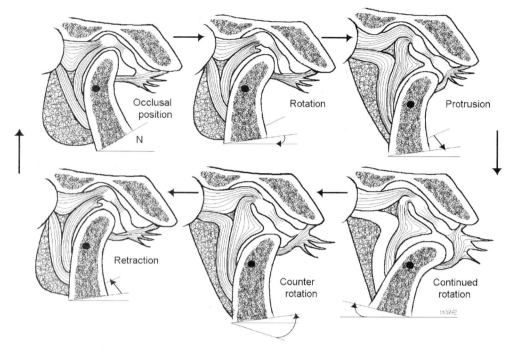

Figure 8.5   The motion characteristics of the temporomandibular joint. N, neutral.

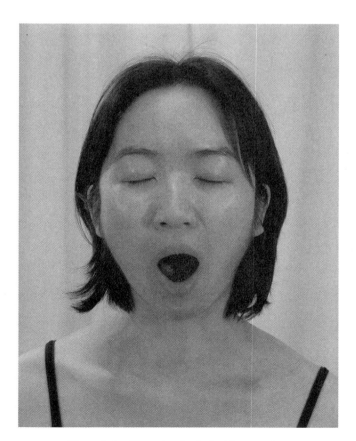

Figure 8.6   Observing for limited jaw opening.

Is there a popping or clicking sound that can be heard of palpated during opening or closing?

Does one mandibular head compress the index finger more than the other?

- Have the patient clench his or her teeth, and palpate the temporalis and masseter muscles for tenderness, atrophy, or hypertrophy.
- Palpate the following counterstrain points for tenderness (Fig. 8.9): anterior first cervical (AC1), internal pterygoid, masseter, sphenoid, squamosal, and posterior auricular.
- The lateral pterygoid muscle on the affected side is palpated for tenderness or hypertonicity in the following manner (e.g., examining the right lateral pterygoid muscle):
  1. With the patient supine, the practitioner stands on the side to be examined.
  2. The practitioner places his or her left hand on the patient's head to prevent rotational or sidebending movement.
  3. The practitioner inserts his or her gloved right little finger into the patient's mouth along the lateral aspect of the right upper teeth, until contact is made with the lateral pterygoid muscle. The muscle typically is exquisitely tender to palpation.
- The myofascial tissues of the jaw for tenderness or hypertonicity are palpated in the following manner (Fig. 8.10):
  1. With the patient supine, the practitioner grasps the anterior and posterior aspects of the rami of the mandible with his or her thumbs and index fingers.
  2. The practitioner moves the mandible superiorly, inferiorly, anteriorly, and posteriorly, observing whether there is symmetry of motion or there is greater ease of motion in one or more directions compared with the others.

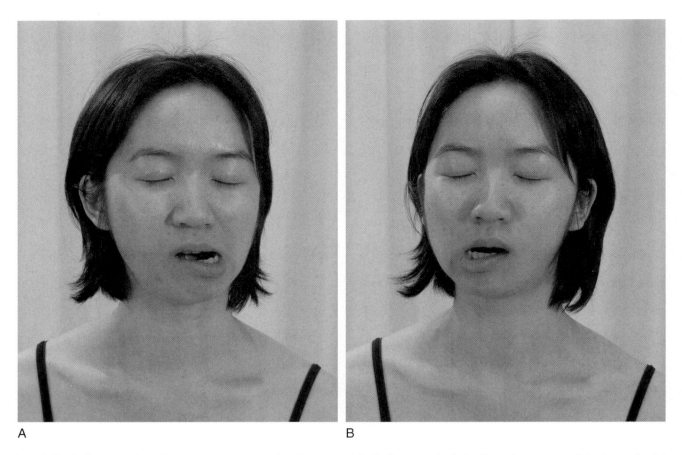

Figure 8.7 **A,** Observing for limited lateral movement of the jaw to the left. **B,** Observing for limited lateral movement of the jaw to the right.

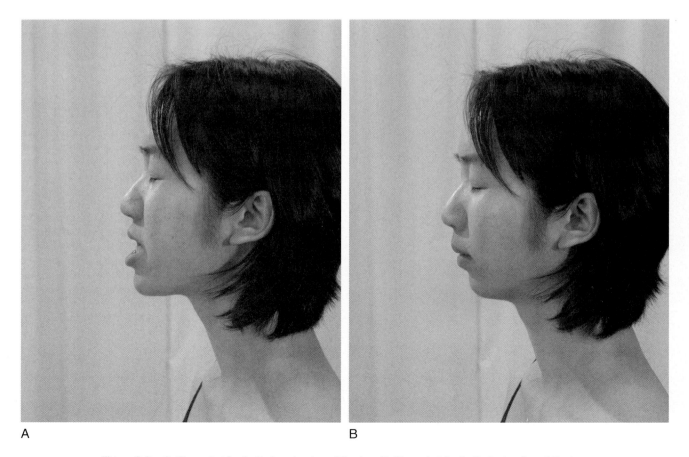

Figure 8.8 **A,** Observing for limited protrusion of the jaw. **B,** Observing for limited retrusion of the jaw.

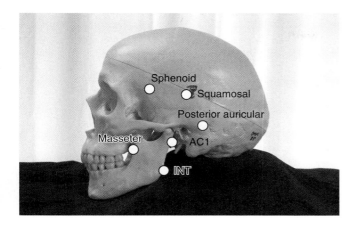

Figure 8.9 Locations of the temporomandibular joint–related counterstrain points. AC1, anterior first cervical counterstrain point; INT, internal pterygoid counterstrain point.

MANUAL MEDICINE TREATMENT PROCEDURES

Muscle Energy Techniques

Muscle Energy Technique for Restricted Temporomandibular Joint Opening

- The procedure is performed as follows:
  1. The patient is seated (Fig. 8.11).
  2. The practitioner stands behind the patient.
  3. The practitioner stabilizes the patient's head with one hand to prevent rotation or sidebending of the patient's head.
  4. The practitioner then places the index or middle finger of his or her other hand on the anterior surface of the patient's mandible and opens the patient's mouth until the motion barrier is engaged.
  5. The patient closes his or her jaw against the practitioner's isometric resistance.
  6. This effort is maintained for 3 to 5 seconds, and the patient then fully relaxes the jaw.

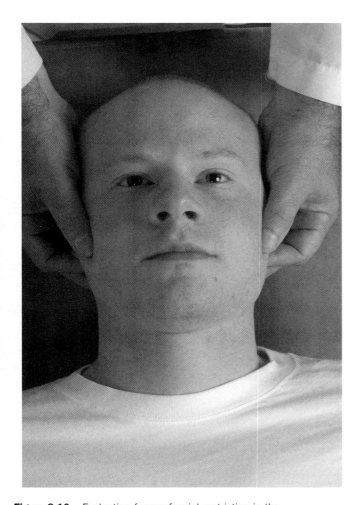

Figure 8.10 Evaluation for myofascial restriction in the temporomandibular joint region.

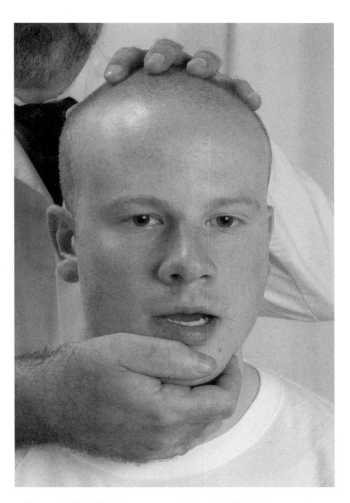

Figure 8.11 Muscle energy technique for limited jaw opening.

7. The practitioner opens the patient's mouth further to engage the next restrictive motion barrier.
8. Steps 3 through 5 are repeated three to five times, followed by a final stretch of the mandible after the last repetition.
9. The practitioner retests the patient.

Muscle Energy Technique for Lateral Deviation of the Mandible

- Example: The mandible deviates to the right on opening the mouth.
- Treatment: The procedure is performed as follows:
  1. The patient is seated (Fig. 8.12).
  2. The practitioner stands behind the patient.
  3. The practitioner places the palm of his or her left hand on the top of the patient's head to prevent rotational or sidebending movement.
  4. The practitioner places the finger pads of his or her right hand over the right lower portion of the patient's mandible and gently moves the mandible to the left to engage the restrictive motion barrier.

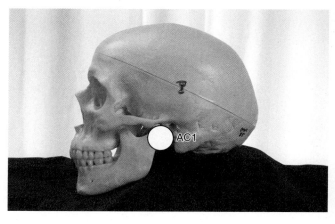

Figure 8.13   Location of the anterior first cervical (AC1) counterstrain point.

5. The patient is instructed to move his or her mandible to the right against the practitioner's isometric resistance.
6. This effort is maintained for 3 to 5 seconds.
7. The patient fully relaxes his or her muscular effort.
8. The practitioner then moves the patient's mandible further toward the left to engage the next restrictive motion barrier.
9. Steps 3 through 7 are repeated three to five times, followed by a final stretch of the mandible after the last repetition.
10. The practitioner retests the patient.

Counterstrain Techniques

Anterior First Cervical

- Location: The anterior first cervical (AC1) counterstrain point is on the tip of the transverse process of C1, in the sulcus between the mastoid process and the mandible (Fig. 8.13).
- Treatment: The procedure is performed as follows (Fig. 8.14):
  1. The patient is supine on the examination table.
  2. The practitioner sits at the head of the table.

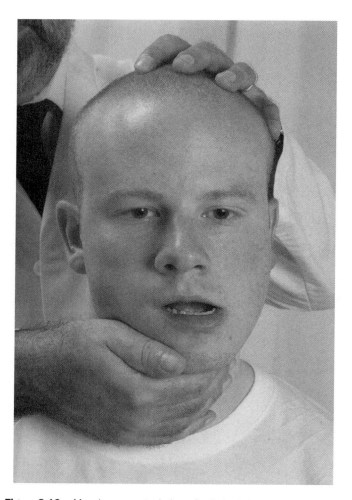

Figure 8.12   Muscle energy technique for limited right lateral jaw movement.

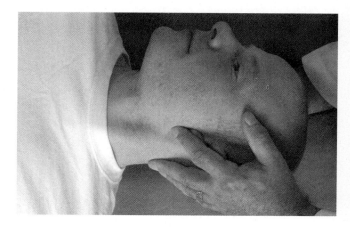

Figure 8.14   Treatment of the anterior first cervical (AC1) counterstrain point.

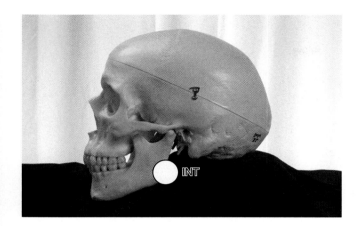

Figure 8.15   Location of the internal pterygoid (INT) counterstrain point.

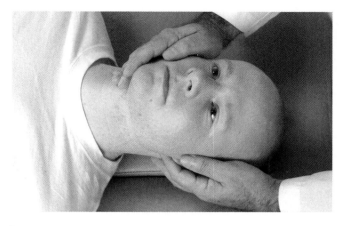

Figure 8.16   Treatment of the internal pterygoid (INT) counterstrain point.

3. While monitoring the tender point, the practitioner sidebends the patient's head toward the tender point until the position of greatest comfort is achieved.
4. This position is held for 90 seconds.
5. The patient's head is slowly returned to the neutral position.
6. The practitioner rechecks the tender point.

Internal Pterygoid
- Location: The internal pterygoid (INT) counterstrain point is on the medial side of the ascending ramus of the mandible, just above the angle of the mandible (Fig. 8.15).
- Treatment: The procedure is performed as follows (Fig. 8.16):
  1. The patient is supine on the examination table.
  2. The practitioner sits at the head of the table.
  3. While monitoring the tender point with the index finger of one hand, the practitioner places his or her other hand on the ascending ramus of the mandible of the opposite side and applies a force medially toward the tender point until the position of greatest comfort is achieved.
  4. This position is held for 90 seconds.
  5. The practitioner slowly releases his or her hand pressure.
  6. The practitioner rechecks the tender point.

Masseter
- Location: The masseter counterstrain point is in the masseter muscle, inferior to the coronoid process of the mandible (Fig. 8.17).
- Treatment: The procedure is performed as follows (Fig. 8.18):
  1. The patient is supine on the examination table.
  2. The practitioner sits at the head of the table on the side opposite the one to be treated.
  3. While monitoring the tender point with the index finger of one hand, the practitioner instructs the patient to open his or her jaw slightly (about 1 cm).
  4. The practitioner places his or her other hand on the top of the patient's head on the side opposite the tender point and applies a force toward the tender point until the position of greatest comfort is achieved.
  5. This position is held for 90 seconds.
  6. The practitioner slowly releases his or her hand pressure.
  7. The practitioner rechecks the tender point.

Sphenoid
- Location: The sphenoid counterstrain point is on the greater wing of the sphenoid (Fig. 8.19).

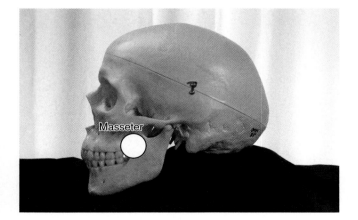

Figure 8.17   Location of the masseter counterstrain point.

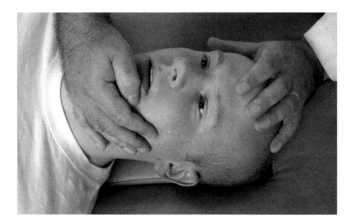

Figure 8.18   Treatment of the masseter counterstrain point.

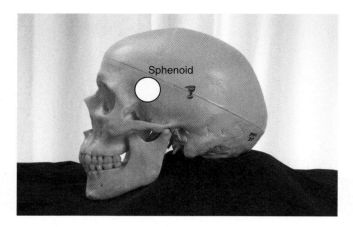

Figure 8.19   Location of the sphenoid counterstrain point.

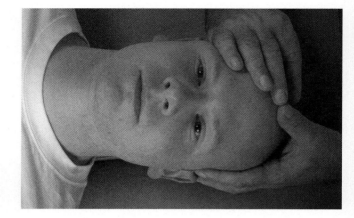

Figure 8.20   Treatment of the sphenoid counterstrain point.

- Treatment: The procedure is performed as follows (Fig. 8.20):
  1. The patient is supine on the examination table.
  2. The practitioner sits at the head of the table on the side opposite the one to be treated.
  3. The practitioner monitors the tender point with the index finger of one hand and uses the rest of this hand to stabilize the patient's head.
  4. The practitioner places his or her other hand over the greater wing of the sphenoid on the side opposite the tender point and applies a force medially toward the tender point until the position of greatest comfort is achieved.
  5. This position is held for 90 seconds.
  6. The practitioner slowly releases his or her hand pressure.
  7. The practitioner rechecks the tender point.

Squamosal
- Location: The squamosal counterstrain point is 2 cm anterior to the top of the pinna of the ear, on the squamous part of the temporal bone (Fig. 8.21).
- Treatment: The procedure is performed as follows (Fig. 8.22):
  1. The patient is supine on the examination table, with the head turned toward the side opposite the tender point.

  2. The practitioner sits at the head of the table.
  3. The practitioner monitors the tender point with the index finger of one hand.
  4. The practitioner places three finger pads of his or her other hand just above the tender point.
  5. Using these three finger pads, the practitioner gently pulls the soft tissues superiorly until the position of greatest comfort is achieved.
  6. This position is held for 90 seconds.
  7. The practitioner slowly releases his or her hand pressure.
  8. The practitioner rechecks the tender point.

Posterior Auricular
- Location: The posterior auricular counterstain point is 1 cm posterior to the top of the pinna of the ear, on the squamous part of the temporal bone (Fig. 8.23).
- Treatment: The procedure is performed as follows (Fig. 8.24)
  1. The patient is supine on the examination table, with his or her head turned toward the side opposite the tender point.
  2. The practitioner sits at the head of the table.
  3. The practitioner monitors the tender point with the index finger of one hand.

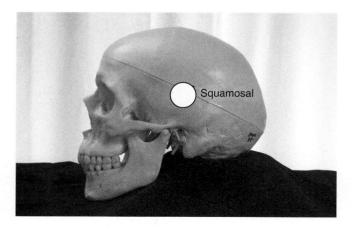

Figure 8.21   Location of the squamosal counterstrain point.

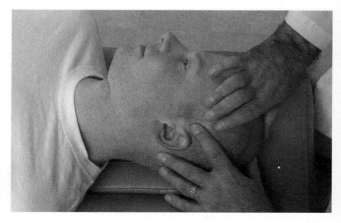

Figure 8.22   Treatment of the squamosal counterstrain point.

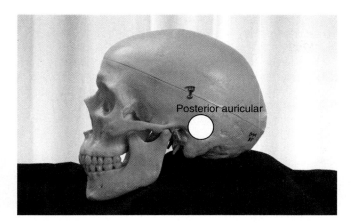

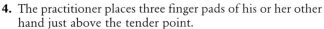

Figure 8.23   Location of the posterior auricular counterstrain point.

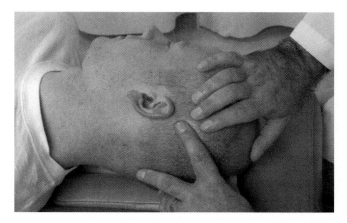

Figure 8.24   Treatment of the posterior auricular counterstrain point.

4. The practitioner places three finger pads of his or her other hand just above the tender point.
5. Using these three finger pads, the practitioner gently pulls the soft tissues superiorly until the position of greatest comfort is achieved.
6. This position is held for 90 seconds.
7. The practitioner slowly releases his or her hand pressure.
8. The practitioner rechecks the tender point.

Pterygoid Muscle Inhibition Release

- Example: right lateral pterygoid muscle restriction
- Treatment: The procedure is performed as follows:
  1. The patient is supine.
  2. The practitioner stands at the patient's right side.
  3. The practitioner places his or her left hand on the patient's head to prevent rotational or sidebending movement.
  4. The practitioner inserts his or her gloved right little finger into the patient's mouth along the lateral aspect of the right upper teeth until contact is made with the lateral pterygoid muscle. The muscle typically is exquisitely tender to palpation.
  5. The practitioner maintains steady digital pressure on the lateral pterygoid muscle within the patient's tolerance level until softening of the fascial tissues and relaxation of the muscle is felt.
  6. The practitioner retests the patient.

Temporomandibular Joint Myofascial Release Technique

- The myofascial release technique is also useful in the case of restricted opening or lateral movement of the jaw (described in the evaluation methods in the previous techniques).
- The procedure is performed as follows:
  1. The patient is supine (Fig. 8.25).
  2. The practitioner sits at the head of the table.

3. The practitioner grasps the patient's mandible bilaterally, using his or her thumbs and index fingers to grasp the anterior and posterior borders of the ramus of the mandible.
4. The practitioner first gently tests the superior and inferior motions of the mandible by moving it passively in these directions. If the mandible moves more easily in one direction or the other, the practitioner observes the direction of ease of motion.
5. The practitioner next tests the anterior and posterior motion of the mandible by moving the mandible bilaterally in these directions. A typical finding is that the mandible moves more easily in an anterior direction on one side and a posterior direction on the opposite side. The practitioner observes these directions of ease of motion.
6. The practitioner then moves the mandible gently as far as possible in the previously observed directions of ease and holds it in this position until softening and relaxation of the myofascial tissues occurs.
7. The practitioner retests the patient.

ADJUNCT TREATMENTS

- Other therapeutic approaches may be helpful in the relief of TMJ dysfunction:
  1. Acupuncture
  2. Hypnosis
  3. Biofeedback
  4. Relaxation therapy
  5. Applied kinesiology[19]

EDUCATION

- The following self-care techniques may provide temporary pain relief:
  1. Local treatment with moist heat or ice
  2. Using soft or blended foods to allow the jaw some temporary rest

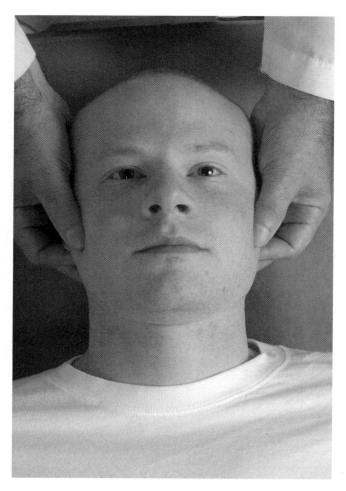

Figure 8.25 Myofascial release technique for the temporomandibular joint region.

3. Avoiding hard, crunchy, and chewy foods
4. Avoiding overstretching the mouth
5. Over-the-counter analgesics
6. Specific jaw exercises to help increase jaw mobility (recommended exercises are found later in this chapter and on the accompanying CD)
7. Relaxation techniques such as slow, deep breathing; meditation; and guided imagery to help reduce or alleviate pain

EXERCISES FOR TEMPOROMANDIBULAR JOINT DYSFUNCTION

- Perform each of the following exercises three times each day.
- For each of the exercises, do the following:
  1. Perform the movement for 10 repetitions and then rest for 30 to 60 seconds.
  2. Repeat step 1 two more times, thereby doing 3 sets of 10 repetitions for each exercise.

Exercise for an Inability to Fully Open the Jaw

- The exercise is performed as follows:
  1. Open your mouth as wide as you can, doing this gently until you begin to feel your jaw muscles stretch.
  2. Place your fingers on the top of your chin.
  3. Close your mouth while you gently resist this movement with your fingers.
  4. Hold this position for 3 to 5 seconds.
  5. Relax your jaw.
  6. Keep your fingers on your chin and open your jaw a little further until you feel your jaw muscles begin to stretch again.
  7. Repeat steps 1 through 6 until you have performed 3 sets of 10 repetitions.

Exercise for Increasing Side-to-Side Movement of the Jaw

The exercise is performed as follows:
  1. With your mouth slightly open, move your jaw to the left as far as you can comfortably (Fig. 8.26).
  2. Place the fingers of your right hand on your right lower jaw.
  3. Move your jaw to the right while you gently resist this movement with your fingers.

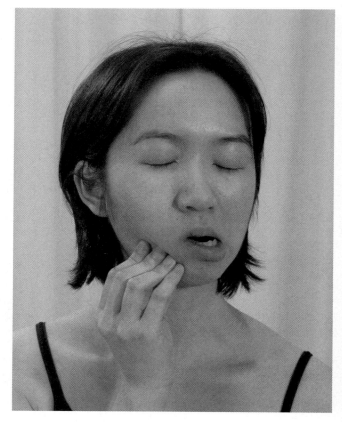

Figure 8.26 Exercise for restricted side-to-side jaw movement.

4. Hold this position for 3 to 5 seconds.
5. Relax your jaw.
6. Keep your fingers on your chin, and move your jaw a little further to the right without forcing it.
7. Repeat steps 1 through 6 until you have performed 3 sets of 10 repetitions.
8. Repeat the entire exercise in the opposite direction.

Exercise for Increasing the Forward and Backward Movement of the Jaw

- The exercise is performed as follows:
  1. With your mouth slightly open, push your jaw forward as far as you can comfortably (Figs. 8.27 and 8.28).
  2. Hold your jaw in this position for 3 to 5 seconds.
  3. Relax your jaw.
  4. Repeat steps 1 through 3 until you have performed 3 sets of 10 repetitions.

CONTROVERSIES

- Numerous theories about the cause of TMJ dysfunction have been proposed. Some, such as nutritional deficiencies and hormonal imbalances, remain unclear and have

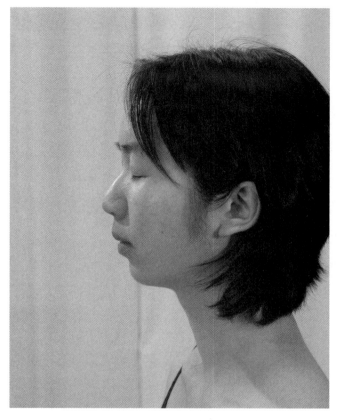

Figure 8.28   Exercise for increasing backward movement of the jaw.

little documentation. There is no universal agreement on the causes of TMJ dysfunction.
- Myriad treatment options have been advocated for TMJ dysfunction. A number of treatment approaches have little evidence base for their use. Controversy exists regarding the effectiveness of some treatment approaches.
- The belief that certain symptoms, such as dizziness or cardiac arrhythmia, may sometimes be part of TMJ dysfunction has engendered much disagreement among various health care practitioners.
- Health care practitioners involved in the care of patients with this problem have not agreed on a standardized approach to the diagnosis of TMJ dysfunction.

OPPORTUNITIES FOR RESEARCH

- Areas for research on TMJ dysfunction include the following:
  1. Collection of precise epidemiologic data on the incidence and prevalence of TMJ dysfunction
  2. Determination of the most effective technologies for the diagnosis of TMJ dysfunction
  3. Studies to scientifically determine the most effective treatments for TMJ dysfunction

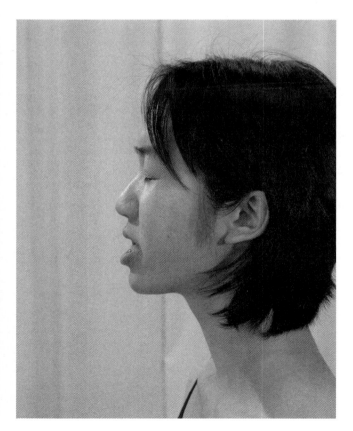

Figure 8.27   Exercise for increasing forward movement of the jaw.

REFERENCES

1. Kraus S (ed): Temporomandibular disorders, 2nd ed. New York, Churchill Livingstone, 1994.
2. Hruby R: The total body approach to the osteopathic management of temporomandibular joint dysfunction. J Am Osteopath Assoc 85:502-510, 1985.
3. Celiker R, Gokce-Kutsal Y, Eryilmaz M: Temporomandibular joint involvement in rheumatoid arthritis: Relationship with disease activity. Scand J Rheumatol 24:22-25, 1995.
4. Garcia R, Arrington JA: The relationship between cervical whiplash and temporomandibular joint injuries: An MRI study. Cranio 14:233-239, 1996.
5. Griffith HW: Complete Guide to Symptoms, Illness and Surgery. New York, Putnam Publishing Group; Electronic rights by Medical Data Exchange. Available at http://www.mdadvice.com/library/symp/illness506.html/ Accessed August 29, 1005.
6. Knight J: Diagnosis and treatment of temporomandibular joint disorders in primary care. Hosp Physician Jun:55-58, 1999.
7. Isberg A: Temporomandibular Joint Dysfunction: A Practitioner's Guide. United Kingdom, Isis Medical Media, 2001.
8. Swanson CE, Hayman LA, Diaz-Marchan PJ, et al: Imaging the temporal fossa. AJR Am J Roentgenol 168:801-806, 1997.
9. Coulter I, Hurwitz E, Adams A, et al: The appropriateness of manipulation and mobilization of the cervical spine. Santa Monica, CA, RAND, 1996.
10. Martini G, Martini M, Carano A: MRI study of a physiotherapeutic protocol in anterior disk displacement without reduction. Cranio 14:216-224, 1996.
11. Chinappi AS Jr, Getzoff H: The dental-chiropractic co-treatment of structural disorders of the jaw and temporomandibular joint dysfunction. J Manipulative Physiol Ther 18:476-481, 1995.
12. Hargreaves AS, Wardle JJ: The use of physiotherapy in the treatment of temporomandibular disorders. Br Dent J 155:121-124, 1983.
13. McCarty WL, Darnell MW: Rehabilitation of the temporomandibular joint through the application of motion. Cranio 11:298-307, 1993.
14. Blood SD: The craniosacral mechanism and the temporomandibular joint. J Am Osteopath Assoc 86:512-519, 1986.
15. Saghafi D, Curl DD: Chiropractic manipulation of anteriorly displaced temporomandibular disk with adhesion. J Manipulative Physiol Ther 18:98-104, 1995.
16. Haldeman SD: Spinal manipulation: When, how, and who? Bull Hosp Joint Dis 55:135-137, 1996.
17. Kuchera ML, DiGiovanna EL, Greenman PE: Efficacy and complications. In Ward RC (ed): Foundations for Osteopathic Medicine, 2nd ed. Philadelphia, Lippincott Williams & Wilkins, 2003, pp 1143-1152.
18. Powell FC, Hanigan WC, Olivero WC: A risk/benefit analysis of spinal manipulation therapy for relief of lumbar or cervical pain. Neurosurgery 33:73-78, 1993.
19. Novey DW (ed): The Clinician's Complete Reference to Complementary/Alternative Medicine. St. Louis, Mosby, 2000, pp 310-314.

SUGGESTED READING

Bates RE, Stewart CM, Atkinson WB: The relationship between internal derangements of the temporomandibular joint and systemic joint laxity. J Am Dent Assoc 109: 446-450, 1984.
Bledsoe WS: Temporomandibular joint space analysis. Cranio 12:177-178, 1994.
Brooks SL, Westesson PL: Temporomandibular joint: Value of coronal MR images. Radiology 188: 17-321, 1993.
Cederberg RA: Temporomandibular joint space analysis. Cranio 12:172-177, 1994.
Chen J, Buckwalter K: Displacement analysis of the temporomandibular condyle from magnetic resonance images. J Biomech 26:1455-1462, 1993.

Dijkstra PU, de Bont LG, van der Weele LT, et al: The relationship between temporomandibular joint mobility and peripheral joint mobility reconsidered. Cranio 12:149-155, 1994.
Dijkstra PU, de Bont LG, de Leeuw R, et al: Temporomandibular joint osteoarthrosis and temporomandibular joint hypermobility. Cranio 11:268-275, 1993.
Friedman MH, Weisberg J: Joint play movements of the temporomandibular joint: Clinical considerations. Arch Phys Med Rehabil 65:413-417, 1984.
Funakoshi M, Fujita N, Takehana S: Relations between occlusal interference and jaw muscle activities in response to changes in head position. J Dent Res 55:684-690, 1976.
Gerard MW, Laughon MM, Colley JL 3rd, et al: Trends in temporomandibular joint surgery. Med Prog Technol 21:171-175, 1996-1997.
Goddard G: Articular disk displacement of TMJ due to trauma. Cranio 11:221-223, 1993.
Graber TM: Craniofacial and dentitional development. In Falkner F (ed): Human Development. Philadelphia, WB Saunders, 1966, pp 510-581.
Gundlach KK: Malformations of the temporo-mandibular joint in laboratory animals and in man. Ann Anat 181:73-75, 1999.
Helland MM: Anatomy and function of the temporomandibular joint. In GP Grieve (ed): Modern Manual Therapy of the Vertebral Column. Edinburgh, Churchill Livingstone, 1986, pp 64-76.
Helms CA: Temporomandibular joint. In TH Berquist (ed): MRI of the Musculoskeletal System, 2nd ed. New York, Raven Press, 1990, pp 75-85.
Hinton RJ: Relationships between mandibular joint size and craniofacial size in human groups. Arch Oral Biol 28:37-43, 1983.
Hodges DC: Temporomandibular joint osteoarthritis in a British skeletal population. Am J Phys Anthropol 85:367-377, 1991.
Hruby R: The total body approach to the osteopathic management of temporomandibular joint dysfunction. J Am Osteopath Assoc 85:502-510, 1985.
Kononen M, Waltimo A, Nystrom M: Does clicking in adolescence lead to painful temporomandibular joint locking? Lancet 347:1080-1081, 1996.
Mintz SS: Craniomandibular dysfunction in children and adolescents: A review. Cranio 11:224-231, 1993.
Muller-Leisse C, Augthun M, Bauer W, et al: Anterior disc displacement without reduction in the temporomandibular joint: MRI and associated clinical findings. J Magn Reson Imaging 6:769-774, 1996.
Nance EP Jr, Powers TA: Imaging of the temporomandibular joint. Radiol Clin North Am 28:1019-1031, 1990.
Piehslinger E, Celar RM, Horejs T, et al: Recording orthopedic jaw movements. Part IV. The rotational component during mastication. Cranio 12:156-160, 1994.
Plesh O, Wolfe F, Lane N: The relationship between fibromyalgia and temporomandibular disorders: Prevalence and symptom severity. J Rheumatol 23:1948-1952, 1996.
Ramieri G, Bonardi G, Morani V, et al: Development of nerve fibres in the temporomandibular joint of the human fetus. Anat Embryol (Berl) 194:57-64, 1996.
Ramos-Remus C, Perez-Rocha O, Ludwig RN, et al: Magnetic resonance changes in the temporomandibular joint in ankylosing spondylitis. J Rheumatol 24:123-127, 1997.
Ramos-Remus C, Major P, Gomez-Vargas A, et al: Temporomandibular joint osseous morphology in a consecutive sample of ankylosing spondylitis patients. Ann Rheum Dis 56:103-107, 1997.
Roessler DM: A management approach for temporomandibular disorders. Aust Fam Physician 21:1271-1282, 1992.
Suenaga S, Hamamoto S, Kawano K, et al: Dynamic MR imaging of the temporomandibular joint in patients with arthrosis: Relationship between contrast enhancement of the posterior disk attachment and joint pain. AJR Am J Roentgenol 166:1475-1481, 1996.
Werner JA, Tillmann B, Schleicher A: Functional anatomy of the temporomandibular joint. A morphologic study on human autopsy material. Anat Embryol (Berl) 183: 89-95, 1991.
Wilkinson TM: Chewing over temporomandibular disorders [editorial]. Med J Aust 167: 117-118, 1997.
Yamada Y, Haraguchi N: Reflex changes in the masticatory muscles with load perturbations during chewing hard and soft food. Brain Res 669:86-92, 1995.
Zonnenberg AJ, Van Maanen CJ, Oostendorp RA, et al: Body posture photographs as a diagnostic aid for musculoskeletal disorders related to temporomandibular disorders (TMD). Cranio 14:225-232, 1996.

CHAPTER 9

Shoulder Pain and Dysfunction

DEFINITION

- The terms *shoulder pain* and *dysfunction* refer to pain and decreased mobility localized to the shoulder region, which usually includes the area between the base of the neck and the elbow, but more specifically refers to the region of the deltoid muscle, the acromioclavicular joint, the superior part of the trapezius muscle, and the scapula.
- Shoulder pain and dysfunction that is treatable with manual medicine is characterized by pain and decreased quality or quantity of motion on active or passive movement of the shoulder, is directly related to the shoulder joints and articulations, and is of musculoskeletal origin.
- The preferred term for the mechanical condition of the shoulder that responds to manual medicine is *shoulder somatic dysfunction*.
- The literature uses the term *shoulder disorder* to describe the mechanical dysfunction or pain of the shoulder joint and its surrounding supportive structures, but it does not distinguish between types of disorders that respond to manipulation and those that do not.
- Several clinic trials have defined the *shoulder girdle* to include the cervicothoracic spine and upper ribs. Shoulder pain and dysfunction stemming from shoulder girdle somatic dysfunction are most amenable to manipulative treatment.

EPIDEMIOLOGY

Age

- All ages are affected by this shoulder pain and dysfunction.
- Peak incidence occurs between the ages of 40 and 60 years.

Gender

- Females are more prone to have shoulder pain and somatic dysfunction than males.

Prevalence

- Shoulder symptoms are one of the most common musculoskeletal disorders.
- In a survey of 4110 people in the United Kingdom, the shoulder (16%) was the third most common site for musculoskeletal pain complaints, following the back (23%) and knee (19%) regions. It was most commonly associated with neck pain.[1]
- The incidence in a Dutch population study of more than 1.5 million patient encounters in a 1-year period in 96 general practices was 19 cases per 1000 person-years. [2]
- The annual incidence of shoulder disorders is estimated at 10 to 25 cases per 1000 persons. [3]
- Point prevalence is estimated at 21%.[4]
- Prevalence estimates vary depending on the definition used: [5]
  1. If the definition of "pain in the shoulder" does not include the upper trunk or neck, the 1-month period prevalence is 31%.
  2. If the definition of "pain in the shoulder" includes the upper trunk and neck, the 1-month period prevalence is 48%.
- Shoulder pain point prevalence (i.e., on the day of the interview) is 32%.
- Shoulder pain plus disability prevalence is 20%.

Natural Clinical Course

- Only about 30% to 50% of patients with shoulder pain or dysfunction seek medical care.[6]
- Most people cope with their shoulder dysfunction without seeking medical care.
- About 50% of all episodes of shoulder disorders presenting in primary care persist for at least 1 year, regardless of treatment.[6]
- Rapid recovery is associated with an acute onset of symptoms, a short interval between onset and initial presentation to a practitioner, recent activities, or slight trauma-related injuries (i.e., sprains and strains of the shoulder).[7]

- Patients with recurrent shoulder problems or increased severity of symptoms and disability at onset tend to have a prolonged clinical course.[6]
- Being female, reporting gradual onset of symptoms, and having a higher baseline disability appear to be independently associated with prolongation of shoulder pain and dysfunction.[8]

Effect on Society

- About 95% of all patients with shoulder disorders are treated in primary health care.[6]
- About 10% of physical therapy referrals are for shoulder disorders.[6]
- Shoulder disorders account for the third largest group of patients with musculoskeletal disorders seen in primary care, following low back and neck disorders.[6]
- Patients with shoulder disorders account for about 6% of health care costs, making them the second most costly diagnostic group.[6]
- Approximately 18% of all sick leave benefit claims for musculoskeletal disorders concern neck and shoulder problems.[6]
- Workers sustaining shoulder injuries are subject to significant lost wages and rehabilitation costs to society, and workers' compensation claims are considerable.
- Female patients older than 60 years have a more prolonged, persistent-recurrent course of illness. [9]

Risk Factors

Common Causes of Shoulder Pain and Decreased Mobility
- Reduced mobility of the cervicothoracic junction has an 84% positive predictive value for shoulder disorder and increases the risk of developing shoulder disorder threefold.[10]
- Other causes include the following[6]:
- Depression
  1. Elderly
  2. Impaired consciousness
  3. Osteophytes
  4. Surgical intervention
  5. Thoracic kyphosis
  6. Trauma

Work-Related Risk Factors
- High levels of distress[11,12]
- Repetitive shoulder motion[11,12]
- High job demands[11,12]
- Force and vibration[12]
- Manufacturing, food processing, lumber, transportation, and other heavy industries, which have the most physical exposures and highest rates of work-related upper extremity disorders[12]

Associated Conditions
- Several conditions are associated with pain and disability.
  1. Ankylosing spondylitis[6]

2. Diabetes mellitus
3. Fibromyalgia
4. Multiple sclerosis
5. Neck dysfunction
6. Osteoarthritis
7. Polymyalgia
8. Polyneuropathy
9. Rheumatoid arthritis
10. Stroke
- Psychosomatic symptoms in adolescents predicted neck and shoulder pain 7 years later as young adults.[13]
- Women sewing machine operators living alone with children, smoking, with low social support, and increased social stress have increased risk of contracting a neck or shoulder disorder.[14]

Perpetuating Factors
- Cervicothoracic spine and upper ribs somatic dysfunction that maintain shoulder dysfunction[6]
- Fear-avoidance behavior
- Psychosocial, cognitive, and behavioral traits

FUNCTIONAL ANATOMY

The Shoulder

Shoulder Joint and Articulations
- The shoulder complex consists of the scapula, clavicle, and humerus[15] (Fig. 9.1).
- The shoulder has three joints: glenohumeral, acromioclavicular, and sternoclavicular. Only the sternoclavicular joint connects the shoulder complex to the axial skeleton; the others are linked by muscles. The main functional unit that is not a joint is the scapulothoracic (ST) articulation.
- The ligamentous structures involved are the acromioclavicular, coracoclavicular, and the glenohumeral capsules (supported by the glenohumeral and coracohumeral ligaments) and the glenoid labrum.[16] The coracoacromial ligament forms an arch, beneath which the supraspinatus muscle tendon passes.
- The *shoulder girdle* classically refers to the two scapulae and two clavicles, but according to some study authors, it also includes the ribs, their costovertebral joints and ligaments, and their costochondral and chondrosternal articulations.

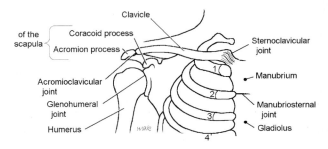

Figure 9.1 Anterior view of the right shoulder complex, composed of the scapula, clavicle, and humerus.

The cervical and thoracic vertebrae and their joints and ligaments are also components of the shoulder girdle.

Shoulder Muscles

- The shoulder muscles and their origins, insertions, actions, innervations, and spinal cord levels are listed in Table 9.1.
- The shoulder muscles may be divided functionally into two groups. An inner group (i.e., inner cone) consists of the supraspinatus, infraspinatus, teres minor, and subscapularis, which are also collectively known as the *rotator cuff* of the shoulder (Fig. 9.2); an outer group (i.e., outer cone) includes the remaining shoulder muscles.
- The rotator cuff muscles all originate from the scapula and insert on the head of the humerus and move the humerus in relation to the scapula. The first letters of these muscles spell the word SITS.
  1. *S*upraspinatus abducts the arm.
  2. *I*nfraspinatus externally rotates the arm.
  3. *T*eres minor externally rotates the arm.
  4. *S*ubscapularis internally rotates the arm.

Table 9.1   Shoulder muscles

Muscle	Origin	Insertion	Action	Innervation (Nerve)	Spinal Cord Level
Biceps brachii (long head)	Supraglenoid tubercle of scapula	Tuberosity of radius and aponeurosis of biceps brachii	Flexes shoulder joint	Musculocutaneous	C5-6
Coracobrachialis	Apex of coracoid process of scapula	Medial surface of middle of humerus shaft	Flexes and adducts the shoulder joint	Musculocutaneous	C6-7
Deltoid	Lateral third of clavicle, acromion process, scapular spine	Deltoid tuberosity of humerus	Abducts shoulder joint from 15 degrees to 90 degrees, involved in all shoulder joint motions	Axillary	C5-6
Infraspinatus	Infraspinous fossa of scapula	Midportion of greater tubercle of humerus and shoulder joint capsule	Externally rotates the shoulder joint	Suprascapular	C5-6
Latissimus dorsi	Spinous processes of lower thoracic vertebrae and ribs, lumbodorsal fascia, crest of ilium, inferior angle of scapula	Intertubercular groove of humerus	Adducts, extends, internally rotates the shoulder joint	Thoracodorsal Anterior thoracic	C6-8 C5-T1
Levator scapulae	Transverse processes of C1-C4	Medial border of scapula, above root of scapular spine	Elevates scapula	Cervical Dorsal scapular	C3-4 C5
Pectoralis major	Sternum, clavicle, cartilages of first 6 or 7 ribs, aponeurosis of external oblique	Crest of greater tubercle of humerus	Adducts and internally rotates shoulder joint	Lateral pectoral	C5-7
Pectoralis minor	Ribs 3-5 and fascia of intercostal muscles	Coracoid process of scapula	Rotates scapula anteriorly and inferiorly	Pectoral	C7-T1
Rhomboid major	Spinous processes of 2nd through 5th thoracic vertebrae	Medial border of scapula, below root of scapular spine	Retracts and elevates the scapula	Dorsal scapular	C5
Rhomboid minor	Spine of 7th cervical and 1st thoracic vertebrae, lower part of nuchal ligament	Medial margin of scapula, at the root of the scapular spine	Retracts and elevates the scapula	Dorsal scapular	C4-5
Serratus anterior	Outer surfaces and superior borders of ribs 1-9	Costal surface of medial border of scapula	Abducts the shoulder joint and protracts the scapula	Long thoracic	C5-8
Subclavius	Sternal end of rib 1	Inferior and lateral aspects of clavicle	Stabilizes sternoclavicular joint	Subclavius	C5-6

Continued

Table 9.1   Shoulder muscles—cont'd

Muscle	Origin	Insertion	Action	Innervation (Nerve)	Spinal Cord Level
Subscapularis	Subscapular fossa of scapula	Lesser tubercle of humerus and shoulder joint capsule	Internally rotates the shoulder joint	Subscapular	C5-7
Supraspinatus	Supraspinous fossa of scapula	Superior aspect of greater tubercle of humerus and shoulder joint capsule	Abducts the shoulder joint (first 15 degrees)	Suprascapular	C4-6
Teres major	Inferior medial border of scapula	Crest of lesser tubercle of humerus	Internally rotates, adducts, and extends shoulder joint	Lower subscapular	C5-7
Teres minor	Lateral border of scapula	Lower aspect of greater tubercle of humerus	Externally rotates and extends shoulder joint	Axillary	C5-6
Trapezius	Superior nuchal line of occipital bone, nuchal ligament, spines of 7th cervical and all thoracic vertebrae	Lateral third of clavicle, median margin of acromion, scapular spine	Upper fibers elevate and lower fibers depress the scapula; both laterally rotate and retract the scapula on thoracic wall	Spinal accessory Cervical	CN XI C2-4
Triceps brachii, long head	Infraglenoid tubercle of scapula	Olecranon process of ulna	Adducts and extends the shoulder joint	Radial	C6-T1

- Most of the remaining shoulder muscles originate from the spine or rib cage and insert on the scapula or humerus.
- The deep muscles of the anterior shoulder region include the subclavius, pectoralis minor, and biceps muscles (Fig. 9.3A).
- The superficial layer anteriorly also entails the pectoralis major muscle, which attaches to the clavicle and to the sternum and upper ribs (see Fig. 9.3B).
- Posteriorly, the superficial trapezius, the latissimus dorsi, and deltoid muscles can be seen overlying the intermediate muscles such as the rhomboids, levator scapulae, and rotator cuff muscles attached to the posterior aspect of the scapula (Fig. 9.4).

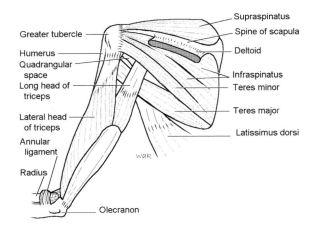

Figure 9.2   Posterior view of three of the four left shoulder rotator cuff muscles: supraspinatus, infraspinatus, and teres minor. Subscapularis can be visualized only from the anterior view of the scapula.

- Each scapula has 17 muscles attached to it:
  1. Posteriorly, from superficial to deep: trapezius, rhomboid major, rhomboid minor, supraspinatus, infraspinatus, levator scapulae, teres minor, teres major, latissimus dorsi, serratus anterior, and subscapularis
  2. Anteriorly, from superficial to deep: deltoid, biceps, coracobrachialis, triceps, pectoralis minor, and omohyoid
  3. Because the shoulder complex has myofascial attachments that extend into the cervical, thoracic, and even pelvic regions, the practitioner needs to be aware that somatic dysfunction in these regions are affected by and can affect shoulder somatic dysfunction.

Shoulder Motions
- The glenohumeral articulation motions include the following:
  1. Flexion: motion in a sagittal plane about a transverse axis through the humeral head, which moves the elbow anteriorly
  2. Extension: motion about the same axis as flexion, which moves the elbow posteriorly
  3. Abduction: motion in a coronal plane about a horizontal anteroposterior axis through the humeral head, which moves the elbow laterally away from the thorax
  4. Adduction: motion about the same axis as for abduction, which moves the elbow medially toward the thorax
  5. External rotation: motion about an axis parallel to the long axis of the humerus, which brings moves the lateral condyle of the elbow posteriorly
  6. Internal rotation: motion about the same axis as for external rotation, which moves the lateral condyle anteriorly
  7. Circumduction: rotation of the arm about a pivot, the glenohumeral articulation[17]

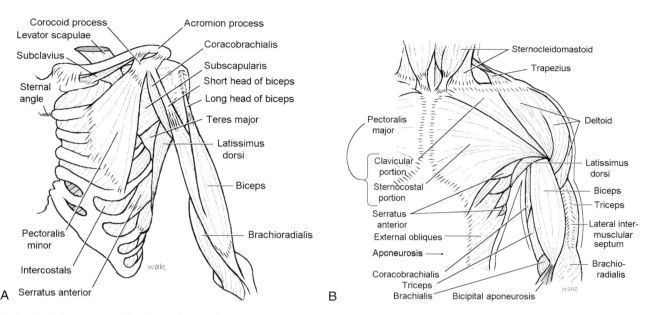

Figure 9.3 **A,** Anterior view of the deep left shoulder muscles. Notice that the fourth rotator cuff muscle, the subscapularis, is visible in this view. **B,** Left shoulder muscles: anterior view of the superficial anterior and deep posterior muscles.

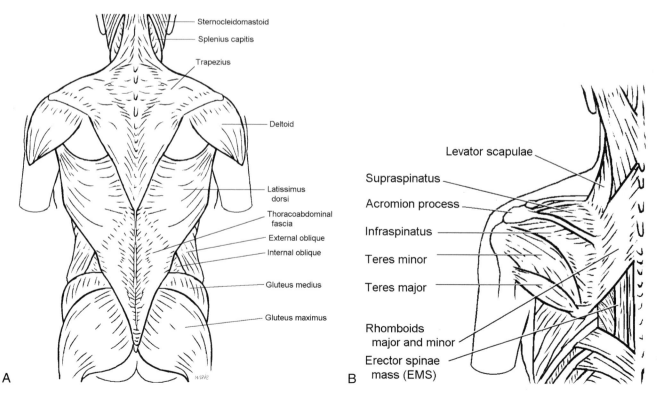

Figure 9.4 **A,** Posterior view of superficial layer of shoulder muscles: trapezius, latissimus dorsi and deltoid muscles. With permission from Gray's Anatomy 35th British Edition, Saunders Co., Philadelphia, 1973:533. **B,** Posterior view of the intermediate layer of the left shoulder muscles.

Table 9.2   Shoulder motions

Movements of the Shoulder Joint	Range of Motion (degrees)	Muscles
Flexion	180	Deltoid (anterior), coracobrachialis, pectoralis major (clavicular head), biceps
Extension	40-60	Latissimus dorsi, teres major, deltoid (posterior), teres minor, triceps (long head)
Abduction	60 (in internal rotation) 180 (in external rotation)	Deltoid (middle), supraspinatus, deltoid (anterior and posterior), serratus anterior
Adduction	35 (with shoulder flexed to 90 degrees)	Pectoralis major, latissimus dorsi, teres major, deltoid (anterior)
External rotation	90	Infraspinatus, teres minor, deltoid (posterior)
Internal rotation	90	Subscapularis, pectoralis major, latissimus dorsi, teres major, deltoid (anterior)

8. Further details regarding motions of the shoulder complex are given in Table 9.2.

• The ST articulation motions include the following:

1. Elevation: superior movement of the distal end of the clavicle, along with concomitant inferior movement of the medial end, around an anteroposterior axis just lateral to the joint at the costoclavicular ligament. The range of elevation is about 45 degrees.

2. Depression: inferior movement of the distal end of the clavicle, along with concomitant superior movement of the medial end, around the same axis as that for elevation. The range of depression is about 15 degrees.

3. Protraction: anterior movement of the distal end of the clavicle about a vertical axis located at the costoclavicular ligament. The range of protraction is about 15 degrees.

4. Retraction: posterior movement of the distal end of the clavicle about the same axis as that for protraction. The range of protraction is about 15 degrees.

5. Rotation: posterior rotation of the clavicle around a longitudinal axis that runs through the clavicle. The range of rotational motion is 30 to 45 degrees.[18]

6. More information regarding these scapular motions is given in Table 9.3.

• The acromioclavicular articulation motions include the following:

1. Scapular rotation: motion around an anteroposterior axis located between the acromioclavicular joint and the coracoclavicular ligament

2. Winging: motion around a vertical axis running through the midline of the body of the scapula

3. Tipping: posterior movement of the inferior angle with a concomitant anterior movement of the superior scapular border around a coronal axis through the middle of the body of the scapula[16]

4. These motions are small and have a wide range of individual differences; degrees of motion are not usually described with these movements.

Scapulohumeral Rhythm

• Normally, elevation of the humerus can be accomplished to about 180 degrees. The glenohumeral articulation contributes about 120 degrees of elevation available to the humerus, with the remaining motion provided by the scapulothoracic articulation through the sternoclavicular and acromioclavicular articular structures.

• This movement is known as the *scapulohumeral rhythm*. It results in the smooth and coordinated maximal amount of motion available to the upper extremity.[17]

Shoulder Bursae

• Two major bursae are associated with the shoulder complex: the subacromial and subdeltoid bursae. They separate the supraspinatus tendon and head of the humerus from the acromion, coracoid process, coracoacromial ligament, and deltoid muscle, and they permit smooth motion between the humerus and supraspinatus tendon and the surrounding structures.[16]

Thoracic (Costal) Cage

Costal Articulations

• The thoracic cage is composed of anterior, posterior, lateral, superior, and inferior elements. These elements include the sternum, thoracic spine, ribs, operculum, and thoracoabdominal diaphragm (Fig. 9.5).

• The heads of the second through the ninth ribs each articulate between the body of its own vertebra and the vertebral body above (e.g., second rib is between the bodies of T2 and T1).

Table 9.3   Scapular motions

Movement of the Scapula	Range of Motion (degrees)	Muscles
Elevation	60	Trapezius (superior), levator scapulae, rhomboid major, and minor
Depression	5-10	Trapezius (inferior), pectoralis minor
Protraction	10	Serratus anterior
Retraction	15	Rhomboid major and minor, trapezius

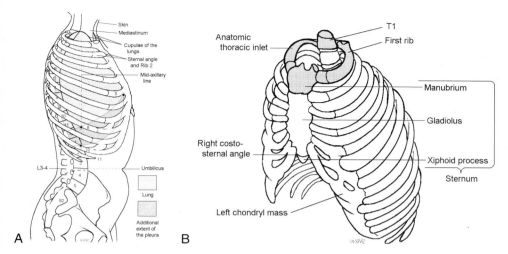

Figure 9.5 **A,** Right lateral view of the thoracic cage. **B,** Left anterolateral view of the costal cage.

- The tubercles of all ribs, except the 11th and 12th, articulate with their own vertebral transverse processes. The first rib head articulates with the body and transverse process of the first thoracic vertebra, but it does not touch the seventh cervical vertebra. Similarly, ribs 10, 11, and 12 have unifacet articulations with their own vertebral bodies.
- Cartilage is interposed between the ribs and the manubrium or sternum.
- The first rib articulates with the manubrium anteriorly by a synchondrosis consisting of a long piece of flexible cartilage that can be palpated near the manubrium for about 2 cm below the inferior margin of the clavicle (Fig. 9.6).
- The second ribs articulate at the junction of the manubrium and the body of the sternum, known as the sternal angle. This is a reliable landmark from which to count ribs. From the manubrium, the second costal cartilage can be traced by palpation lateral about 6 cm before it passes posterosuperiorly behind the clavicle (see Fig. 9.6).

Costal Muscles
- The scalene muscles originate from the C2 to C7 transverse processes and act as secondary muscles of respiration. The anterior and middle scalene muscles insert onto the first ribs, and the posterior scalene muscles insert onto the second ribs (Fig. 9.7). They are used in muscle energy procedures to elevate these ribs to improve their motion.

Figure 9.6 Right first and second rib articulations with the manubrium and sternal angle, respectively. Notice the costoclavicular ligaments between the first rib and clavicle.

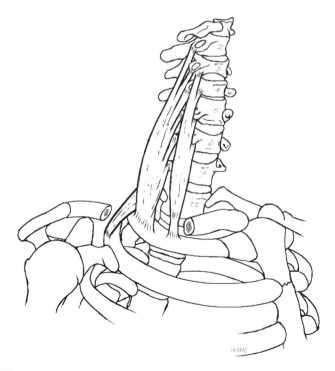

Figure 9.7 Right scalene muscles. With permission from Simons DG, Travel JG, Simons LS. Myofascial Pain and Dysfunction. Volume I. Upper Half of the Body. Second Edition. Baltimore: Williams and Wilkins 1999:507.

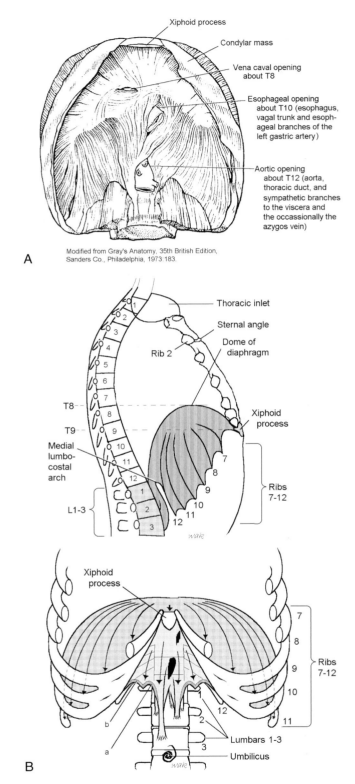

Modified from Gray's Anatomy, 35th British Edition, Sanders Co., Philadelphia, 1973:183.

Figure 9.8 **A,** Inferior surface of the thoracic diaphragm, showing its attachments. **B,** Lateral and anterior views of the thoracic diaphragm. With permission from Kapandji IA. The Physiology of the Joints. Volume III. The Trunk and the Vertebral Column. 2nd Edition. New York: Churchill Livingstone, 1974; Elsevier Science Limited 2002, page 147.

- The pectoralis major and minor muscles act as secondary muscles of inhalation in addition to their roles in shoulder motion. They are used in muscle energy procedures to improve upper rib mobility.
- The serratus anterior muscles attach to the superior aspects of ribs 1 through 9 and stabilize the scapulae. They are used in muscle energy manipulation procedures to improve the motion of these ribs.
- The intercostal muscles assist in exhalatory movement of the ribs.
- The thoracoabdominal diaphragm is the primary muscle of inhalation. It attaches to the lower six ribs, as well as the first three lumbar vertebral bodies (Fig. 9.8). The diaphragm is used in muscle energy rib manipulation and during functional techniques throughout the body to increase the effectiveness of these procedures.
- The quadratus lumborum muscles stabilize the 12th rib and act as secondary muscles of inhalation. They are used in muscle energy techniques to improve the motion of the 12th ribs.

Thoracic Cage Motions
- A line drawn from the head of the rib through its costotransverse joint approximates the axis of its respiratory movement. Each set of transverse processes projects more and more posteriorly from T1 through T12. As a result of this anatomic arrangement, the rib motion in the upper ribs mainly has a pump-handle character and that in the lower ribs mainly has a bucket-handle character (Fig. 9.9A).
- Ribs 11 and 12, however, are commonly described as having caliper action (see Fig. 9.9B).

PATHOPHYSIOLOGY

- Intrinsic shoulder pain can be caused by dysfunctions or inflammation within any of the previously described structures, but most commonly, pain is generated from the articulations, muscles, tendons, or ligaments of the shoulder complex and shoulder girdle.
- Pain on movement is often associated with an entrapment of subacromial soft tissue under the coracoacromial complex.
- Reduced range of motion is often associated with fibrosis and adhesions of the glenohumeral joint capsule and surrounding soft tissue structures.
- Loss of muscle strength occurs most often with tears of the rotator cuff muscles or biceps tendon.
- Whether these shoulder disorders are a continuum as part of the evolution of an initial strain or sprain is unclear.
- The impingement syndrome entails a series of pathologic changes in the supraspinatus tendon[19]:
  1. Stage I: hemorrhage and edema
  2. Stage II: tendonitis and fibrosis
  3. Stage III: tendon degeneration of the rotator cuff and biceps, bony changes, and tendon rupture
- Table 9.4 lists the various pathologic processes and diagnoses that can underlie shoulder pain and dysfunction.
- Although about 80% of patients with shoulder pain have a primary shoulder cause, the remaining 20% likely have cervical spine abnormalities on radiographs and normal

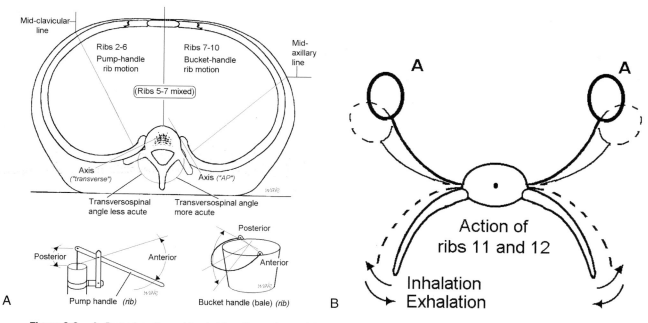

Figure 9.9 **A,** Pump-handle and bucket-handle motions of the ribs. **B,** Caliper or pincer motions of the 11th and 12th ribs.

Table 9.4   Differential diagnosis for shoulder pain and dysfunction

Pathophysiology*	Diagnosis	Characteristics
Vascular	Ischemia Hemarthrosis Avascular necrosis Thoracic outlet syndrome	History: acute pain at rest; hemophilia (hemarthrosis) Physical findings: pain, motion loss; hypertonic scalene muscles on affected side; hand is cold, pale; muscles fatigue on sustained muscle challenge; diminished brachial and radial pulses and blood pressure with subclavian artery compression in thoracic outlet syndrome Radiology: radiograph is normal unless pathology is caused by bony displacement or there is disintegration of joint due to necrosis; ultrasound shows accumulation of blood in hemarthrosis; technetium bone scan and MRI can detect necrosis in early stages
Inflammatory	Septic joint Tendonitis Bursitis Ligament sprain Adhesive capsulitis (acute) Traumatic arthritis	History: overuse; pain with movement; immobilization after inflammation followed by severe motion loss in adhesive capsulitis Physical findings: warmth, swelling, tender over inflamed structures; motion loss typically in abduction, external rotation, and some internal rotation Radiology: radiograph is normal Aspiration: white blood cells; organisms if infected
Neurologic (referred pain)	Cervical radiculopathy Internal organ disease	History: no shoulder trauma or motion loss; pain radiates beyond elbow in lower cervical radiculopathies Physical findings: normal shoulder movement and tissue feel Radiology: normal shoulder anatomy
Neurologic (lesion)	Cerebral vascular accident (CVA; i.e., stroke) Cervical lesion Axillary nerve palsy Subscapular nerve palsy Brachial plexus palsy Multiple sclerosis	History: no shoulder trauma or motion loss; CVA; cervical trauma or injury to nerve root or brachial plexus; excessive giggling or familial history may indicate multiple sclerosis Physical findings: painless weakness, muscle atrophy; flaccid paralysis after CVA; scalene muscle hypertonicity may be present with brachial plexus palsy (elevating first rib to compress brachial plexus as it traverses between first rib and clavicle) Radiology: radiograph shows normal shoulder skeletal structures, although cervical spine may show degenerative changes; brain CT may show hemorrhage; brain MRI may show ischemia or multiple sclerosis

Continued

Table 9.4   Differential diagnosis for shoulder pain and dysfunction—cont'd

Pathophysiology*	Diagnosis	Characteristics
Degenerative	Osteoarthritis	History: may have had past trauma Physical findings: motion loss Radiology: radiograph shows degenerative changes
Iatrogenic	After surgery	History: surgical repair Physical findings: motion loss, pain with movement, contractures Radiology: shows repaired structures; negative if soft tissue repair
Cancer	Primary tumor Metastasis	History: no trauma, no overuse; pain at rest, at night, or with movement; weakness Physical findings: normal or restricted motion, tenderness; muscle atrophy; extreme pain and weakness on muscle testing Radiology: radiograph may show loss of bony structure; MRI shows tumor
Autoimmune	Rheumatoid arthritis Systemic lupus Ankylosing spondylitis Gouty arthritis	History: bilateral joint pain, swelling Physical findings: warmth, swelling, tenderness; motion loss typically in abduction, external rotation, and some internal rotation. Radiology: radiograph may show deformation of joint; ultrasound shows inflammation of soft tissues Aspiration: white blood cells; urate crystals if gout
Trauma	Fracture Dislocation Muscle tear Labrum tear Capsular tear Instability (also atraumatic)	History: trauma, overuse Physical findings: displaced structures, motion loss, painful weakness in abduction and external rotation, extreme tenderness, swelling if acute, laxity if chronic after inflammation and muscle guarding have subsided; drop arm and empty can test results positive in rotator cuff tears; apprehension and relocation test results positive with instability or dislocation Radiology: radiograph is diagnostic for fracture and dislocation; ultrasound and MRI show soft tissue disruptions
Endocrine	Diabetes mellitus	History: no shoulder trauma or overuse; polydipsia, polyphagia, polyuria Physical findings: warmth, swelling, tender, motion loss, pain and weakness Radiology: normal Aspiration: white blood cells; organisms
Somatic	Somatic dysfunction Muscle imbalance Impingement Tendinosis Adhesive capsulitis (chronic)	History: trauma, overuse, pain with movement, stiffness, motion loss; pain worse at night may indicate impingement Physical findings: abnormalities of tissue texture, landmark asymmetry, restricted range of motion, sensitivity to digital pressure Radiology: normal or nonspecific

*Using the VINDICATES mnemonic.

shoulder radiographs. Tenderness on digital provocation of shoulder muscle motor points was associated with the cervical spondylosis in 407 patients complaining of shoulder pain.[20]

- Short leg; pronated foot; and lumbar, thoracic, cervical, and cranial somatic dysfunction may underlie development of a thoracic outlet syndrome or shoulder somatic dysfunction.[21]

DIFFERENTIAL DIAGNOSIS

- The practitioner of manual medicine should determine whether the shoulder pain and dysfunction is related to muscle imbalance, shoulder girdle dysfunction, inflammation, referred pain from systemic or internal organ disease, or disruption of anatomic structures.
- As with any pain complaint or neurologic dysfunction, the practitioner needs to discern the degree to which signs and symptoms are related to central or peripheral nervous system

pathophysiology. For example, a patient may have sprained her shoulder, but the recovery can be complicated if she has an underlying central nervous system disease such as multiple sclerosis.

- Table 9.4 lists differential diagnoses for shoulder pain and dysfunction and their distinguishing characteristics.

HISTORY

- When evaluating the patient with shoulder pain, information about the location, quality, radiation, aggravating or relieving factors, age, dominant hand, and sport or work activities are important determinants of several shoulder disorders.[22]
- For patients with pain in the upper arm or deltoid region and no history of fracture, dislocation, or systemic diseases as causes of the pain, a longer duration of symptoms, gradual onset of pain, and high pain intensity at presentation are predictors of

prolongation of symptoms for at least 6 months under conservative care (i.e., medications, steroid injections, and physical therapy).[23]

- A history of shoulder corticosteroid injections leads the practitioner to consider osteopenia and rotator cuff tendon atrophy as potential causes of persistent pain and dysfunction.
- A history of shoulder instability, stiffness, locking, catching, and swelling, along with a history of acute trauma, should be obtained.
- Cervical or thoracic spine and costal cage symptoms should be elicited.
- Pain worse at rest or at night and not related to movement is not shoulder girdle or joint specific and indicates further evaluation for systemic causes of the shoulder symptoms and dysfunction.
- Shoulder dysfunction that is treatable by manual medicine typically stems from overuse or trauma.
- Disuse of the shoulder from inflammation or pain caused by overuse or trauma can lead to contractures and frozen shoulder syndrome. The longer the duration of the condition, the higher the likelihood of a prolonged course of rehabilitation.
- The historical characteristics of shoulder somatic dysfunction are as follows:
  1. Intensity: Pain is sharp and severe when from acute muscle spasm, and it is dull and achy when chronic, as occurs after inflammatory processes subside.
  2. Precipitating factors
     Overuse or trauma, which usually entails inflammation of soft tissue structures, leads to muscle imbalance and shoulder dysfunction.

Movement makes the pain worse.
Cervical, thoracic, or costal somatic dysfunction or pain can precipitate or accompany shoulder pain and dysfunction.
  3. Location: Pain and motion abnormalities can be localized to specific shoulder structures and can include the lower cervical spine, upper thoracic spine, and upper ribs.
  4. Radiation: There may be radiation to the upper arm or back from shoulder somatic dysfunction.
  5. Characteristics: Motion loss, weakness, muscle imbalance, pain worse with movement, and tenderness to palpation are most common.
  6. Associated symptoms: Cervicothoracic and upper rib pain and dysfunction often accompany shoulder somatic dysfunction amenable to manipulation.

PHYSICAL FINDINGS

- There are essentially two groups of patients that complain of shoulder pain: those with limitations in range of motion and those without limitations in range of motion.[24,25]
- Results of the physical examination, including central and peripheral nervous system evaluations, should be negative for systemic or internal organ disease as causes of the shoulder pain and dysfunction.
- The shoulder region physical examination includes inspection, palpation, range of motion, strength, and sensation assessment, along with provocative special tests such as those listed in Table 9.5.

Table 9.5 Special tests

Test	Procedure	Positive Sign	Interpretation
Adson's	Practitioner passively slightly abducts and slightly extends patient's arm on affected side and palpates patient's radial pulse while patient turns head toward or away from the affected arm and inhales deeply.	Diminished pulse	Compression or occlusion of the subclavian artery as it traverses between the anterior and middle scalene muscles (thoracic outlet syndrome)
Apley's scratch	Patient touches superior and inferior aspects of opposite scapula.	Decreased range	Rotator cuff dysfunction
Apprehension	Practitioner abducts affected arm to 90 degrees, externally rotates and applies anterior pressure on the humerus.	Pain or apprehension about impending subluxation	Anterior glenohumeral instability
"Clunk"	With patient supine, practitioner passively rotates and flexes the affected shoulder through its range.	A "clunk" sound or clicking sensation is heard or felt	Glenoid labrum disorder (tear)
Cross-arm	Patient actively flexes the affected arm to 90 degrees and actively adducts across his or her trunk.	Pain at acromioclavicular joint	Acromioclavicular joint inflammation
Drop arm	Passively abduct patient's affected arm to at least 90 degrees and ask patient to lower it slowly down to the side.	Arm drops without control to the side	Rotator cuff tear; supraspinatus weakness
Empty can	Patient attempts to elevate arms against resistance with shoulder flexed to 90 degrees and internally rotated, elbow extended, and forearm pronated (thumb pointing inferiorly).	Weakness	Rotator cuff tear; suprascapular nerve entrapment or neuropathy

Continued

Table 9.5   Special tests—cont'd

Test	Procedure	Positive Sign	Interpretation
Hawkin's	Practitioner passively forward flexes patient's shoulder to 90 degrees and internally rotates it.	Subacromial pain	Supraspinatus tendon impingement or rotator cuff tendonitis
Neer's	Patient's arm is passively flexed and forearm pronated.	Subacromial pain	Subacromial impingement
Relocation	Practitioner performs this after a positive apprehension test result with patient supine. Practitioner applies a posterior force on patient's humerus while externally rotating the arm.	Decrease in pain or apprehension	Anterior glenohumeral joint instability
Scapula winging	Patient pushes against the wall with practitioner behind patient observing scapulae for symmetry and degree of "winged" appearance of medial border.	Medial scapula border displays posterior displacement	Serratus anterior weakness or injury
Speed's	Patient's elbow is passively flexed to 20-30 degrees and forearm is supinated with the shoulder flexed to 60 degrees. The practitioner resists patient's active attempts to further flex the affected shoulder while palpating with the other hand the proximal biceps tendon at the shoulder.	Pain or lateral or medial movement of the biceps tendon	Biceps tendon instability or tendonitis
Spurling's	With patient seated, patient actively extends his or her spine, and practitioner passively rotates patient's head to the side of the affected shoulder while pressing down on the top of patient's head.	Radicular pain or paresthesias in a dermatomal pattern	Cervical nerve root impingement or inflammation
Sulcus sign	With patient's elbow flexed to 90 degrees, practitioner pulls downward on patient's elbow or wrist and observes the shoulder for a sulcus or depression lateral or inferior to the acromion.	Shoulder depression or sulcus upon provocation	Inferior glenohumeral joint instability
Yergason's	Patient's elbow is flexed to 90 degrees with the forearm pronated. Practitioner holds patient's wrist and resists patient's attempt to actively supinate and flex the elbow fully.	Pain in the biceps tendon (long head)	Biceps tendon instability or tendonitis

- Results of the special tests for joint and soft tissue integrity are typically negative in patients with shoulder somatic dysfunction. However, some muscle weakness may be found in, for example, the serratus anterior, supraspinatus, or deltoid muscles.
- Shoulder impingement is characterized by pain on active or passive movement and reduced passive range of motion, and it can be accompanied by loss of muscle strength during abduction and flexion.[6]
- Cervical and thoracic spine restriction of motion and tenderness may be present.[25,26]
- Reliable tests useful for determining treatment approaches in primary care are the active and passive abduction and passive external rotation tests (kappa > 0.4).[7] Pain with movement commonly indicates impingement, muscle spasm, or inflammatory disorders, whereas painless movement is indicative of chronic disorders typically requiring rehabilitation and possibly repair of damaged structures.
- Painful movement and restricted range of motion in all directions is found in adhesive capsulitis; external rotation is particularly decreased, and there is less decrease in abduction range of motion.
- Signs of a short leg; pronated foot; sacral base asymmetry; scoliosis; lumbar, thoracic, cervical, or elbow tenosynovitis; carpal tunnel syndrome; or cranial somatic dysfunction may be present.[21]

LABORATORY AND RADIOGRAPHIC FINDINGS

- Radiographs and laboratory test results are typically normal in cases of shoulder somatic dysfunction.
- Plain radiographs can detect congenital abnormalities, degenerative joint changes, dislocations, fractures, and separations.
- Ultrasound is useful to identify torn muscles or ligaments as well as swollen bursa or joint capsules.
- Magnetic resonance imaging (MRI) is useful in identifying torn muscles and ligaments, cancers, and atrophic changes in muscles.

- Diagnostic ultrasound, computed tomography (CT), and MRI are most commonly used for diagnosis of shoulder disorders refractory to conservative care.

MANUAL MEDICINE

Best Evidence

- The first randomized clinical trial evaluating the effectiveness of shoulder manipulation as an addition to standard care (i.e., nonsteroidal medication) compared with physiotherapy and corticosteroid injection was reported in the *British Medical Journal* by Winter and colleagues 1997.[27] There were three types of diagnostic categories, and subjects in each were randomly assigned to receive one of the three adjunct therapies:
  1. The synovial group consisted of patients with pain or limited movement in one or several directions of the glenohumeral joint. The pain was thought to originate from disorders of the subacromial structures, the acromioclavicular joint, the glenohumeral joint, or combinations of these synovial structures.
  2. The shoulder girdle group consisted of patients with pain and sometimes with slightly limited range of active movement of the glenohumeral joint. The pain was thought to originate from functional disorders of the cervical or upper thoracic spine or the upper ribs.
  3. The combination group consisted of patients with pain and sometimes slightly limited range of active or passive movements in the glenohumeral joint together with pain or limited range of movement of the cervical or upper thoracic spine or upper ribs. The synovial structures and the shoulder girdle were thought to have caused the pain.
  4. A total of 172 subjects were randomized to receive one of the adjunct therapies after a standard 1-week treatment with anti-inflammatory medication.
  5. Results were stratified according to diagnostic group. The 58 patients in the shoulder girdle dysfunction group that received manipulation had a shorter duration of complaints and fewer reports of treatment failure than those that received physiotherapy (e.g., exercise, modalities, massage). However, corticosteroid injection had better outcomes in the synovial group of patients than manipulation in other patients.
- Two randomized, controlled trials showed promising results for the application of manipulation and physiotherapy in the management of shoulder pain.
- In a follow-up to the trial reported by Winters and colleagues, Bergman and coworkers,[26] recruited 150 patients with shoulder symptoms and dysfunction of the shoulder girdle from general practices in the Netherlands.
  1. Subjects were randomly assigned into usual care versus usual care plus manipulative therapy (up to six treatment sessions in a 12-week period).
  2. At the end of the study period of 12 weeks, 21% of the usual care group and 43% of the intervention group reported full recovery.
  3. This significant difference in improvement was also observed at 52 weeks of follow-up.[26]

- In a trial by Hay and associates,[28] 207 patients with shoulder pain recruited from primary care clinics in the United Kingdom were randomly divided into a physiotherapy group and a corticosteroid injection group.
  1. Their baseline characteristics appear to be similar.
  2. At 6 months, 60% in the physiotherapy group and 53% in the injection group reported a minimum 50% drop in their disability scores.[28]
- Two randomized clinical trials of manipulation under anesthesia were conducted for patients with frozen shoulder syndrome refractory to conservative care.[29,30] They both showed benefit with no complications or adverse events, and they demonstrated improved outcomes compared with conservative care. Sustained improvement has been demonstrated for at least 15 years after the procedure.[31]
- A systematic review of randomized, controlled clinical trials evaluating the effectiveness of therapeutic exercise and orthopedic manual therapy for impingement syndrome concluded that there was positive but limited evidence to support their use. More methodologically sound studies were recommended.[32]

Risks

- Complications or adverse events occurring after manipulation of the shoulder have not been reported in the literature. None of the clinical trials evaluating this modality has reported any complications or adverse events in patients with shoulder somatic dysfunction.
- The manual treatment procedures in this chapter have no known risks associated with their use in patients with shoulder somatic dysfunction.
- Risks of increasing shoulder pain, dislocation, and disability may occur if there is a misdiagnosis and the practitioner manipulates a hypermobile shoulder that is already unstable due to loss of integrity (i.e., tear) of the rotator cuff, labrum, or other primary shoulder structure.

Benefits

- Manual medicine is used to treat somatic dysfunction. Manual procedures can increase motion, strengthen weak muscles, lyse adhesions, and decrease pain.
- Manipulative therapy for the shoulder girdle in addition to usual care by a general practitioner accelerates recovery of shoulder symptoms and reduces their severity.[26]

Practice Recommendations

- Evidence-based practice recommendations can be found in Table 9.6.
- Manipulation of the shoulder, cervicothoracic spine, and upper ribs is indicated in patients with shoulder somatic dysfunction accompanied by cervical, thoracic, and costal cage somatic dysfunctions[26,27,33,34] (grade A evidence).

Table 9.6   Evidence-based medicine practice recommendations

Level of Evidence*	Recommendation	Studies
A	Manipulation should be used in addition to usual care for patients with shoulder somatic dysfunction.	Hay et al, 2003[28] Bergman et al, 2004[26]
A	Manipulation under anesthesia should be used for frozen shoulder that is refractory to conservative treatments.	Kivimäki and Pohjolainen, 2001[30] Farrell et al, 2005[31]
A	Manipulation plus exercise should be used for rotator cuff dysfunction.	Green et al, 1998[39]
A	Manipulation plus exercise should be used for shoulder impingement syndrome.	Desmeules et al, 2003[32]

*Evidence levels: A, randomized, controlled trials, meta-analyses, and systematic reviews; B, case-control or cohort studies, retrospective studies, and certain uncontrolled studies; C, consensus statements, expert guidelines, usual practice, and opinion.

- Manipulation of the shoulder is indicated in patients with adhesive capsulitis (i.e., frozen shoulder), which may need to be done under anesthesia[30,35] (grade A evidence).
- The Dutch College of General Practitioners developed practice guidelines that were last revised in May 1999.[7] They can be accessed at http://nhg.artsennet.nl/upload/104/guidelines2/E08.htm. In summary, they recommended that conservative care with education, advice, and analgesics should be used in the first 2 to 4 weeks of treatment, followed by a intra-articular glenohumeral corticosteroid injection for severely limited external rotation (three times, 2 weeks apart), subacromial corticosteroid injection when there is pain on abduction, and after 6 weeks, physical therapy if there is loss of function and limitation of daily activities.

DIAGNOSTIC PROCEDURES

- The ICD-9 diagnostic code for shoulder somatic dysfunction is the same as for upper extremity somatic dysfunction: 739.7.

Observation

- Observe the patient in the standing position as in the screening examination performed in Chapter 3.
- Notice any asymmetries of shoulder levels, scapula levels, spinal curvatures, or deformities, such as scoliosis or increased thoracic kyphosis.
- Notice if there is any evidence of muscle wasting, atrophy, or fasciculations.

Neurologic Evaluation

- Evaluate deep tendon reflexes to the upper extremities, dermatome sensation, and muscle strength of all shoulder muscles.
- Spurling's maneuver can be used to determine whether cervical radiculopathy is present.
- Central nervous system evaluation can help to rule out presence of cerebrovascular accident or other pathology that may affect shoulder function.

Vascular Evaluation

- Assess distal pulses and blood pressure.
- Adson's test can help to determine whether thoracic outlet syndrome, with accompanying subclavian artery compression, is present.
- Notice any signs of swelling of the shoulder.

Active Motion

- The patient is instructed to abduct and raise his or her hands overhead and place the hands palm to palm, internally rotate the shoulders, and pronate the forearms to bring the backs of the hands together. The practitioner observes any asymmetries in the range or quality of motion.
- Patients with subacromial bursitis, calcium deposits, peritendinitis, or tendinosis of the rotator cuff muscles may have pain between 60 and 120 degrees of abduction because these structures can be pinched under the acromion process and coracoacromial ligament, called the *painful arc.*[36]
- The practitioner tests active range and quality of motion in flexion, extension, abduction, adduction, and internal and external rotation.
- The Apley's scratch test is useful to test a combination of motions together. The patient is instructed to touch the superior and then the inferior aspects of the opposite scapula with each hand. This test assesses internal rotation, adduction, and extension when the patient touches the inferior aspect of the opposite scapula and external rotation, abduction, and flexion when touching the superior aspect.
- Other special tests to assess shoulder function are listed in Table 9.5.
- The practitioner notices movement of the scapula in relation to movement of the humerus. The scapula should move one-half as much as the humerus in abduction.
- The sternoclavicular joint is examined for superior and inferior mobility as follows:
  1. The patient is supine on the table, with the arms resting comfortably at the side.

2. The practitioner stands at the side of the table and places his or her index fingers over the superior medial aspects of each clavicle.

3. The patient is asked to actively shrug the shoulders by raising the shoulders toward the ears.

4. The practitioner observes and palpates the movement at the medial ends of the clavicles.

5. The normal finding is equal movement of the medial ends of the clavicles in an inferior direction.

6. A positive finding is the failure of one clavicle to move inferiorly compared with the opposite one.

- The sternoclavicular joint is examined during shoulder horizontal flexion as follows:

1. The patient is supine.

2. The practitioner stands at the side of the table and places his or her index fingers over the anterior aspect of the medial end of each clavicle.

3. The patient reaches toward the ceiling, extending the elbows of each arm with the shoulders flexed to 90 degrees.

4. The normal finding is for each clavicle to move symmetrically in a posterior direction as the lateral ends of the clavicles move anteriorly.

5. A positive finding is the failure of one clavicle to move in a posterior direction during the reaching effort.

- Trapezius muscle strength can be tested by resisting the patient's shoulder shrug; this tests integrity of cranial nerve XI, which innervates the trapezius muscles.

- The cervical spine and thoracic spine are examined as in Chapters 3 and 6.

- The costal cage is assessed as in Chapter 3.

- Ribs 1 through 4 (pump handle predominant) are examined as follows:

1. The patient is supine.

2. The practitioner stands to the side of the patient with the dominant eye over the midline of the patient's body.

3. While facing the patient, the practitioner places the distal fingertips at the inferior boarder of the patient's clavicles. The index fingers are palpating rib one under the medial end of the clavicle while the palms are spread over the anterior aspects of ribs 2 through 4.

4. Pump-handle motion is assessed by having the patient inhale and exhale deeply.

5. The practitioner compares the motion of the two sides.

- Ribs 5 through 7 (i.e., mixed pump-handle and bucket-handle motion) are examined as follows:

1. The patient is supine.

2. The practitioner stands to the side of the patient with the dominant eye over the midline of the patient's body.

3. The practitioner places his or her hands on the anterolateral aspect of the patient's ribs 5 through 7. (A female patient should be asked if she feels more comfortable when the practitioner assesses the motion of ribs 5 through 7 with her hands covering her breasts and the practitioner palpating over the patient's hands instead of directly on the breasts. Some practitioners put their finger pads on the ribs lateral to the breast tissue in the anterior axillary line instead of using his or her palms over the midclavicular line.)

4. The mixed pump-handle and bucket-handle motion is assessed by having the patient inhale and exhale.

5. The practitioner compares motion of the two sides.

- Ribs 8 through 10 (i.e., bucket-handle motion predominant) are examined as follows:

1. The patient is supine.

2. The practitioner stands to the side of the patient with the dominant eye over the midline of the patient's body.

3. The practitioner places his or her hands on the lateral aspect of the patient's ribs 8 through 10.

4. Bucket-handle motion is assessed by having the patient inhale and exhale.

- Ribs 11 and 12 (i.e., caliper motion predominant) are examined as follows:

1. The patient is prone.

2. The practitioner stands to the side of the patient with the dominant eye over the midline of the patient's body.

3. The practitioner places the thenar eminences on each of the costal vertebral junctions, with the palms and fingers over the shafts of ribs 11 and 12.

4. Caliper motions are evaluated by having the patient inhale and exhale.

- Interpretation of costal cage motion tests

1. The side that lags in inhalation motion compared with the opposite side is considered to be *restricted in inhalation*.

2. In a group that has an inhalation restriction, one of the more superior ribs in the group is likely dysfunctional and resists superior movement during inhalation, preventing the entire group from moving into inhalation (i.e., superiorly in the case of pump-handle motion, laterally for bucket-handle motion, and posteriorly for caliper-type motion). Conversely, the dysfunctional rib moves easiest into exhalation (i.e., the anterior aspect moves easiest in the inferior direction).

3. The practitioner then needs to assess each rib compared with its counterpart on the normal side, starting with the most superior in the group and working inferiorly until the abnormal rib is located.

4. The side that lags in exhalation motion is *restricted in exhalation*.

5. In a group that has an exhalation restriction, one of the more inferior ribs in the group is likely the dysfunctional one and resists inferior movement during exhalation, preventing the entire group from moving into exhalation (i.e., inferiorly in the case of pump-handle motion, medially for bucket-handle motion, and anteriorly for caliper-type motion). Conversely, the dysfunctional rib moves easiest into inhalation (i.e., the anterior aspect moves easiest in the superior direction).

6. The practitioner then assesses each rib compared with its counterpart on the normal side, starting with the most inferior in the group and working superiorly until the abnormal rib is located.

7. For an inhalation or an exhalation restriction, the rib that is not moving properly is called the *key rib* in the group, and after it is mobilized, the group should move normally.

Passive Motion

- The practitioner evaluates passive shoulder range and quality of motion, assesses pain during or at the end range of a movement, and compares the resistance or compliance at the end of the range of motion in all directions.
- Special tests listed in Table 9.5 can help distinguish among muscle imbalance, weakness, and dislocation or muscle, tendon, or ligamentous rupture or tears.
- The acromioclavicular joint is examined for restriction in abduction or adduction as follows:
  1. The patient is seated.
  2. The practitioner stands behind the patient.
  3. The practitioner palpates the medial superior aspect of the acromioclavicular joint with one hand and grasps the patient's proximal forearm with the other hand.
  4. The practitioner introduces adduction and external rotation of the patient's forearm while palpating for gapping motion at the acromioclavicular joint.
  5. Comparison is made with the opposite acromioclavicular joint. Absence of gapping motion is evidence of restriction of adduction.
  6. The practitioner then introduces abduction movement while monitoring for motion at the acromioclavicular joint.
  7. Comparison is made with the opposite acromioclavicular joint.
  8. Absence of palpable motion at the acromioclavicular joint is evidence for restricted abduction.
- The acromioclavicular joint is examined for restriction in internal or external rotation as follows:
  1. The patient is seated.
  2. The practitioner stands behind the patient and uses one hand to monitor the superior aspect of the acromioclavicular joint.
  3. The practitioner uses his or her other hand to move the patient's upper extremity on the restricted side into about 30 degrees of horizontal flexion and then abduction until a motion barrier is reached.
  4. The practitioner then introduces internal and external rotation to determine which of these two motions is restricted.
  5. Comparison is made with the opposite side.
- The glenohumeral articulation is examined as follows:
  1. The patient is seated.
  2. The practitioner stands behind the patient.
  3. The practitioner uses one hand to stabilize the shoulder complex, with the fingers on the coracoid process, the palm of the hand over the acromioclavicular joint, and the thumb over the spine of the scapula.
  4. The practitioner uses his or her other hand to induce the following motions in the patient's upper extremity:
     Flexion
     Extension
     External rotation
     Internal rotation with the patient's forearm in front and behind of the torso
     Adduction
     Abduction

5. The practitioner observes the range and quality of each motion.
6. Comparison is made with the patient's opposite shoulder. The practitioner observes any specific motion restrictions of the glenohumeral joint.

Palpation

- The bony and soft tissues of the shoulder are palpated, assessing each bone, joint, ligament, tendon, bursa, and muscle for integrity, tenderness, swelling, or warmth.
- The most common tender points amenable to counterstrain manipulation treatment are assessed (Fig. 9.10).
  1. Lateral coracoid (LCO): on the superolateral aspect of the coracoid process
  2. Short head of the biceps (SH): on the inferolateral aspect of the coracoid process
  3. Long head of the biceps (LH): in the bicipital groove of the humerus
  4. Subscapularis (SUB): on the anterior surface of the scapula, in the posterior axillary fold
  5. Supraspinatus (SUP): in the belly of the supraspinatus muscle (along the spine of the scapula)
  6. Teres minor (TMI): on the lateral border of the scapula at the origin of the teres minor muscle
- Tissue tension is assessed along the cervical and thoracic spine for evidence of somatic dysfunction.
- The practitioner assesses for any palpable asymmetry of rib angles posteriorly with the patient seated or supine.
- The practitioner assesses for tenderness anteriorly along the chondrosternal and costochondral articulations when the patient is seated or supine.
- The practitioner assesses for the most common anterior rib (AR) tender points with patient seated or supine (Fig. 9.11A):
  1. AR1: on the first costal cartilage, beneath the clavicle, adjacent to the sternum
  2. AR2: in the midclavicular line, on the inferior margin of the second rib
  3. AR3: in the anterior axillary line on the inferior margin of the third rib
  4. AR4: in the anterior axillary line on the inferior margin of the fourth rib
  5. AR5: in the anterior axillary line on the inferior margin of the fifth rib
  6. AR6: in the anterior axillary line on the inferior margin of the sixth rib
- The practitioner assesses for the most common posterior rib (PR) tender points with the patient seated or supine (see Fig. 9.11B):
  1. PR1: on the posterolateral aspect of the first rib, beneath margin of the trapezius muscle at the angle of the neck and shoulder
  2. PR2: on the superior margin of the second rib angle
  3. PR3: on the superior margin of the third rib angle
  4. PR4: on the superior margin of the fourth rib angle
  5. PR5: on the superior margin of the fifth rib angle
  6. PR6: on the superior margin of the sixth rib angle

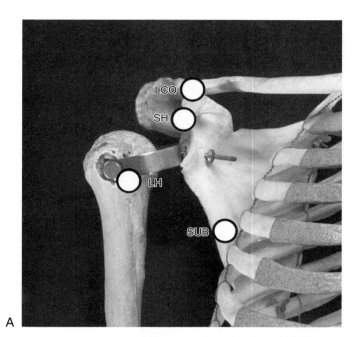

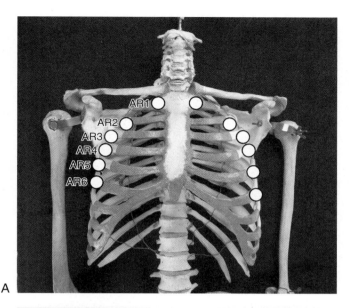

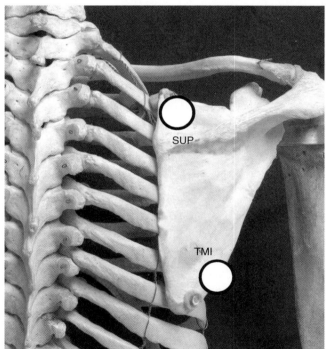

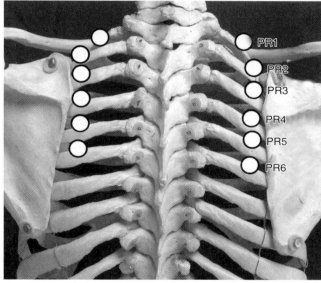

Figure 9.11 **A,** Anterior view of common rib tender points on a skeletal model. **B,** Posterior view of common rib tender points on a skeletal model. AR, anterior rib; PR, posterior rib.

Figure 9.10 **A,** Anterior view of common right shoulder tender points on a skeletal model. **B,** Posterior view of common right shoulder tender points on a skeletal model. LCO, lateral coracoid; LH, long head of the biceps; SH, short head of the biceps; SUB, subscapularis; SUP, supraspinatus; TMI, teres minor.

TREATMENT PROCEDURES

Shoulder Treatment Procedures

Shoulder Articulatory Technique

- Example: articulatory technique for the right shoulder
- The procedure is performed as follows:
  1. The patient lies on the left side (Fig. 9.12).
  2. The practitioner stands at the side of the table and faces the patient.

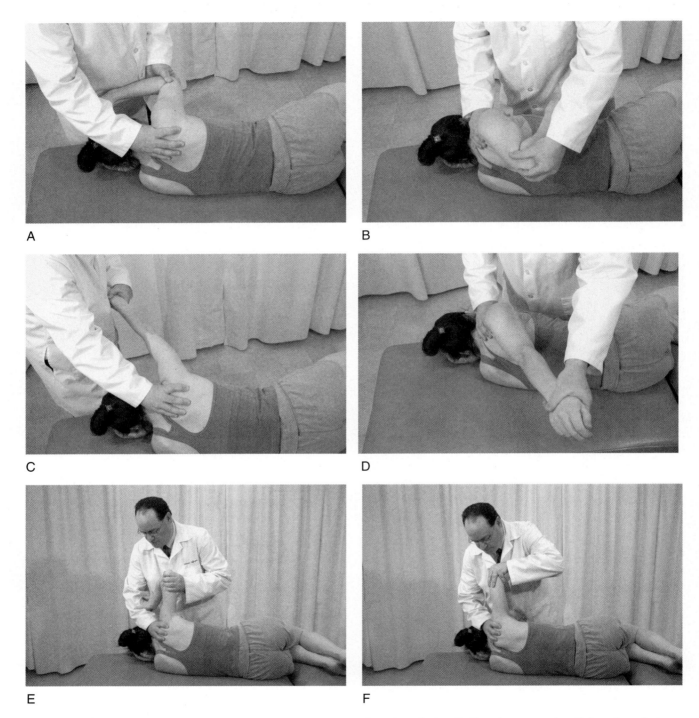

Figure 9.12   Articulatory treatment for right shoulder restricted motion. **A,** Short lever flexion. **B,** Short lever extension. **C,** Long lever flexion. **D,** Long lever extension. **E,** Short lever abduction. **F,** Short lever circumduction.

The following sequence has been demonstrated clinically to be well tolerated, although it can be performed in a different sequence or some directions of motion not necessarily addressed if there is no restriction in that particular direction. The sequence can be determined according to the needs of the patient and the restrictions discovered on assessment at any particular office visit.

- To improve flexion and extension motion
  3. The practitioner stabilizes the patient's right shoulder complex with his or her right hand and grasps the patient's right elbow with his or her left hand.
  4. Keeping patient's elbow flexed, the practitioner gently, passively flexes and extends the patient's right arm repeatedly

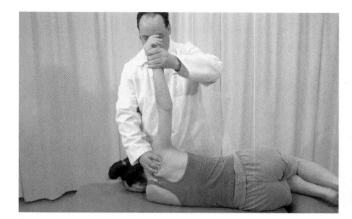

G

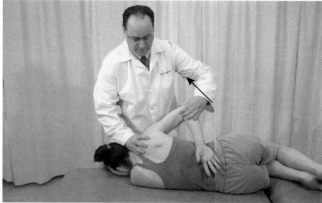

H

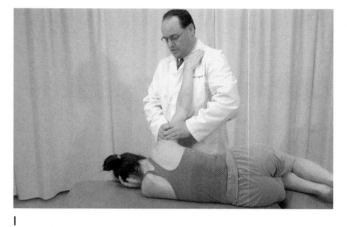

I

Figure 9.12, cont'd   **G,** Long lever circumduction. **H,** Internal rotation. **I,** Distraction of right shoulder by "scooping" the humerus away from the glenoid fossa.

to the restrictive barrier without inducing pain. This motion is repeated several times to stretch the soft tissues and increase the passive range of motion (see Fig. 9.12A and B).

5. The practitioner then grasps the patient's right wrist with his or her left hand. With the patient's elbow extended, the practitioner gently, passively flexes and extends the arm repeatedly as in step 4 (see Fig. 9.12C and D).

• To improve abduction motion

6. The practitioner grasps the patient's right wrist with his or her left hand with the patient's right elbow flexed and the patient's right hand rests on the practitioner's right forearm.

7. The practitioner slowly abducts the patient's humerus to the restrictive barrier (see Fig 9.12E).

8. The humerus is then returned to the neutral position, and the motions are repeated several times until an increase in range of motion is attained.

• To improve circumduction motion

9. The practitioner grasps the patient's left elbow with his or her left hand with the patient's elbow flexed. The practitioner abducts the humerus to 90 degrees. The practitioner gently circumducts the humerus slowly clockwise and then counterclockwise in small circles. The radii of the circles

are gradually increased as permitted without inducing pain (see Fig. 9.12F).

10. The practitioner then grasps the patient's wrist with the patient's elbow extended. The practitioner repeats circumduction maneuvers as in step 6 (see Fig. 9.12G).

• To improve internal and external rotation

11. The practitioner passively places the patient's right hand posterior to the patient's ipsilateral lower ribs (see Fig. 9.12H).

12. The patient's right elbow is abducted slightly, and the practitioner passively internally rotates the humerus, engages the restrictive barrier, and then relaxes this position. This motion is repeated several times.

• To improve glenohumeral capsular compliance

13. The practitioner extends the patient's right elbow fully and passively places the patient's right hand on the practitioner's left shoulder.

14. The practitioner then grasps the patient's right shoulder with both hands and interlaces his or her fingers around the patient's glenohumeral joint, with the hypothenar eminences placed just distal to the acromioclavicular joint and glenoid labrum and just proximal to the head of the humerus.

15. The practitioner then slowly and repeatedly applies medial to lateral traction to the patient's deltoid muscles lateral to the scapula.

16. The practitioner then exerts a lateral traction of the humerus in a scooping motion. This is best performed by rocking his or her weight from the front foot to the back foot in a rhythmic fashion. This motion is repeated several times until improved compliance is observed (see Fig. 9.12I).

• Reassessment

17. The practitioner then rechecks the overall range of motion of the shoulder.

Shoulder Myofascial Release
Myofascial Scapular Release

• Example: myofascial release of the right scapula (Fig. 9.13)

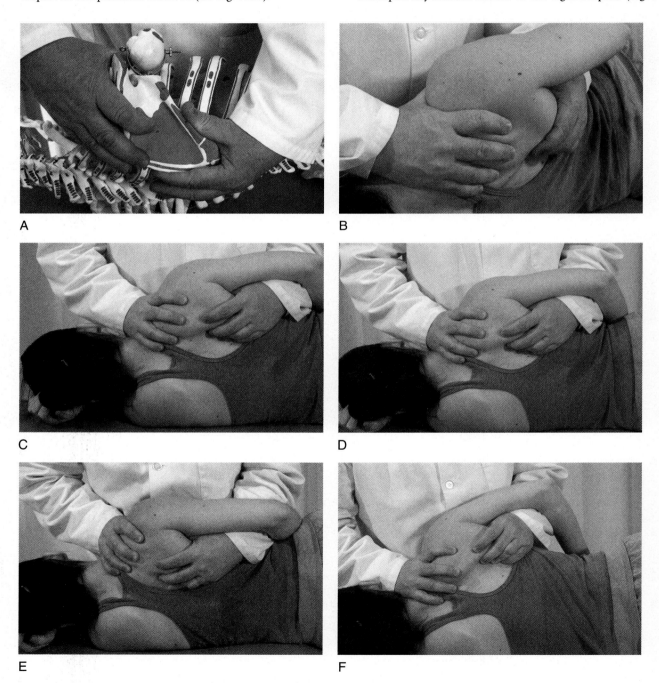

A

B

C

D

E

F

Figure 9.13 **A,** Hand position on a skeletal model in preparation for right scapula myofascial release (MFR). **B,** MFR of the right scapula: superoposterior view of hand positions. **C,** Right scapula MFR passive motion testing: superior direction. **D,** Right scapula MFR passive motion testing: inferior direction. **E,** Right scapula MFR passive motion testing: protraction. **F,** Right scapula MFR passive motion testing: retraction.

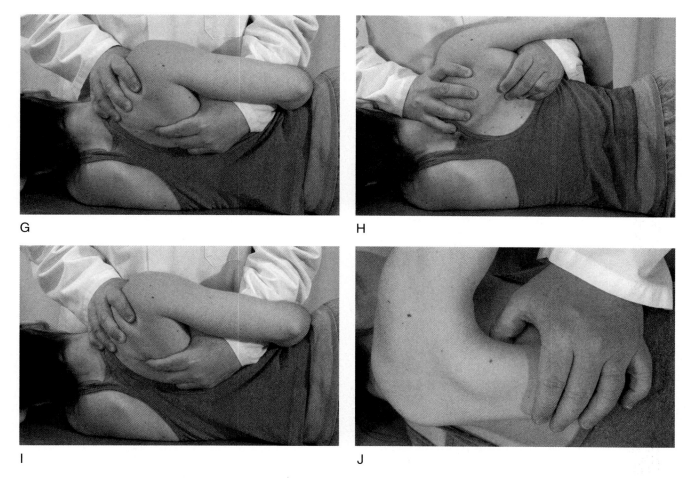

Figure 9.13, cont'd   **G,** Right Scapula MFR passive motion testing: medial translation. **H,** Right scapula MFR passive motion testing: lateral translation. **I,** Right scapula MFR treatment using all directions of ease combined. **J,** Right subscapula MFR thumb position. The practitioner pushes the scapula away from the thorax to release subscapularis myofascial tension.

- The procedure is performed as follows:
  1. The patient lies on his or her left side.
  2. The practitioner stands at the side of the table and faces the patient.
  3. The practitioner grasps the upper portion of the right scapular with his or her right hand. At the same time, the practitioner places he left forearm underneath the patient's right arm and grasps the lower portion of the right scapular with the left hand (see Fig. 9.13A and B).
  4. The practitioner tests the passive motion of the scapula to find the direction of ease of motion in all directions: superior or inferior, protraction or retraction, and medial or lateral (see Fig. 9.13C to H).
  5. Combining, or stacking, all the directions toward which there is compliance, or relative ease of motion, the practitioner finds the scapular position of maximum ease and holds the scapula in this position until the surrounding soft tissues relax and allow free scapular gliding motion over the costal cage (see Fig. 9.13I).

  6. As the soft tissues relax, the scapula can be moved to new positions of maximal ease.
  7. The practitioner allows this unwinding to continue until it resolves and the scapula comes to a resting state.
  8. The practitioner retests motion in all directions.

Subscapularis Release
- The procedure is performed as follows:
  1. The patient is sidelying with the affected shoulder freely mobile. For the right shoulder dysfunction, the patient lies on the left side.
  2. The practitioner stabilizes the patient's shoulder with his or her right hand by grasping the shoulder anteriorly and superiorly, placing the thumb over the patient's coracoid process as for the scapular release.
  3. The practitioner places his or her left thumb underneath the patient's right scapula inferior to the axilla, pushing posteriorly until the subscapularis muscle is engaged (see Fig. 9.13J).

4. Using direct pressure with the thumb fingertip, the practitioner maintains sustained pressure in an anteroposterior direction, as if lifting the scapula off the patient's back.
5. The practitioner tests scapula passive motion compliance superiorly, inferiorly, medially, laterally, protracted, and retracted and combines the motions that are most compliant, holds the scapula in that position, and waits for further release of tension.

6. As the soft tissues relax, the scapula can be moved to new positions of maximal ease.
7. The practitioner allows this unwinding to continue until it resolves and the scapula comes to a resting state.
8. The practitioner retests motion in all directions. There should be complete relaxation of the muscles attached to the scapula, and it should be able to be passively moved freely in all directions, gliding over the costal cage without resistance.

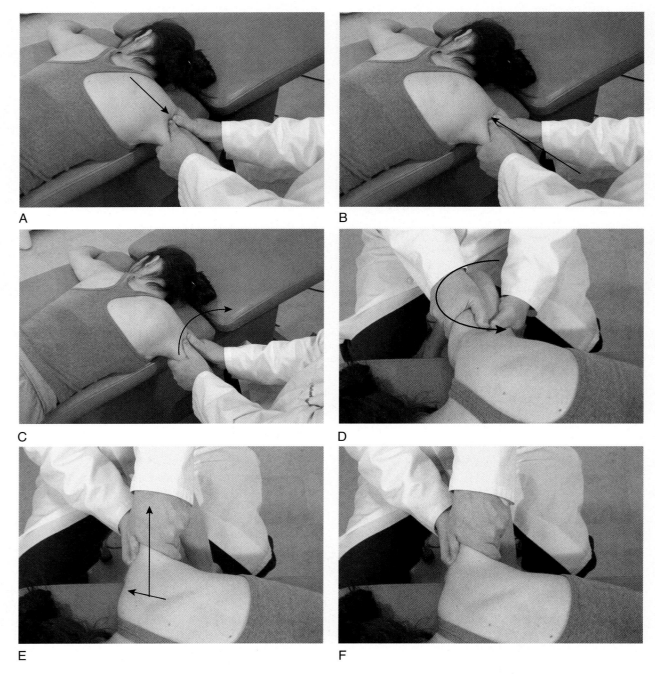

Figure 9.14   Prone right shoulder passive myofascial motion testing. **A,** Traction. **B,** Compression. **C,** Internal rotation. **D,** External rotation. **E,** Prone right shoulder myofascial release (MFR) treatment combining all motions in the directions of ease or greatest compliance. **F,** Further MFR in the directions of ease, following the response of the myofascial tissues until "unwinding" begins.

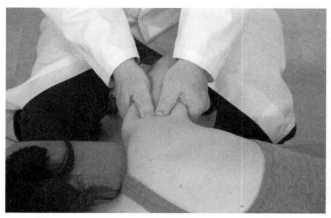

G

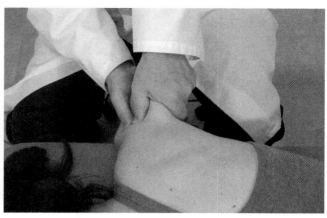

H

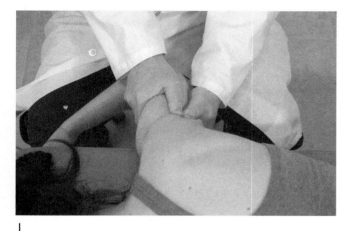

I

Figure 9.14, cont'd G, For prone right shoulder MFR, the practitioner follows the unwinding of the myofascial tissue back toward the original restrictive barrier. **H,** For prone right shoulder MFR, the practitioner follows the unwinding of the myofascial tissue again back toward the direction of ease. **I,** For prone right shoulder MFR, after unwinding ceases, the practitioner rechecks passive myofascial motion in all planes.

Shoulder Myofascial Release with the Patient Prone

- Example: myofascial release of the right shoulder (Fig. 9.14)
- The procedure is performed as follows:
  1. The patient lies on his or her left side.
  2. The practitioner sits at the side of the table and faces the patient.
  3. The practitioner grasps the upper portion of the right humerus with both hands.
  4. The practitioner tests the passive motion of the scapula to find the direction of ease of motion in the following planes: distraction or compression and internal or external rotation (see Fig. 9.14A to D).
  5. Combining, or stacking, all the motions of ease, the practitioner finds the position of maximum ease of all the affected shoulder motions and holds the shoulder in this position until the soft tissues relax and allow free glenohumeral motion (see Fig. 9.14E).
  6. As the soft tissues relax, the shoulder can be moved to new positions of maximal ease (see Fig. 9.14F).
  7. The practitioner allows this unwinding to continue until it resolves and the shoulder comes to a resting state (see Fig. 9.14G and H). The unwinding process often entails following the shoulder from its position of ease back toward its restrictive barrier and then back to its position of ease because of the asynchrony in the release of the various hypertonic shoulder muscles. The hypertonic muscles that are pulling the shoulder toward them relax when the practitioner shortens the distance between their origins and insertions, enabling movement back toward the restrictive barrier. A new restrictive barrier is felt as each group of muscles relaxes. The tight muscles that are still restricting movement pull the shoulder back toward them, and the practitioner follows this pull and does not resist it, essentially moving the shoulder into the direction of ease. After all the muscles have relaxed, compliant passive motion is felt in all directions.
  8. The practitioner retests motion in all directions (see Fig. 9.14I).

Shoulder Muscle Energy: Isometric and Isotonic Techniques
Rotation

- Example: internally rotated right shoulder, restriction of external rotation (Fig. 9.15)
  1. The patient lies on the left side with the right hand behind the back.
  2. The practitioner stands at the side of the table and faces the patient.
  3. The practitioner grasps the patient's right elbow and distal arm with his or her left hand and stabilizes the patient's shoulder with his or her right hand.

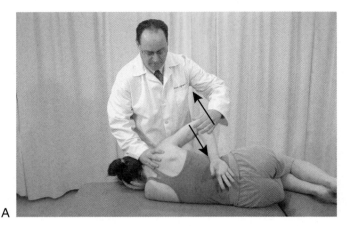

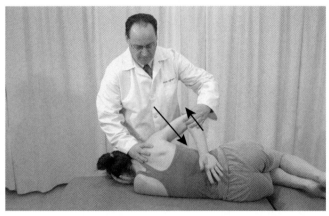

Figure 9.15 **A,** Right shoulder sidelying isometric muscle energy treatment (MET) for external rotation restriction. **B,** Right shoulder sidelying isotonic MET for external rotation restriction entails external rotator muscle weakness strengthening and reciprocal inhibition of tight internal rotators. The practitioner resists but allows motion into external rotation.

- Treatment: isometric procedure to decrease tone of the hypertonic internal rotators (see Fig. 9.15A)
  1. The practitioner externally rotates the patient's right shoulder to the restrictive barrier.
  2. The practitioner instructs the patient to internally rotate his or her right humerus against the practitioner's unyielding counterforce.
  3. The patient maintains the effort for 3 to 5 seconds and then relaxes his or her right arm for 2 to 3 seconds.
  4. The practitioner repositions the patient's right arm into a new restrictive barrier by increasing the external rotation.
  5. Steps 3 and 4 are repeated three to five times.
  6. The practitioner performs a final stretch into the restrictive barrier after the final repetition.
  7. The practitioner retests the external rotation motion.
- Treatment: isotonic procedure to strengthen the weak external rotators of the right shoulder or decrease the resting tone of the hypertonic internal rotators using reciprocal inhibition (see Fig. 9.15B). The procedure is performed as follows:
  1. The practitioner internally rotates the patient's right shoulder.

2. The practitioner instructs the patient to externally rotate his or her right humerus.
3. The practitioner provides resistance but allows the patient to move his or her right shoulder into external rotation up to the restrictive motion barrier.
4. The practitioner repositions the patient's right arm into internal rotation.
5. Steps 2 through 4 are repeated three to five times.
6. The practitioner retests the range and quality of motion of passive and active external shoulder rotation.
- Example: externally rotated right shoulder, restriction of internal rotation (Fig. 9.16)
  1. The patient lies on the left side.
  2. The practitioner stands at the side of the table and faces the patient.
  3. The practitioner grasps the patient's right elbow and distal arm with his or her left hand and stabilizes the patient's right shoulder with his or her right hand.
- Treatment: isometric procedure to decrease the tone of the hypertonic external rotators (see Fig. 9.16A)

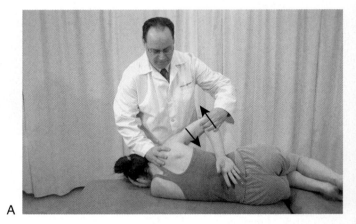

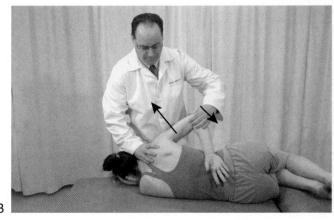

Figure 9.16 **A,** Right shoulder sidelying isometric muscle energy treatment (MET) for internal rotation restriction. **B,** Right shoulder sidelying isotonic MET for internal rotation restriction entails internal rotator muscle weakness strengthening and reciprocal inhibition of tight external rotators. The practitioner resists but allows motion into internal rotation.

1. The practitioner internally rotates the patient's right shoulder to the restrictive barrier.
2. The practitioner instructs the patient to externally rotate his or her right humerus against the practitioner's unyielding counterforce.
3. The patient maintains the effort for 3 to 5 seconds and then relaxes his or her right arm for 2 to 3 seconds.
4. The practitioner repositions the patient's right arm into the new restrictive barrier by increasing internal rotation.
5. Steps 3 through 5 are repeated three to five times.
6. The practitioner performs a final stretch into the restrictive barrier after the final repetition.
7. The practitioner retests the internal rotation motion.

- Treatment: isotonic procedure to increase the tone of the hypotonic internal rotators and employ reciprocal inhibition to decrease the tone of the hypertonic external rotators (see Fig. 9.16B)
  1. The practitioner externally rotates the patient's right shoulder to the restrictive barrier.
  2. The practitioner instructs the patient to internally rotate his or her right humerus.
  3. The practitioner provides resistance but allows the patient to move his or her right shoulder into internal rotation.
  4. The practitioner repositions the patient's right arm into external rotation.
  5. Steps 2 through 4 are repeated three to five times.
  6. The practitioner retests the range and quality of motion of passive and active internal shoulder rotation.

Flexion

- Example: extended right shoulder, restriction of flexion (Fig. 9.17)
  1. The patient lies on the left side.
  2. The practitioner stands at the side of the table and faces the patient.
  3. The practitioner grasps the patient's right elbow and distal arm with his or her left hand and stabilizes the patient's right shoulder with his or her right hand.

- Treatment: isometric procedure to decrease the resting tone of the hypertonic extensor muscles (see Fig. 9.17A)
  1. The practitioner flexes the patient's arm into the restrictive barrier.
  2. The practitioner instructs the patient to extend his or her right humerus against the practitioner's unyielding counterforce.
  3. The patient maintains the effort for 3 to 5 seconds and then relaxes his or her right arm for 2 to 3 seconds.
  4. The practitioner repositions the patient's right arm into the new restrictive barrier by increasing flexion.
  5. Steps 3 through 5 are repeated three to five times.
  6. The practitioner performs a final stretch into the restrictive barrier following the final repetition.
  7. The practitioner retests the flexion motion.

- Treatment: isotonic procedure to increase the strength of weak flexors and employ reciprocal inhibition to decrease the resting tone of hypertonic extensors (see Fig. 9.17B)
  1. The practitioner extends the patient's right shoulder to the restrictive barrier.
  2. The practitioner instructs the patient to flex his or her right shoulder.
  3. The practitioner provides resistance but allows the patient to move his or her right shoulder into flexion.
  4. The practitioner repositions the patient's right arm into extension.
  5. Steps 2 through 4 are repeated three to five times.
  6. The practitioner retests the range and quality of active and passive shoulder flexion motion.

- Example: flexed right shoulder, restriction of extension (Fig. 9.18)
  1. The patient lies on the left side.
  2. The practitioner stands at the side of the table and faces the patient.
  3. The practitioner grasps the patient's right elbow and distal arm with his or her left hand and stabilizes the patient's right shoulder with his or her right hand.

- Treatment: isometric procedure to decrease the resting tone of hypertonic shoulder flexor muscles (see Fig. 9.18A)

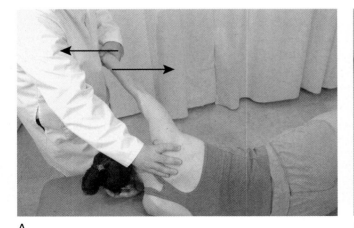
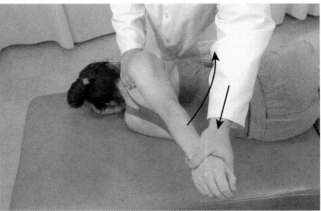

A

B

Figure 9.17 **A,** Right shoulder isometric muscle energy treatment (MET) for flexion restriction. **B,** Right shoulder sidelying isotonic MET for flexion restriction entails flexor muscle weakness strengthening and reciprocal inhibition of tight extensors. The practitioner resists but allows motion into flexion.

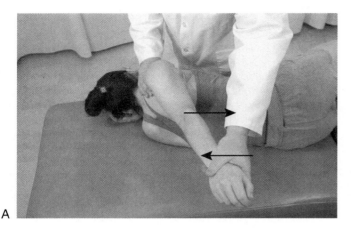

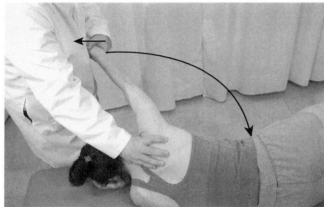

Figure 9.18 A, Right shoulder isometric muscle energy treatment (MET) for extension restriction. **B,** Right shoulder sidelying isotonic MET for extension restriction entails extensor muscle weakness strengthening and reciprocal inhibition of tight flexors. The practitioner resists but allows motion into extension.

1. The practitioner extends the patient's arm into the restrictive barrier.
2. The practitioner instructs the patient to flex his or her right humerus against the practitioner's unyielding counterforce.
3. The patient maintains the effort for 3 to 5 seconds and then relaxes his or her right arm for 2 to 3 seconds.
4. The practitioner repositions the patient's right arm into the new restrictive barrier by increasing extension.
5. Steps 2 through 4 are repeated three to five times.
6. The practitioner performs a final stretch into the restrictive barrier after the final repetition.
7. The practitioner retests the extension motion.
- Treatment: isotonic procedure to increase the strength of weak extensor muscles and employ reciprocal inhibition to decrease the resting tone of hypertonic flexor muscles (see Fig. 9.18B)
  1. The practitioner flexes the patient's right shoulder.
  2. The practitioner instructs the patient to extend his or her right shoulder.
  3. The practitioner provides resistance but allows the patient to move his or her right shoulder into extension.

4. The practitioner repositions the patient's right arm into flexion.
5. Steps 2 through 4 are repeated three to five times.
6. The practitioner retests the range and quality of active and passive shoulder extension motion.

Adduction and Abduction

- Example: adducted right shoulder, restriction of abduction (Fig. 9.19)
  1. The patient lies on the left side.
  2. The practitioner stands at the side of the table and faces the patient.
  3. The practitioner grasps the patient's right elbow and distal arm with his or her left hand and stabilizes the patient's right shoulder with his or her right hand.
- Treatment: isometric procedure to decrease the resting tone of hypertonic adductors (see Fig. 9.19A)
  1. The practitioner engages the restrictive barrier by gently bringing the patient's right shoulder into abduction.

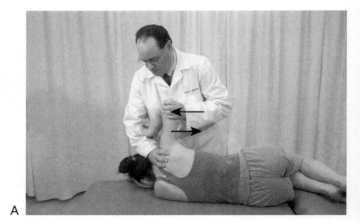

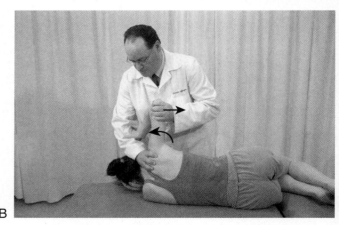

Figure 9.19 A, Right shoulder isometric muscle energy treatment (MET) for abduction restriction. **B,** Right shoulder isotonic MET for abduction restriction entails abductor muscle weakness strengthening and reciprocal inhibition of hypertonic adductors. The practitioner resists but allows motion into abduction.

2. The practitioner instructs the patient to adduct his or her right humerus against the practitioner's unyielding counterforce.

3. The patient maintains the effort for 3 to 5 seconds and then relaxes his or her right arm for 2 to 3 seconds.

4. The practitioner repositions the patient's right arm into the new restrictive barrier by increasing abduction.

5. Steps 2 through 4 are repeated three to five times.

6. The practitioner performs a final stretch into the restrictive barrier after the final repetition.

7. The practitioner retests the abduction motion.

- Treatment: isotonic procedure to strengthen the weak abductors and employ reciprocal inhibition to decrease the resting tone of hypertonic adductors (see Fig. 9.19B)

1. The practitioner engages the restrictive barrier by gently bringing the patient's right shoulder into adduction.

2. The practitioner instructs the patient to abduct his or her right humerus.

3. The practitioner provides resistance but allows the patient to move his or her right shoulder into abduction.

4. The practitioner repositions the patient's right arm into adduction.

5. Steps 2 through 4 are repeated three to five times.

6. The practitioner retests the range and quality of active and passive shoulder abduction motion.

- Example: right shoulder, restricted adduction (Fig. 9.20)

1. The patient lies on the left side.

2. The practitioner stands at the side of the table and faces the patient.

3. The practitioner grasps the patient's right elbow and distal arm with his or her left hand and stabilizes the patient's right shoulder with his or her right hand.

- Treatment: isometric procedure to decrease the resting tone of the hypertonic abductors (see Fig. 9.20A)

1. The practitioner engages the restrictive barrier by gently bringing the patient's right shoulder into adduction.

2. The practitioner instructs the patient to abduct his or her right humerus against the practitioner's isometric counterforce.

3. The patient maintains the effort for 3 to 5 seconds and then relaxes his or her right arm for 2 to 3 seconds.

4. The practitioner repositions the patient's right arm into the new restrictive barrier by increasing adduction.

5. Steps 2 through 4 are repeated three to five times.

6. The practitioner performs a final stretch into the restrictive barrier following the final repetition.

7. The practitioner retests the adduction motion.

- Treatment: isotonic procedure to strengthen weak adductor muscles and employ reciprocal inhibition to decrease the resting tone of hypertonic abductors (see Fig. 9.20B)

1. The practitioner engages the restrictive barrier by gently bringing the patient's right shoulder into abduction.

2. The practitioner instructs the patient to adduct his or her right humerus.

3. The practitioner provides resistance but allows the patient to move his or her right shoulder into adduction.

4. The practitioner repositions the patient's right arm into abduction.

5. Steps 2 through 4 are repeated three to five times.

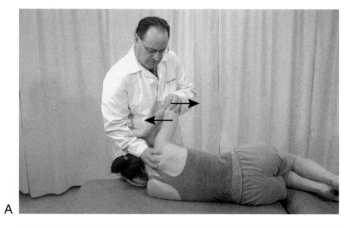

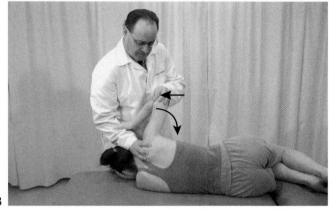

Figure 9.20   A, Right shoulder isometric muscle energy treatment (MET) for adduction restriction. **B,** Right shoulder isotonic MET for adduction restriction entails adduction muscle weakness strengthening and reciprocal inhibition of tight abductors. The practitioner resists but allows motion into adduction.

6. The practitioner retests the range and quality of active and passive shoulder adduction motion.

Shoulder Functional Technique

- Example: right shoulder somatic dysfunction
- The procedure is performed as follows:

1. The patient is lying on the left side (Fig. 9.21).

2. The practitioner stands to the side of the patient with the patient's right arm overhead in abduction and supported by the practitioner's right forearm. The practitioner's left finger pads contact the patient's medial right scapular border to monitor the soft tissue changes in response to passive right shoulder motion (see Fig. 9.21A and B).

3. The practitioner then introduces the following paired motions, noticing the directions that cause relative ease (or bind) of the soft tissues being monitored at the right scapula's medial border: extension (see Fig. 9.21C), flexion (see Fig. 9.21D), abduction (see Fig. 9.21E), adduction (see Fig. 9.21F), distraction (see Fig. 9.21G), and compression (see Fig. 9.21H).

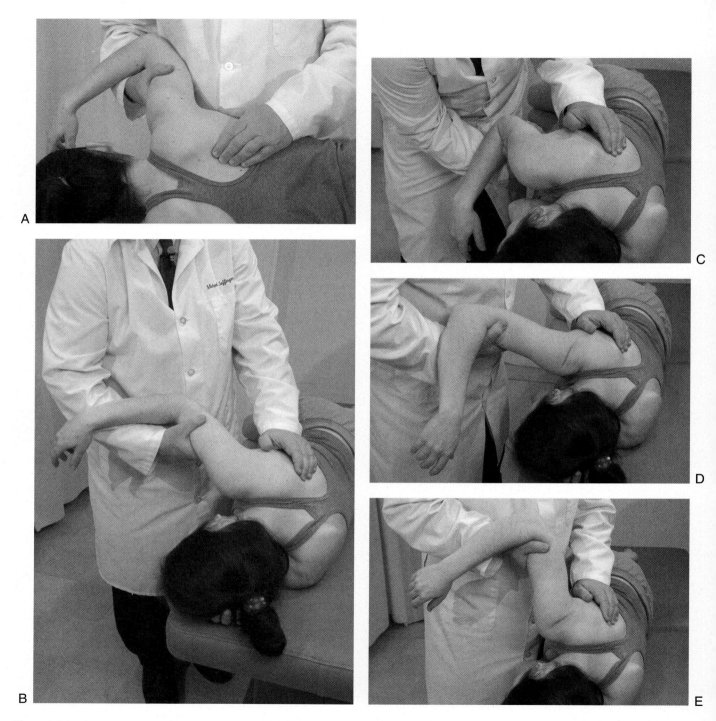

Figure 9.21 Sidelying functional technique for the right shoulder. **A,** Functional technique for the scapula uses the arm as a lever to induce a response to motion along the medial scapular border. The practitioner's left finger pads monitor tension in the soft tissues in response to shoulder motion. **B,** Reverse angle view. **C,** Assessing the medial border of the right scapular soft tissue response to passive shoulder extension. **D,** Assessing the medial border of the right scapular soft tissue response to passive shoulder flexion. **E,** Assessing the medial border of the right scapular soft tissue response to passive shoulder abduction.

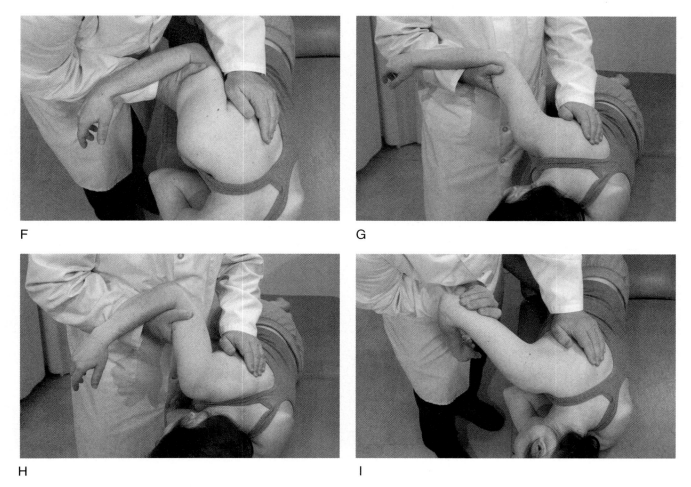

F, Assessing the medial border of the right scapular soft tissue response to passive shoulder adduction. **G,** Assessing the medial border of the right scapular soft tissue response to passive shoulder distraction. **H,** Assessing the medial border of the right scapular soft tissue response to passive shoulder compression. **I,** The practitioner stacks all planes of motion, eliciting a response of ease or relaxation of the medial scapular border soft tissues while the patient inhales or exhales—whichever increases the sense of ease.

4. The practitioner then asks the patient to inhale, and exhale and determines which phase of respiration causes increased ease of the soft tissues being monitored at the medial scapular border.
5. The practitioner then combines all directions of motion to which the soft tissues responded with ease or relaxation while the patient takes a breath in the phase that also increased ease or relaxation. This stacking of motions leads to a vector, a distinct direction of motion that induces relaxation of the soft tissues (see Fig. 9.21I).
6. The practitioner retests the response of the periscapular soft tissues to passive shoulder motions. There should be no soft tissue binding or resistance with any passive motion of the shoulder.

Shoulder Counterstrain
Supraspinatus
- Location: in the belly of the supraspinatus muscle (along the spine of the scapula) (Fig. 9.22)

- The procedure is performed as follows (Fig. 9.23):
  1. The patient is supine.
  2. The practitioner flexes the humerus to 45 degrees, abducts it to 45 degrees, and externally rotates it to 45 degrees.
  3. This position is maintained for 90 seconds.
  4. The patient's shoulder is slowly and passively returned to the neutral position.
  5. The practitioner retests the counterstrain point for tenderness.

Teres Minor
- Location: on the lateral border of the scapula at the origin of the teres minor muscle (Fig. 9.24)
- The procedure is performed as follows (Fig. 9.25):
  1. The patient is supine.
  2. The practitioner induces marked external rotation of the humerus, with slight flexion and abduction as needed.
  3. This position is maintained for 90 seconds.

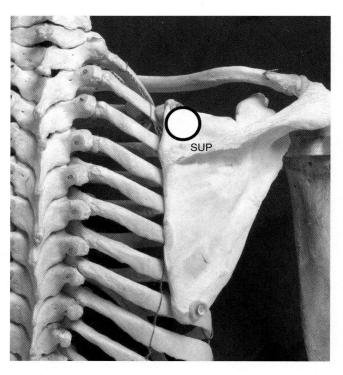

Figure 9.22 Right supraspinatus (SUP) tender point on a skeletal model.

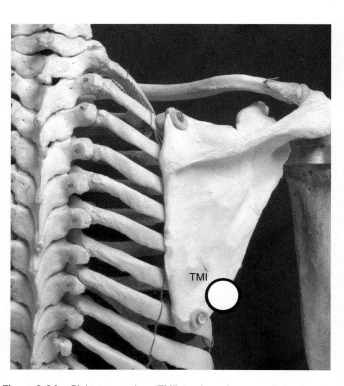

Figure 9.24 Right teres minor (TMI) tender point on a skeletal model.

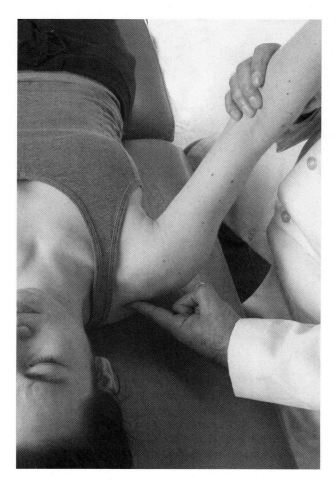

Figure 9.23 Counterstrain treatment position for the right supraspinatus tender point.

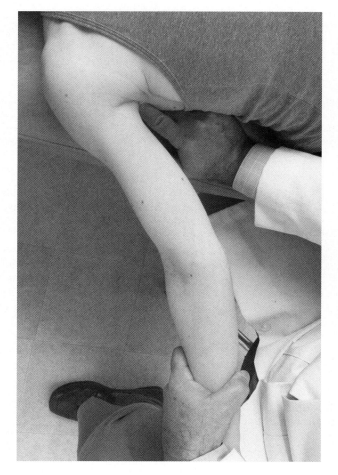

Figure 9.25 Counterstrain treatment position for the right teres minor tender point.

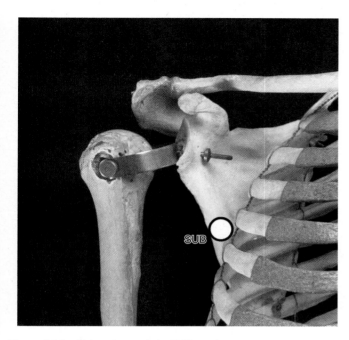

Figure 9.26 Right subscapularis (SUB) tender point on a skeletal model.

4. The patient's shoulder is slowly and passively returned to the neutral position.
5. The practitioner retests the counterstrain point for tenderness.

Subscapularis
- Location: on the anterior surface of the scapula, in the posterior axillary fold (Fig. 9.26)
- The procedure is performed as follows (Fig. 9.27):
  1. The patient is supine.
  2. The practitioner extends the patient's affected arm 45 degrees off the table with marked internal rotation of the humerus, adding adduction or abduction as needed.
  3. This position is maintained for 90 seconds.
  4. The patient's shoulder is slowly and passively returned to the neutral position.
  5. The practitioner retests the counterstrain point for tenderness.

Long Head of the Biceps
- Location: in the bicipital groove of the humerus (Fig. 9.28)
- The procedure is performed as follows (Fig. 9.29):
  1. The patient is supine.
  2. The practitioner supinates the patient's forearm, then flexes the humerus with the palmar aspect of wrist placed on the patient's forehead, and adds internal or external rotation as needed.
  3. This position is maintained for 90 seconds.
  4. The patient's shoulder is slowly and passively returned to the neutral position.
  5. The practitioner retests the counterstrain point for tenderness.

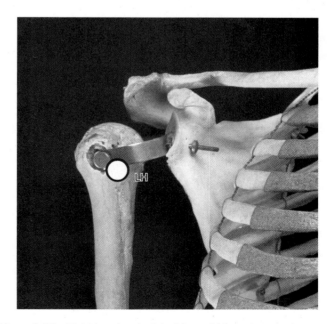

Figure 9.27 Counterstrain treatment position for the right subscapularis tender point.

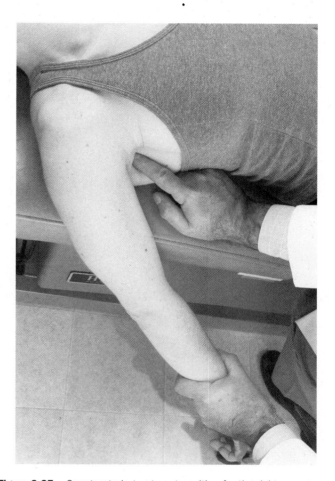

Figure 9.28 Right long head of the biceps (LH) tender point on a skeletal model.

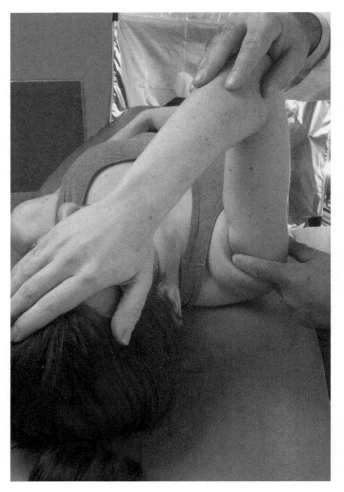

Figure 9.29 Counterstrain treatment position for the right long head of the biceps tender point.

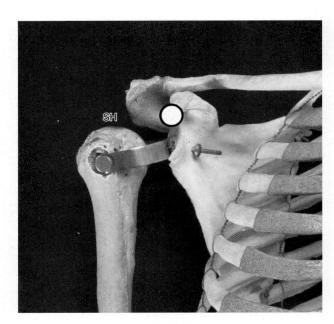

Figure 9.30 Right short head of the biceps (SH) tender point on a skeletal model.

Short Head of the Biceps
- Location: on the inferolateral aspect of the coracoid process (Fig. 9.30)
- The procedure is performed as follows (Fig. 9.31):
  1. The patient is supine.
  2. The practitioner supinates the patient's forearm, flexes the humerus to 90 degrees, and adducts the humerus across the patient's body.
  3. This position is maintained for 90 seconds.
  4. The patient's shoulder is slowly and passively returned to the neutral position.
  5. The practitioner retests the counterstrain point for tenderness.

Lateral Coracoid
- Location: on the superolateral aspect of the coracoid process (Fig. 9.32)
- The procedure is performed as follows (Fig. 9.33):
  1. The patient is supine.
  2. The practitioner extends the patient's head off the table and rotates the head toward and sidebends the head away from the tender point.

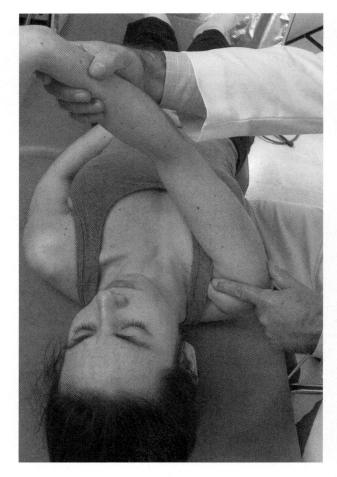

Figure 9.31 Counterstrain treatment position for the right short head of the biceps tender point.

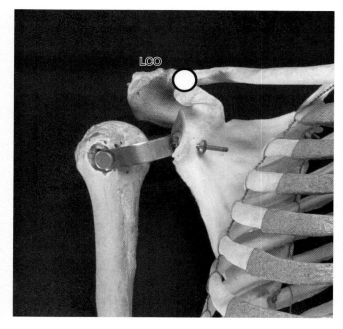

Figure 9.32 Right superolateral coracoid process (LCO) tender point on a skeletal model.

3. This position is maintained for 90 seconds.
4. The patient's shoulder is slowly and passively returned to the neutral position.
5. The practitioner retests the counterstrain point for tenderness.

Thoracic (Costal) Cage Treatment Procedures

Thoracic Spine Soft Tissue Procedures
Prone Pressure Soft Tissue Technique

- Example: left thoracic paraspinal muscle hypertonicity (Fig. 9.34)
- This technique is commonly performed bilaterally for hypertonic thoracic paraspinal soft tissues, because relaxing the hypertonic side often reveals hypertonicity in the contralateral side, although to a lesser degree.
- The procedure is performed as follows:
  1. The patient is prone on the examination table, with his or her head turned toward the practitioner.
  2. The practitioner stands at the side of the table opposite the hypertonic paraspinal muscles that he or she will be treating.
  3. The practitioner places his or her thumb and thenar eminence of one hand on the far side of the thoracic spine between the spinous and transverse processes and over the paravertebral muscles (see Fig. 9.34A).
  4. The practitioner places his or her other hand on top of the first, working in conjunction with it along the spine (see Fig. 9.34B).
  5. The practitioner applies an anterolateral pressure, moving his or her hands in a lateral direction and using continuous pressure until the tissue is taken to its restrictive barrier.

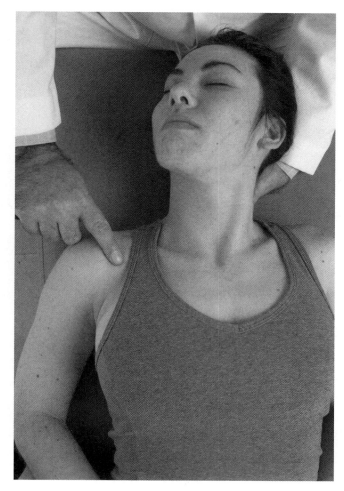

Figure 9.33 Counterstrain treatment position for the right superolateral coracoid process tender point.

6. The practitioner holds the soft tissues at the restrictive barrier until further relaxation of the tissues is observed, allowing a slight increase in lateral motion.
7. The soft tissues are then allowed to passively return to the starting position.
8. Steps 4 through 7 are repeated in a rhythmic fashion until increased soft tissue compliance is achieved.
9. The process is repeated on the opposite side.
10. The practitioner retests the compliance of the soft tissues.

Lateral Recumbent Thoracic Soft Tissue Technique

- Example: hypertonic right thoracic paraspinal soft tissues (Fig. 9.35)
- The procedure is performed as follows:
  1. The patient is in the left lateral recumbent position.
  2. The practitioner stands at the side of the table and faces the patient.
  3. The patient flexes his or her hips and knees slightly.
  4. The practitioner contacts the right uppermost thoracic paravertebral muscles with the finger pads of both hands, avoiding the spinous processes.

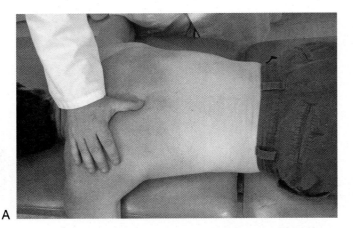

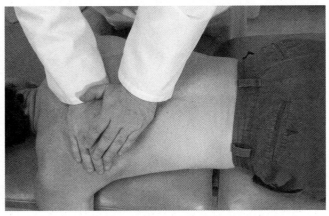

Figure 9.34 Soft tissue paraspinal muscle lateral stretch for left shoulder dysfunction. **A,** Bottom hand treatment position. **B,** Top hand treatment position.

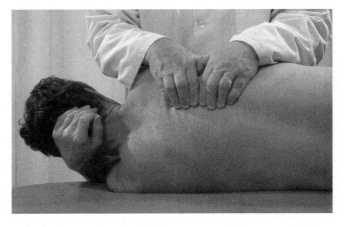

Figure 9.35 Right thoracic paraspinal muscle lateral stretch for right shoulder dysfunction with the patient in the left lateral recumbent position.

5. The practitioner drapes the patient's right arm over his or her right arm (while treating the upper thoracic spine) or over the left arm (while treating the middle and lower thoracic spine).
6. The practitioner moves the paravertebral muscles and associated soft tissues anterolaterally with his or her finger pads until the restrictive barrier is engaged.
7. The practitioner continues to apply lateral traction until the tissues relax, soften, and lengthen. The lateral traction is then slowly released.
8. Steps 6 and 7 are repeated until increased compliance in the thoracic soft tissues is observed.
9. The practitioner applies this technique along the spinal region from the cervicothoracic junction to the lower thoracic spine.
10. The process is repeated on the opposite side.
11. The practitioner retests the compliance of the thoracic soft tissues.

Diaphragm Myofascial Release Technique
Seated Thoracic Diaphragm Myofascial Release Technique
- The procedure is performed as follows:
  1. The patient is seated.
  2. The practitioner stands behind the patient.
  3. The practitioner places his or her hands around the thoracic cage under the patient's arms, with the fingertips or the fifth finger edge and hypothenar eminence underneath the patient's costal margins.
  4. The practitioner passively rotates the diaphragm to the left and right until diaphragm tension is felt under the fingers. The practitioner observes whether there is symmetry of motion or there is greater ease of motion in one direction or the other.
  5. Using the same hand position, the practitioner rotates the diaphragm in the direction of ease as far as comfortably possible.
  6. This position is maintained until increased compliance and relaxation of the diaphragm is observed, and the diaphragm is moving freely in a rhythmic, symmetric motion.
  7. The practitioner then allows the diaphragm and associated myofascial tissues to passively return to neutral.
  8. The practitioner rechecks the motion and compliance of the diaphragm.

Supine Thoracic Diaphragm Myofascial Release Technique
- The procedure is performed as follows:
  1. The patient is supine.
  2. The practitioner stands at the patient's side.
  3. The practitioner places his or her hands and fingers on the outer aspect of the inferior border of the lower ribs, with the thumbs pointed toward each other medially and positioned directly inferior to the xiphoid process of the sternum (Fig. 9.36).
  4. The practitioner passively assesses the lower costal cage for compliance or resistance to clockwise and counterclockwise motion in the coronal and vertical planes (Fig. 9.37).
  5. The practitioner finds the position of maximal compliance and holds this position while the patient exhales and holds his or her breath out as long as possible (see Fig. 9.37B).

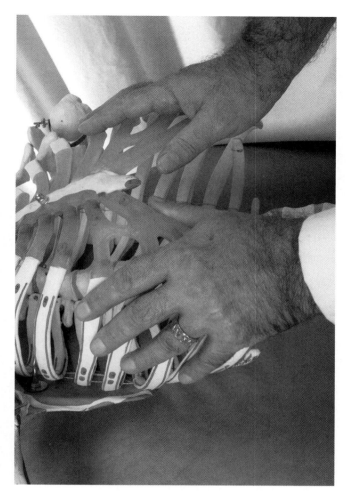

Figure 9.36 Supine diaphragm myofascial assessment, with the hand position shown on a skeletal model.

6. The practitioner follows the unwinding of the lower costal cage as the diaphragm tension releases (see Fig. 9.37C).
7. Just before the patient has to inhale, the practitioner feels a release of tension and increase in ease of motion.
8. The practitioner reassesses compliance of the lower costal cage to active (inhalation) and passive motion (see Fig. 9.37D).

Pectoralis Minor Direct Myofascial Release Technique
• This technique is performed bilaterally for hypertonic pectoralis minor muscles (Fig. 9.38).
• The procedure is performed as follows:
  1. The patient is supine.
  2. The practitioner is seated at the head of the table.
  3. The practitioner gently and firmly grasps the myotendinous insertion of the pectoralis minor muscles at right angles to the direction of their fibers.
  4. The practitioner then slowly leans back to put gentle traction on the muscles and engage the restrictive barrier.
  5. The practitioner holds this position until relaxation of the tissues is observed.
  6. The practitioner retests the compliance of the pectoralis minor myofascial tissues.

Costal Cage Articulatory Techniques
Costal Cage Supine Articulatory Technique
• Example: restriction of motion of right rib 8 (Fig. 9.39)
• The procedure is performed as follows:
  1. The patient is supine.
  2. The practitioner stands on the right side of the patient.
  3. The practitioner grasps the patient's right wrist with his or her left hand.
  4. The practitioner contacts the lateral aspect of the angle of the dysfunctional right rib 8 with his or her right index finger and hand.
  5. The practitioner then stabilizes and places lateral traction on the patient's right rib 8 while passively abducting the patient's right arm to meet and exceed the restrictive barrier.

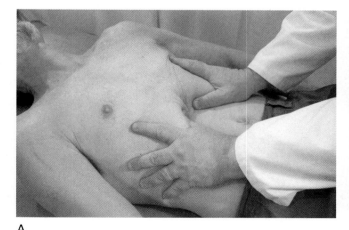

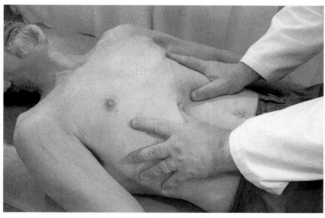

A   B

Figure 9.37 Supine diaphragm myofascial release. **A,** Supine diaphragm myofascial assessment: clockwise versus counterclockwise motion in the coronal plane. **B,** The practitioner finds the direction of ease, which is counterclockwise in this photograph.

Continued

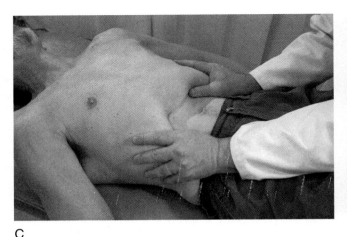
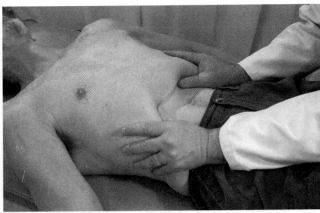

C

D

Figure 9.37, cont'd **C,** The practitioner follows the release of tension of the tissues into the clockwise direction. **D,** The practitioner follows the tissues as the restrictive barrier gives way and symmetric ease is restored.

6. The practitioner returns the patient's shoulder to neutral position and then repeats step 5 three to five times or until improved rib 8 motion occurs.
7. Active (inhalation) rib 8 motion is reassessed.

Alternative Supine Costal Cage Articulatory Technique
- Example: dysfunctional right sided rib with exhalation somatic dysfunction
- The procedure is performed as follows:
  1. The patient is supine.
  2. The practitioner stands on the right side of the patient.
  3. The practitioner grasps the patient's right wrist with his or her left hand.
  4. The practitioner stabilizes the rib below the key rib (i.e., most dysfunctional rib) of the group anteriorly by placing the thenar or hypothenar eminence of his or her right hand on the anterosuperior surface of the specific rib.
  5. For ribs 2 through 5, the practitioner simultaneously brings the arm into flexion while the patient inhales deeply to stretch the intercostal space above the stabilized rib and

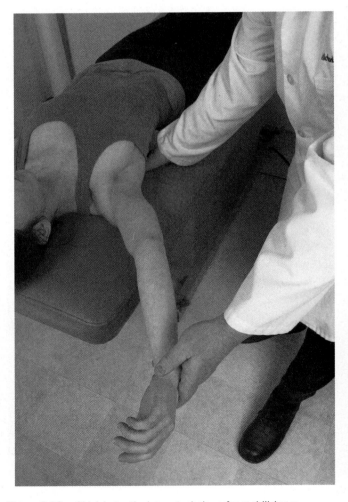

Figure 9.39 Sidelying articulatory technique for mobilizing a dysfunctional rib.

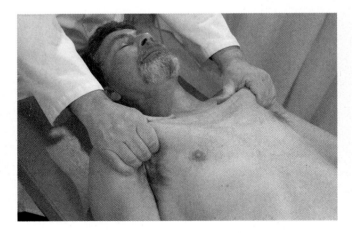

Figure 9.38 Myofascial release treatment for the pectoral muscles.

engage the restrictive barrier for 3 to 5 seconds and then returns the arm to neutral during exhalation.

6. For ribs 6 through 10, the practitioner simultaneously brings the arm into abduction while the patient inhales deeply to stretch the intercostal space above the stabilized rib and engage the restrictive barrier for 3 to 5 seconds and then returns the arm to neutral during exhalation.

7. The practitioner repeatedly engages this restrictive barrier in a rhythmic fashion until there is increased range of motion toward the physiologic barrier.

8. The practitioner retests the rib cage motion.

Costal Cage Sidelying Articulatory Technique

- Example: exhalation rib somatic dysfunction of ribs 6 through 10 (i.e., bucket-handle motion restriction)
- The procedure is performed as follows:
  1. The patient lies in the lateral recumbent position on the side opposite the rib restriction.
  2. The practitioner stands in front of the patient.
  3. The practitioner grasps the patient's elbow on the side of rib restriction.
  4. The practitioner stabilizes the rib below the key dysfunctional rib along the midaxillary line with his or her thumb and thenar eminence.
  5. For ribs 6 through 10, the practitioner simultaneously brings the arm into abduction while the patient inhales deeply to stretch the intercostal space above the stabilized rib and engage the restrictive barrier for 3 to 5 seconds and then returns the arm to neutral during exhalation.
  6. The practitioner repeatedly engages this restrictive barrier in a rhythmic fashion until there is increased range of motion toward the physiologic barrier.
  7. The practitioner retests the rib cage motion.

Costal Cage Seated Articulatory Technique

- Example: somatic dysfunction of any rib or group of ribs (Figs. 9.40 and 9.41)
- The procedure is performed as follows:
  1. The patient is seated.
  2. The practitioner stands in front of the patient.
  3. The patient crosses his or her fully extended arms and places both arms over the practitioner's shoulder (see Fig. 9.40A).
  4. The patient's head rests on his or her arms (see Fig. 9.40B).
  5. The practitioner reaches behind the patient with both arms to contact the rib angles medially with the finger pads as a fulcrum for extension of the patient's spine (see Fig. 9.40C).
  6. The practitioner simultaneously applies anterolateral traction on the contacted rib angles and extends the patient's spine by shifting the practitioner's center of gravity posteriorly and pulling the patient toward the practitioner to engage the restrictive barrier (see Fig. 9.41).
  7. This position is held for 3 to 5 seconds, and the patient then is returned to the neutral position.
  8. The practitioner repeatedly engages this restrictive barrier in a rhythmic fashion until there is increased range of motion toward the physiologic barrier.
  9. The practitioner retests the motion of the rib cage.

Muscle Energy Techniques for Costal Cage Somatic Dysfunction
Muscle Energy Technique for Rib Inhalation Somatic Dysfunction: Rib 1

- Example: inhalation somatic dysfunction of the right first rib, exhalation restriction (Fig. 9.42)
- The procedure is performed as follows:
  1. The patient is supine.
  2. The practitioner stands or sits at the head of the table.
  3. The practitioner contacts the angle of the patient's right first rib in the supraclavicular fossa, just anterior to the superior trapezius muscle border at the base of the neck with his or her right thumb.
  4. The practitioner applies gentle pressure to the first rib with his or her right thumb, moving the rib inferiorly until the restrictive barrier is engaged.
  5. The practitioner uses his or her left hand to flex the patient's head until motion is felt at the first rib.
  6. The patient inhales and exhales deeply. As the patient exhales, the practitioner uses his or her right thumb to move the first rib further inferiorly and engage a new restrictive barrier.
  7. The patient holds his or her breath in exhalation for 3 to 5 seconds. During this time, the practitioner instructs the patient to push his or her head backward against the practitioner's left hand, which provides an unyielding counterforce. This isometric contraction should last for the 3 to 5 seconds that the patient is holding his or her breath.
  8. When the patient inhales, the practitioner uses his or her right thumb to resist the natural tendency of the rib to rise with inhalation.
  9. Steps 4 through 8 are repeated three to five times.
  10. After the final repetition, a final stretch is performed further into the restrictive barrier.
  11. The practitioner retests the motion of the right first rib compared with the opposite side.
- After the dysfunctional rib is treated, it often moves better than its counterpart on the opposite side. During reassessment, the untreated side then seems to be restricted and should also be treated until symmetric and nonrestricted rib motion on inhalation and exhalation is attained.

Muscle Energy Technique for Rib Inhalation Somatic Dysfunction: Ribs 2 to 5

- Example: inhalation somatic dysfunction of the right third rib, exhalation restriction (Fig. 9.43)
- The procedure is performed as follows:
  1. The patient is supine.
  2. The practitioner stands or sits at the head of the table.
  3. The practitioner places the web space formed by the thumb and index finger of his or her right hand in the second intercostal space above the dysfunctional right rib (rib 3) on its anterosuperior surface.
  4. The practitioner uses his or her right hand to move rib 3 inferiorly and engage the restrictive barrier.
  5. Using his or her left hand, the practitioner flexes the patient's head until motion is felt at rib 3.

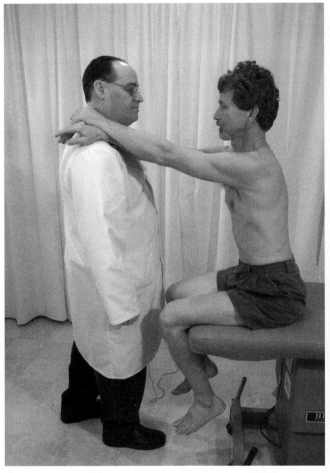

A

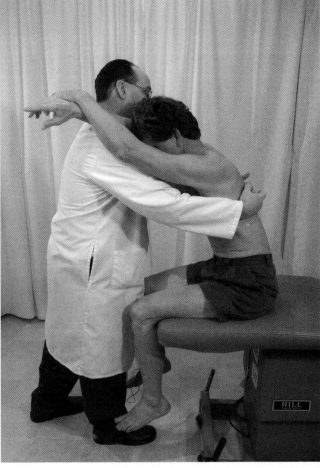

B

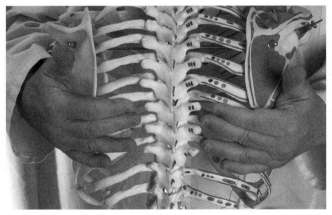

C

Figure 9.40   **A,** Seated rib articulatory technique starting position with the patient's arms crossing at the wrists and resting on the practitioner's shoulder. **B,** Seated rib articulatory technique treatment position with practitioner's hands around the patient's back and palpating the rib angles. **C,** Posterior view of practitioner's hand position on the rib angles of a skeletal model.

6. The patient inhales and exhales deeply. As the patient exhales, the practitioner moves the third rib further inferiorly and engages a new restrictive barrier.
7. The patient holds his or her breath in exhalation for 3 to 5 seconds. As the patient holds his or her breath in exhalation, he or she performs an isometric contraction by

extending the head and neck against the practitioner's left hand, which provides an unyielding counterforce.
8. As the patient inhales, the practitioner uses his or her right hand to resist the natural tendency of the rib to rise during inhalation.
9. Steps 4 through 8 are repeated three to five times.

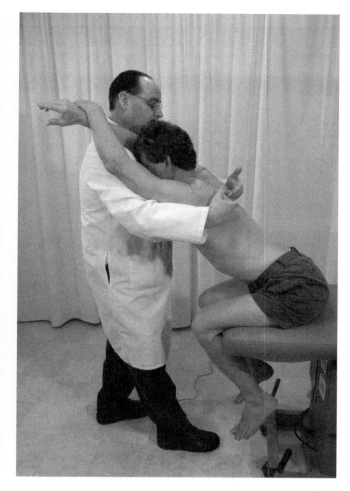

Figure 9.41 Seated articulatory rib treatment. The practitioner leans back to extend the patient's spine and elevate the ribs.

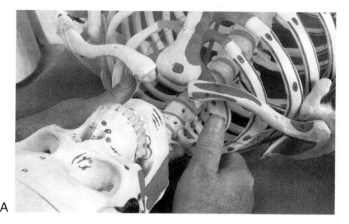

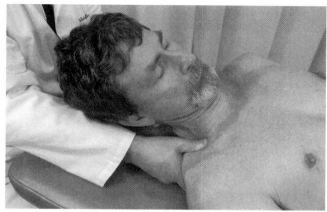

Figure 9.42   A, Thumb position used for a right first rib inhalation somatic dysfunction muscle energy treatment (MET) is demonstrated on a skeletal model. **B,** MET position for the right first rib inhalation somatic dysfunction.

10. After the final repetition, a final stretch is performed further into the restrictive barrier.
11. The practitioner retests the motion of the treated rib.

Muscle Energy Technique for Rib Inhalation Somatic Dysfunction: Ribs 6 to 10

- Example: inhalation somatic dysfunction of left rib 8, exhalation restriction (Fig. 9.44)
- The procedure is performed as follows:
  1. The patient is supine.
  2. The practitioner stands on the side of the dysfunctional rib near the head of the supine patient
  3. The practitioner places the web space between the index finger and thumb of his or her left hand in the seventh intercostal space on the superior border of patient's left rib 8 in the midaxillary line.
  4. The practitioner applies gentle pressure to rib 8 to move it inferiorly and engage the restrictive barrier.
  5. Using his or her right hand, the practitioner flexes and sidebends the patient's head to the left until he or she detects motion at the level of rib 8.

6. The practitioner instructs the patient to inhale and exhale fully. As the patient exhales, the patient also reaches toward his or her left foot with the left hand.
7. The patient holds his or her breath in exhalation for 3 to 5 seconds while isometrically contracting the head and neck against the practitioner's right hand, which provides an unyielding counterforce.
8. As the patient inhales the practitioner uses his or her left hand to resist the natural tendency of the rib to rise (i.e., bucket-handle motion) during inhalation.
9. Steps 4 through 8 are repeated three to five times.
10. After the final repetition, a final stretch is performed further into the restrictive barrier.
11. The practitioner retests the motion of the treated rib.

Muscle Energy Technique for Rib Inhalation Somatic Dysfunction: Ribs 11 and 12

- Example: inhalation somatic dysfunction of the left 12th rib, exhalation restriction (Fig. 9.45)
- The procedure is performed as follows:
  1. The patient is prone.
  2. The practitioner stands at the right side of the patient.

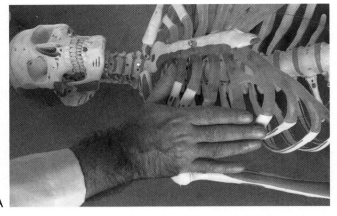

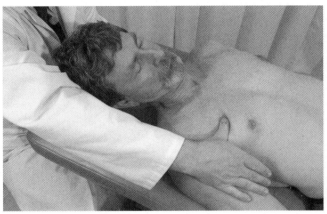

Figure 9.43 **A,** Muscle energy treatment (MET) hand position for a right second rib inhalation somatic dysfunction is demonstrated on a skeletal model. **B,** MET position for a right third rib inhalation somatic dysfunction.

3. The practitioner places the thenar eminence of his or her right hand on the superior border of the patient's left 12th rib.
4. The practitioner moves the rib inferiorly and laterally to engage the restrictive barrier.

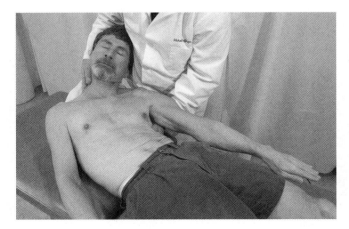

Figure 9.44 Muscle energy treatment (MET) position for a left eighth rib inhalation somatic dysfunction.

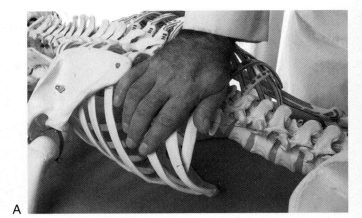

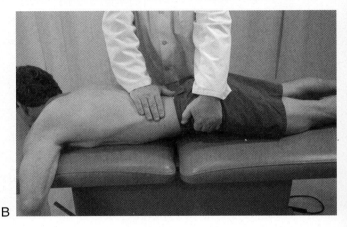

Figure 9.45 **A,** Hand position on a skeletal model in preparation for a left 12th rib inhalation somatic dysfunction muscle energy treatment (MET). **B,** MET position for a left 12th rib inhalation somatic dysfunction.

5. The practitioner's right hand grasps the patient's left anterosuperior iliac spine (ASIS) and lifts the left side of the patient's pelvis toward the ceiling.
6. The patient is instructed to attempt to pull his or her left hip toward the table for 3 to 5 seconds against the practitioner's unyielding counterforce.
7. The patient then relaxes, and the practitioner releases his or her counterforce.
8. The practitioner raises the left side of the patient's pelvis further toward the ceiling to engage the next restrictive barrier.
9. Steps 6 through 8 are repeated three to five times.
10. After the final repetition, a final stretch is performed further into the restrictive barrier.
11. The practitioner retests the motion of the treated rib.

Muscle Energy Technique for Rib Exhalation Somatic Dysfunction: Rib 1
- Example: exhalation somatic dysfunction of the right first rib, inhalation restriction (Fig. 9.46)
- The procedure is performed as follows:
  1. The patient is supine.
  2. The practitioner stands at the patient's left side.

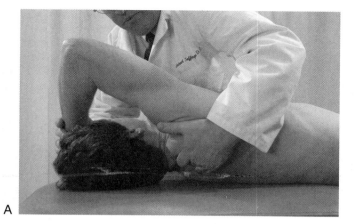

A

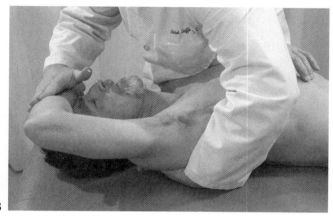

B

Figure 9.46 **A,** Muscle energy treatment (MET) for a right rib 1 exhalation somatic dysfunction: posterior view of the hand position with practitioner's fingertips of the left hand curled around the superior aspect of the first rib angle exerting an inferior force. **B,** MET for a left rib 1 exhalation somatic dysfunction: lateral view of the true treatment position.

3. The practitioner places his or her left hand under the patient's left shoulder and grasps the rib angle of the dysfunctional left first rib with his or her fingertips (see Fig. 9.46A).
4. The practitioner exerts an inferior force on the patient's right first rib angle to engage the restrictive barrier, titling the anterior portion of the first rib superiorly (i.e., in its pump-handle motion).
5. The practitioner places the dorsum of the patient's right wrist on the patient's forehead (see Fig. 9.46B).
6. The practitioner places his or her right hand on the patient's right wrist.
7. The patient inhales and holds his or her breath for 3 to 5 seconds while attempting to lift the head toward the ceiling against the practitioner's unyielding counterforce.
8. The patient then exhales and relaxes his or her head and neck muscles.
9. Steps 6 through 8 are repeated three to five times.
10. After the final repetition, a final stretch is performed further into the restrictive barrier.

11. The practitioner retests the motion of the right first rib compared with the opposite side during inhalation and exhalation. The left first rib may also need to be treated.

Muscle Energy Technique for Rib Exhalation Somatic Dysfunction: Rib 2

- Example: exhalation somatic dysfunction of the right second rib, inhalation restriction (Fig. 9.47)
- The procedure is performed as follows:
  1. The patient is supine.
  2. The practitioner stands at the patient's left side.
  3. The practitioner places his or her left hand under the patient' right shoulder and grasps the superior aspect of the rib angle of the dysfunctional second rib with his or her fingertips (see Fig. 9.47A).
  4. The practitioner exerts an inferior force on the patient's right second rib with his or her left hand to engage the restrictive barrier.
  5. The practitioner places the dorsum of the patient's right wrist on the patient's forehead.

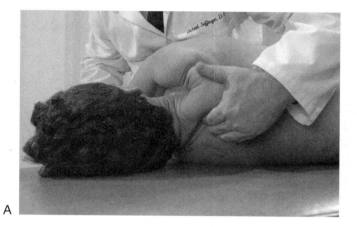

A

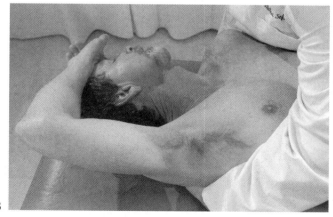

B

Figure 9.47 **A,** Muscle energy treatment (MET) for an exhalation somatic dysfunction of the right rib 2: posterior view of practitioner's left hand position with fingertips on the superior aspect of the second rib angle exerting an inferior force. **B,** MET for a right rib 2 exhalation somatic dysfunction.

6. The practitioner places his or her right hand on the patient's right wrist.
7. The patient's head is rotated 30 degrees to the left for better contraction of the right posterior scalene muscle.
8. The patient inhales and holds his or her breath for 3 to 5 seconds while at the same time attempting to lift the head toward the ceiling against the practitioner's unyielding counterforce.
9. The patient then exhales and relaxes his or her head and neck muscles.
10. Steps 7 through 9 are repeated three to five times.
11. After the final repetition, a final stretch is performed further into the restrictive barrier.
12. The practitioner retests the motion of the second rib compared with the other side during inhalation and exhalation. The opposite side may also need to be treated to obtain symmetric and unrestricted motion.

Muscle Energy Technique for Rib Exhalation Somatic Dysfunction: Ribs 3 to 5

• Example: exhalation somatic dysfunction of right rib 4, inhalation restriction (Fig. 9.48)
• The procedure is performed as follows:
  1. The patient is supine.
  2. The practitioner stands at the left side of the patient.
  3. The practitioner places his or her left hand under the patient's right shoulder and grasps the superior aspect of the rib angle of the dysfunctional rib 4.
  4. The practitioner exerts an inferior force on the rib to engage the restrictive barrier.
  5. The practitioner flexes the patient's right elbow to 90 degrees and abducts and flexes the patient's right shoulder, placing the hand above the head of the patient with the elbow adjacent to the patient's head and the arm resting on the table.
  6. The practitioner places his or her right hand on the patient's right elbow.
  7. The patient inhales and holds his or her breath for 3 to 5 seconds while at the same time attempting to bring the right elbow toward the left ASIS against the practitioner's unyielding counterforce.

8. The patient then exhales and relaxes his or her right arm.
9. Steps 6 through 8 are repeated three to five times.
10. After the final repetition, a final stretch is performed further into the restrictive barrier.
11. The practitioner retests the motion of the treated rib compared with the opposite side during inhalation and exhalation.

Muscle Energy Technique for Rib Exhalation Somatic Dysfunction: Ribs 6 to 10

• Example: exhalation somatic dysfunction of the left 8th rib, inhalation restriction (Fig. 9.49)
  1. The patient is supine.
  2. The practitioner stands at the left side of the patient.
  3. The practitioner places his or her left hand under the patient and grasps the rib angle of the dysfunctional rib 8 with his or her fingertips.
  4. The practitioner abducts the patient's left arm to 90 degrees and places his or her right leg against the patient's distal left forearm.
  5. The practitioner exerts an inferior force on the patient's eighth rib to engage the restrictive barrier.
  6. The patient inhales and holds his or her breath for 3 to 5 seconds while attempting to adduct his or her left arm against the practitioner's unyielding counterforce provided by the practitioner's right leg.
  7. The patient then exhales and relaxes his or her left arm.
  8. Steps 5 through 7 are repeated three to five times.
  9. After the final repetition, a final stretch is performed further into the restrictive barrier.
  10. The practitioner retests the motion of the treated rib compared with the opposite side during inhalation and exhalation.

Muscle Energy Technique for Rib Exhalation Somatic Dysfunction: Ribs 11 and 12

• Example: exhalation somatic dysfunction of the left 12th rib, inhalation restriction (Fig. 9.50)
• The procedure is performed as follows:
  1. The patient is prone.

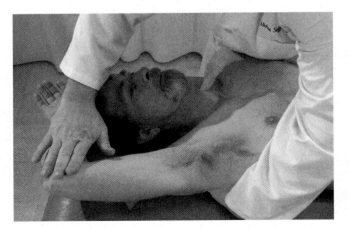

Figure 9.48 Muscle energy treatment (MET) for right ribs 3 through 5 exhalation somatic dysfunction.

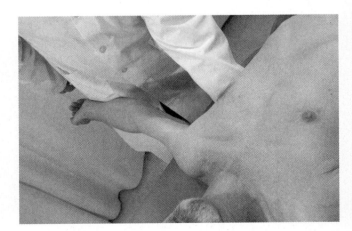

Figure 9.49 Muscle energy treatment (MET) for left ribs 6 through 10 exhalation somatic dysfunction.

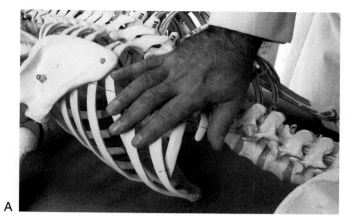

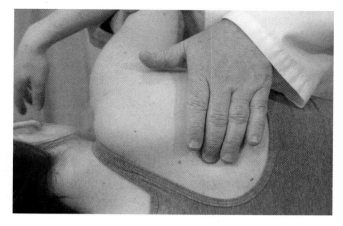

Figure 9.51 Hand position for monitoring the soft tissues overlying the dysfunctional right rib angle during the functional technique.

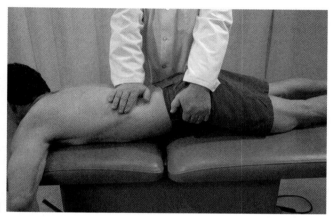

Figure 9.50 **A,** Left 12th rib exhalation somatic dysfunction hand position on a skeletal model. **B,** Muscle energy treatment (MET) for a 12th rib exhalation somatic dysfunction.

2. The practitioner stands at the patient's right side.
3. The practitioner pulls the patient's legs 15 to 20 degrees to the right, away from the dysfunctional rib.
4. The practitioner places the thenar eminence of his or her right hand inferior and medial to the angle of the dysfunctional 12th rib (see Fig. 9.50A).
5. The practitioner's left hand grasps the patient's left ASIS and raises the left side of the patient's pelvis toward the ceiling to engage the restrictive barrier (see Fig. 9.50B).
6. The patient is instructed to attempt to pull his or her left hip toward the table for 3 to 5 seconds against the practitioner's unyielding counterforce.
7. The patient then relaxes, and the counterforce is ceased.
8. The practitioner moves the left side of the patient's pelvis further toward the ceiling to engage the next restrictive barrier.
9. Steps 6 through 8 are repeated three to five times.
10. After the final repetition, a final stretch is performed further into the restrictive barrier.
11. The practitioner retests the motion of the treated rib compared with the opposite side during inhalation and exhalation.

Costal Cage Functional Techniques
- Example: right rib 7 somatic dysfunction (Fig. 9.51)
- The procedure is performed as follows:
  1. The patient is sidelying in the left lateral recumbent position.
  2. The practitioner stands in front of the patient.
  3. The practitioner grasps the patient's elbow with his or her right hand and monitors the soft tissues overlying the rib angle of the dysfunctional rib with his or her left finger pads.
  4. The practitioner passively moves the patient's shoulder through its normal motions, observing which directions decrease the tissue tension palpated around the angle of the affected rib: flexion, extension, abduction, adduction, external rotation, and internal rotation and compression and distraction of the glenohumeral joint.
  5. The practitioner stacks the motion directions that elicited a sense of ease or compliance in the soft tissue overlying the affected rib and asks the patient to breathe in and out slowly and deeply.
  6. While the patient is breathing in the phase of respiration that further elicits relaxation in the monitored soft tissues, the practitioner fine-tunes the shoulder motions in the directions of ease to maximize the relaxation of the monitored tissues.
  7. At the end of the single breath, the practitioner reassesses the response of the soft tissues overlying the affected rib angle to passive shoulder motions.

Rib Counterstrain
Anterior Rib Counterstrain Points
- The anterior rib 1 (AR1) location is on the first costal cartilage, beneath the clavicle and adjacent to the sternum (Fig. 9.52). The procedure is performed as follows (Fig. 9.53):
  1. The patient is seated.
  2. The practitioner's knee is placed under the patient's axilla on the side opposite the tender point.

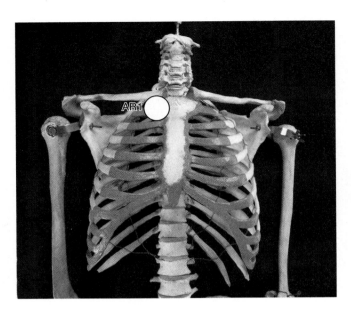

Figure 9.52 Location of the right anterior rib 1 (AR1) tender point on a skeletal model.

3. The practitioner flexes the patient's head and neck and then rotates and markedly sidebends the patient's head toward the tender point.
• Alternate treatment position for AR1
  1. The patient is supine.
  2. The practitioner flexes the patient's head and neck and then rotates and sidebends the patient's head toward the counterstrain point.

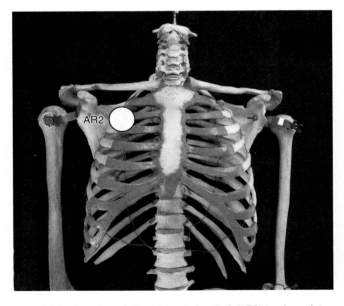

Figure 9.54 Location of the right anterior rib 2 (AR2) tender point on skeletal model.

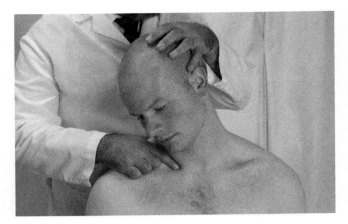

Figure 9.53 Counterstrain treatment position for the right anterior rib 1 tender point.

• The anterior rib 2 (AR2) location is in the midclavicular line, on the inferior margin of the second rib (Fig. 9.54). The procedure is performed as follows (Fig. 9.55):
  1. The patient is seated.
  2. The practitioner flexes the patient's head and then rotates and markedly sidebends the patient's head toward the counterstrain point.
• Alternate treatment position for AR2
  1. The patient is supine.
  2. The practitioner flexes the patient's head and neck and then rotates and sidebends the patient's head toward the counterstrain point.
• Locations of anterior ribs 3 through 6
  1. AR3: in the anterior axillary line on the inferior margin of the third rib
  2. AR4: in the anterior axillary line on the inferior margin of the fourth rib (Fig. 9.56)

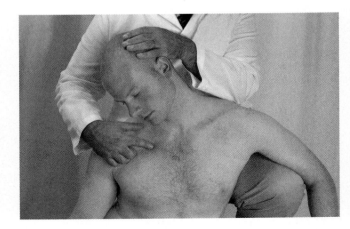

Figure 9.55 Counterstrain treatment position for the right anterior rib 2 tender point.

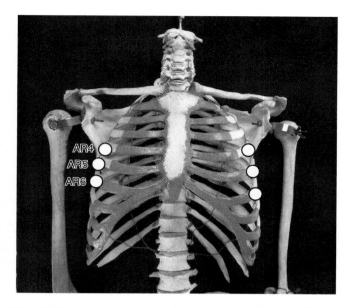

Figure 9.56   Location of the anterior rib 4 through 6 (AR4 to AR6) tender points on a skeletal model.

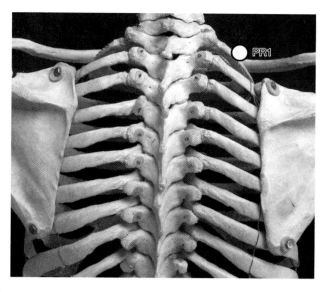

Figure 9.58   Location of the right posterior rib 1 (PR1) tender point on a skeletal model.

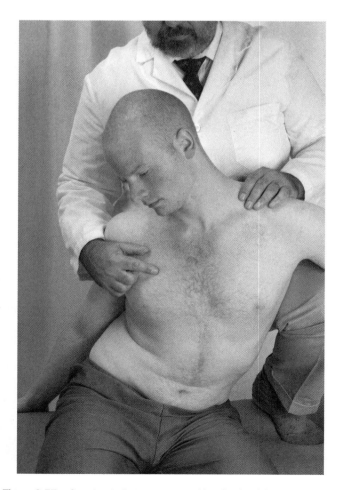

Figure 9.57   Counterstrain treatment position for the right anterior rib 4 tender point.

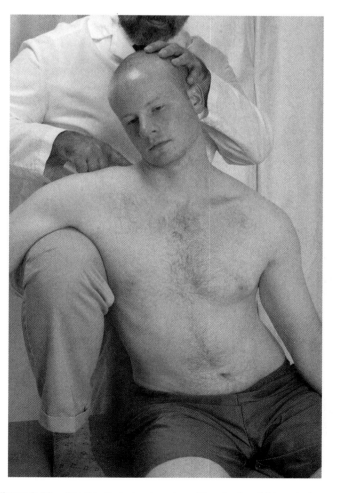

Figure 9.59   Counterstrain treatment position for the right posterior rib 1 tender points.

3. AR5: in the anterior axillary line on the inferior margin of the fifth rib (see Fig. 9.56)
4. AR6: in the anterior axillary line on the inferior margin of the sixth rib (see Fig. 9.56)
- The procedure is performed as follows (Fig. 9.57):
  1. The patient is seated.
  2. The practitioner's knee is placed under the patient's axilla in the side opposite the tender point.
  3. The patient's arm on the side of the affected rib is suspended behind the patient's back.
  4. The practitioner induces slight flexion of the torso and rotation and sidebending of the torso toward the tender point.

Posterior Rib Counterstrain

- The posterior rib 1 (PR1) location is on the posterolateral aspect of the first rib, beneath margin of the trapezius muscle at the angle of the neck and shoulder (Fig. 9.58).
- The procedure is performed as follows (Fig. 9.59):
  1. The patient is seated.
  2. The practitioner places his or her foot on the treatment table on the same side as the rib to be treated.
  3. The patient's axilla on the same side of the tender point is placed over the practitioner's thigh.
  4. The practitioner extends the patient's head slightly and then sidebends the patient's head away from and rotates the patient's head toward the tender point.
- Locations of posterior ribs 2 through 6 (PR2 through PR6) (Fig. 9.60)
  1. PR2: on the superior margin of the second rib angle
  2. PR3: on the superior margin of the third rib angle

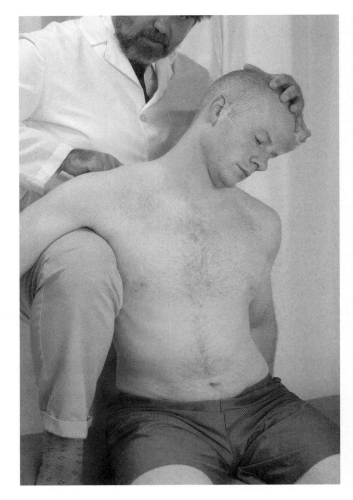

Figure 9.61 Counterstrain treatment position for the right posterior rib 2 tender point.

3. PR4: on the superior margin of the fourth rib angle
4. PR5: on the superior margin of the fifth rib angle
5. PR6: on the superior margin of the sixth rib angle
- The procedure is performed as follows (Fig. 9.61):
  1. The patient is seated.
  2. The practitioner places his or her foot on the treatment table on the same side as the rib to be treated.
  3. The patient's axilla on the same side of the tender point is placed over the practitioner's thigh.
  4. The patient's arm on the opposite side of the tender point is suspended behind his or her back to induce slight extension of the patient's torso with sidebending and rotation away from the tender point.

ADJUNCT TREATMENTS

Results of randomized clinical trials have provided evidence about the benefits and lack of benefits for various adjunct treatments.

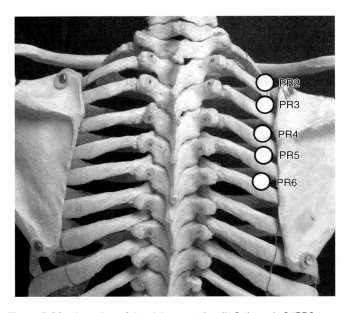

Figure 9.60 Location of the right posterior rib 2 through 6 (PR2 to PR6) tender points on a skeletal model.

- Beneficial
  1. Nonsteroidal anti-inflammatory drugs (NSAIDs)[6]
  2. Subacromial corticosteroid injection[6]
  3. Individualized exercise therapy[6,37]
  4. Acupuncture[38]
- Not likely to be beneficial
  1. Ultrasound[6]
  2. Transcutaneous electric neural stimulation[6]

EDUCATION

- Patients should be informed about proper postural support for the shoulder and should be advised to refrain from movements that aggravate the pain and, for prevention of further injury, to avoid repetitive or violent activities.
- Patients should gradually increase activities as the pain decreases, without waiting until the pain disappears entirely.
- For adhesive capsulitis, encourage patients to move through the restrictive barrier during passive range of motion exercises, even if it is painful.

EXERCISES

Exercise 1

- The exercise to improve shoulder flexion motion is performed as follows:
  1. Starting position: Stand facing a wall, so that when you reach forward with your arm, your fingertips touch the wall (Fig, 9.62A).
  2. Walk your fingers up the wall toward the ceiling.
  3. Move closer to the wall as your fingers move higher (see Fig. 9.62B and C).
  4. Move your fingers as far as you can and then return to the starting position.
  5. Repeat this exercise until you can comfortably do 3 sets of 10 repetitions.

Exercise 2

- The exercise to improve shoulder abduction motion is performed as follows:
  1. Starting position: Stand next to a wall, so that when you reach to the side with your arm, your fingertips touch the wall (Fig. 9.63A).
  2. Walk your fingers up the wall toward the ceiling (see Fig. 9.64B).
  3. Move closer to the wall as your fingers move higher (see Fig. 9.63C).
  4. Move your fingers as far as you can and then return to the starting position.
  5. Repeat this exercise until you can comfortably do 3 sets of 10 repetitions.

Exercise 3

- The exercise to improve external rotation motion is performed as follows:
  1. Starting position: Hold a strap of leather (e.g., a belt) or a towel with both hands behind your back, with one hand behind your head and the other behind your low back (Fig. 9.64A).
  2. Pull downward with the lower hand to accentuate external rotation of the opposite shoulder (see Fig. 9.64B).
  3. Meet and exceed the restrictive barrier and then return to the starting position.
  4. Repeat this exercise until you can comfortably do 3 sets of 10 repetitions.

Exercise 4

- The exercise to improve internal rotation motion is performed as follows:
  1. Starting position: Hold a strap of leather (e.g., a belt) or a towel with both hands behind your back, with one hand behind your head and the other behind your low back (Fig. 9.65A).
  2. Pull upward with the upper hand to accentuate internal rotation of the opposite shoulder (see Fig. 9.65B).
  3. Meet and exceed the restrictive barrier and then return to starting position.
  4. Repeat this exercise until you can comfortably do 3 sets of 10 repetitions.

CONTROVERSIES

- The greatest controversy regarding manipulation for shoulder pain and dysfunction is the definition of the problem. Very few practitioners take into consideration the effects of the cervicothoracic spine and adjacent ribs on shoulder pain and dysfunction. According to the evidence from randomized clinical trials, practitioners should consider shoulder somatic dysfunction as a dysfunction inclusive of the upper back, neck, and ribs and should treat the shoulder complex accordingly to improve at least short-term outcomes.
- Which practitioners should be allowed to perform shoulder manipulation under anesthesia is always a controversy, because so few practitioners are adequately trained to do so in any particular profession.

OPPORTUNITIES FOR RESEARCH

- More clinical trials on the effectiveness of manipulative therapy for shoulder disorders are needed. In particular, patients with shoulder girdle dysfunction need to be studied further.
- The quality of randomized clinical trials assessing treatment efficacy for shoulder pain and dysfunction needs

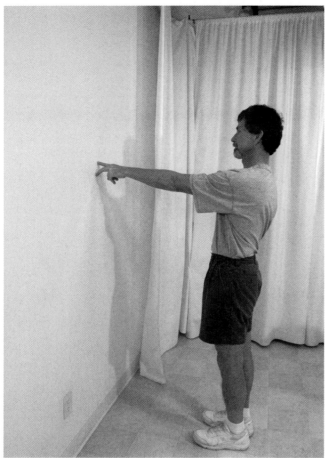

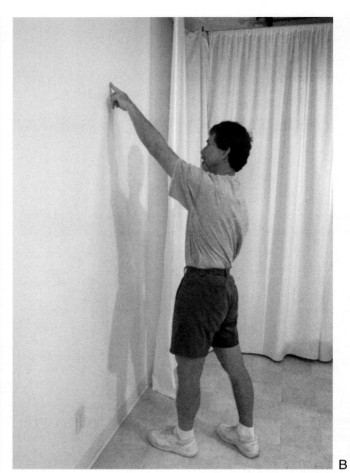

A

B

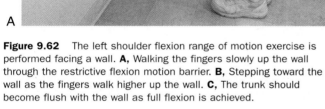

Figure 9.62 The left shoulder flexion range of motion exercise is performed facing a wall. **A,** Walking the fingers slowly up the wall through the restrictive flexion motion barrier. **B,** Stepping toward the wall as the fingers walk higher up the wall. **C,** The trunk should become flush with the wall as full flexion is achieved.

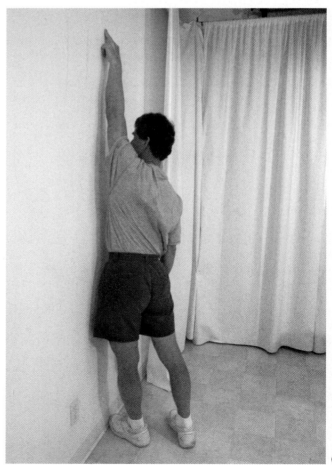

C

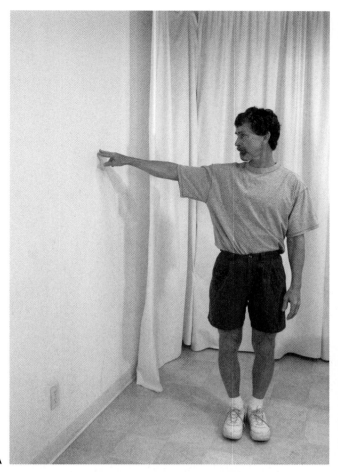

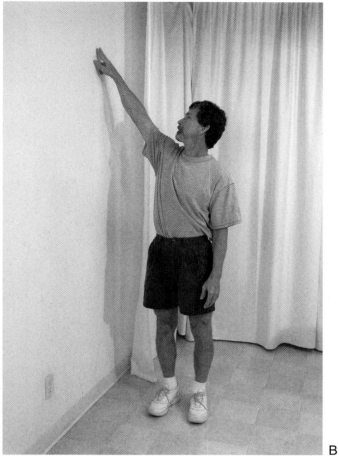

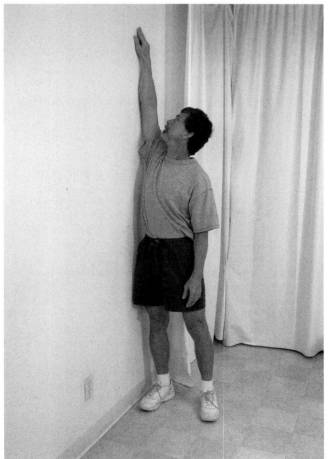

Figure 9.63 The right shoulder abduction range of motion exercise uses a wall. **A,** Walking the fingers slowly up the wall through the restrictive abduction motion barrier. **B,** Stepping closer to the wall as the fingers walk higher. **C,** The trunk should become flush with the wall as full abduction is achieved.

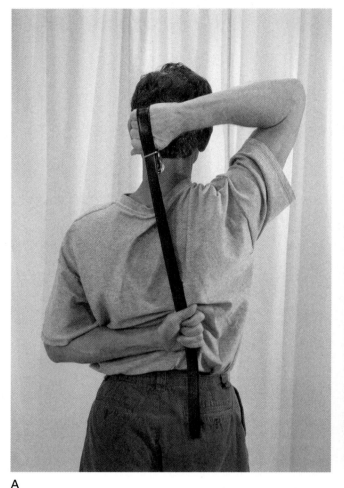 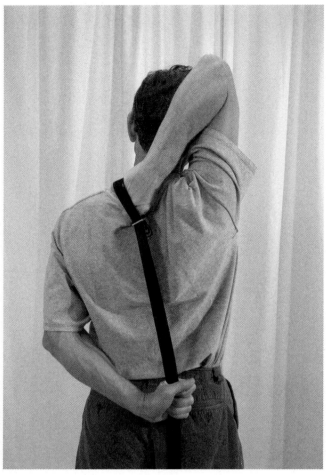

A   B

Figure 9.64   A, Starting position for passive stretching of the right shoulder to improve flexion, abduction, and external rotation. **B,** Pulling downward with the left hand improves right shoulder passive flexion, abduction, and external rotation.

to be improved. There should be an adoption of a uniform method of labeling and defining shoulder disorders and incorporation of a standard set of outcome measures to facilitate evaluation of efficacy of treatment approaches for shoulder pain and dysfunction through statistical pooling and meta-analysis of randomized clinical trials.[39]

- The Revision Panel for the (United States National) Clinical Guideline on Shoulder Pain believes that additional outcome studies, which assess outcomes resulting from the use of specific guidelines, are necessary and beneficial. The further refinement and defining of "best practice patterns"—improving the evidence on which guideline recommendations are based—may then serve as an improved model for further guideline revision and improvement. The Revision Panel recommends the following three additional studies be designed and initiated using the best scientific methodology:

1. Indications and efficacy for shoulder rehabilitation (rotator cuff and scapular stabilizer strengthening with restoration

of range of motion) as initial treatment of shoulder impingement syndrome

2. Indications and efficacy for steroid injection to treat patients presenting with shoulder pain

3. Evaluation and critique of the American Academy of Orthopaedic Surgeons' clinical guidelines for shoulder pain—methods of dissemination, application, and efficacy

- The Revision Panel recommends that the American Academy of Orthopedic Surgery develop a clinical guideline on acute shoulder injury to address issues related to acute shoulder trauma.[40]

- The Dutch College of General Practitioners practice guidelines need to be assessed for validity in other countries as well.

- Osteopathic researchers recommend future studies should focus on specific shoulder dysfunction and use three groups: (1) osteopathic manipulation treatment group; (2) manipulation sham treatment group; (3) a group receiving no treatment.

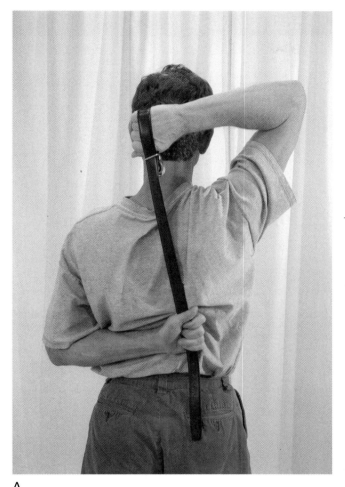 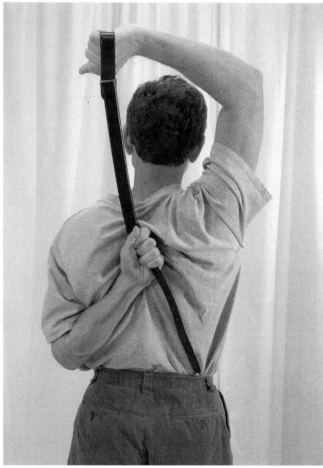

A   B

Figure 9.65 **A,** Starting position for passive stretching of the left shoulder to improve extension, adduction, and internal rotation. **B,** Pulling upward with the right hand improves left shoulder passive extension, adduction, and internal rotation.

REFERENCES

1. Urwin M, Symmons D, Allison T, et al: Estimating the burden of musculoskeletal disorders in the community: The comparative prevalence of symptoms at different anatomical sites, and the relation to social deprivation. Ann Rheum Dis 57:649-655, 1998.
2. Bot SD, van der Waal JM, Terwee CB, et al: Incidence and prevalence of complaints of the neck and upper extremity in general practice. Ann Rheum Dis 64:118-123, 2005.
3. Luime JJ, Koes BW, Hendriksen IS, et al: Prevalence and incidence of shoulder pain in the general population: A systemic review. Scand J Rheumatol 33:73-81, 2004.
4. Picavet HS, Schouten JS: Musculoskeletal pain in the Netherlands: Prevalence, consequences and risk groups: The DMC(3) study. Pain 102:167-178, 2003.
5. Pope DP, Croft PR, Pritchard CM, et al: Prevalence of shoulder pain in the community: The influence of case definition. Ann Rheum Dis 56:308-312, 1997.
6. van der Heijden GJMG: Shoulder disorders: A state-of-the-art review. Baillieres Best Pract Res Clin Rheumatol 13:287-309, 1999.
7. Winters JC, de Jongh AC, van der Windt DAWM, et al: Guidelines for Shoulder Complaints of the Dutch College of General Practitioners (May 1999). Available at http://nhg.artsennet.nl/upload/104/guidelines2/E08.htm/ Accessed May 2, 2006.
8. Thomas E, van der Windt DA, Hay EM, et al: Two pragmatic trials of treatment for shoulder disorders in primary care: Generalisability, course, and prognostic indicators. Ann Rheum Dis 64:1056-1061, 2005.
9. Zheng X, Simpson JA, van der Windt DA, et al: Data from a study of effectiveness suggested potential prognostic factors related to the patterns of shoulder pain. J Clin Epidemiol 58:823-830, 2005.
10. Norlander S, Gustavsson BA, Lindell J, et al: Reduced mobility in the cervico-thoracic motion segment. A risk factor for musculoskeletal neck-shoulder pain: A two-year prospective follow-up study. Scand J Rheum Med 29:167-174, 1997.
11. Andersen JH, Kaergaard A, Mikkelsen S, et al: Risk factors in the onset of neck/shoulder pain in a prospective study of workers in industrial and service companies. Occup Environ Med 60:649-654, 2003.
12. Institute of Medicine: Musculoskeletal disorders and the workplace: Low back and upper extremities. Washington, DC, National Academy Press, Institute of Medicine, 2001.
13. Siivola SM, Levoska S, Latvala K, et al: Predictive factors for neck and shoulder pain: A longitudinal study in young adults. Spine 29:1662-1669, 2004.
14. Kaergaard A, Andersen JH: Musculoskeletal disorders of the neck and shoulders in female sewing machine operators: Prevalence, incidence, and prognosis. Occup Environ Med 57;528-534, 2000.
15. Greenman PE: Principles of Manual Medicine. Philadelphia, Lippincott Williams & Wilkins, 2003.
16. Norkin CC, Levangie PK: Joint Structure and Function: A Comprehensive Analysis, 2nd ed. Philadelphia, FA Davis, 1992.
17. Kappler RA, Ramey KA: Upper Extremities. In Ward RC (ed): Foundations for Osteopathic Medicine. Philadelphia, Lippincott Williams & Wilkins, 2003.
18. Sandring S (ed): Gray's Anatomy, 39th ed. London, Elsevier Churchill Livingstone, 2005.
19. Woodward TW, Best TM: The painful shoulder. Part II. Acute and chronic disorders. Am Fam Physician 61:3291-3300, 2000.

20. Gunn CC, Milbrandt WE: Tenderness at motor points: An aid in the diagnosis of pain in the shoulder referred from the cervical spine. J Am Osteopath Assoc 77:196-212, 1977.
21. Sucher BM, Heath DH: Thoracic outlet syndrome—A myofascial variant. Part 3. Structural and postural considerations. J Am Osteopath Assoc 93:334, 340-345, 1993.
22. Woodward TW, Best TM: The painful shoulder. Part I. Clinical evaluation. Am Fam Physician 61:3079-3088, 2000.
23. Kujipers T, van der Windt DA, Boeke AJP, et al: Clinical prediction rules for the prognosis of shoulder pain in general practice. Pain 120:276-285, 2006.
24. Groenier KH, Winters JC, de Jong BM: Classification of shoulder complaints in general practice by means of nonmetric multidimensional scaling. Arch Phys Med Rehabil 84:812-817, 2003.
25. Groenier KH, de Winter AF, Winters JC, et al: Complaint severity and cervical spine problems successfully classified patients with shoulder complaints. J Clin Epidemiol 57:730-736, 2004.
26. Bergman GJD, Winters JC, Groenier KH, et al: Manipulative therapy in addition to usual medical care for patients with shoulder dysfunction and pain. Ann Intern Med 141:432-439, 2004.
27. Winters JC, Sobel JS, Groenier KH: Comparison of physiotherapy, manipulation, and corticosteroid injection for treating shoulder complaints in general practice: Randomized, single blind study. BMJ 314:1320-1325, 1997.
28. Hay EM, Thomas E, Paterson SM, et al: A pragmatic randomized controlled trial of local corticosteroid injection and physiotherapy for the treatment of new episodes of unilateral shoulder pain in primary care. Ann Rheum Dis 62:394-399, 2003.
29. Griggs SM, Ahn A, Green A: Idiopathic adhesive capsulitis. A prospective functional outcome study of nonoperative treatment. J Bone Joint Surg Am 82:1398-1407, 2000.
30. Kivimäki J, Pohjolainen T: Manipulation under anesthesia for frozen shoulder with and without steroid injection. Arch Phys Med Rehabil 82:1188-1190, 2001.
31. Farrell CM, Sperling JW, Cofield RH: Manipulation for frozen shoulder: Long-term results. J Shoulder Elbow Surg 14:480-484, 2005.
32. Desmeules F, Cote CH, Fremont P: Therapeutic exercise and orthopedic manual therapy for impingement syndrome: A systematic review. Clin J Sports Med 13:176-182, 2003.
33. Winters JC, Jorritsma W, Groenier KH: Treatment of shoulder complaints in general practice: Long term results of a randomized, single blind study comparing physiotherapy, manipulation, and corticosteroid injection. BMJ 318:1395-1396, 1999.
34. Winters JC, Sobel JS, Groenier KH, et al: The long term course of shoulder complains: A prospective study in general practice. Rheumatology (Oxford) 38:160-163, 1999.
35. Dias R, Cutts S, Massoud S: Frozen shoulder. BMJ 331:1453-1456, 2005.
36. Magee DJ: Orthopedic Physical Assessment, 4th ed. Philadelphia, Elsevier, 2002.
37. Ginn KA, Cohen ML: Exercise therapy for shoulder pain aimed at restoring neuromuscular control: A randomized comparative clinical trial. J Rehabil Med 37:115-122, 2005.
38. Green S, Buchbinder R, Hetrick S: Acupuncture for shoulder pain. Cochrane Database Syst Rev (2):CD004258, 2005.
39. Green S, Buchbinder R, Glazier R, et al: Systematic review of randomized controlled trials of interventions for painful shoulder: Selection criteria, outcome assessment, and efficacy. BMJ 316:354-360, 1998.
40. American Academy of Orthopedic Surgeons: AAOS clinical guideline on shoulder pain: Support document. Rosemont, IL, American Academy of Orthopedic Surgeons; 2001. Available at www.guidelines.gov (National Guidelines Clearinghouse): http://www.guideline.gov/summary/summary.aspx?ss=15&doc_id=2998&nbr=2224/ Accessed December 31, 2005.
41. Knebl JA, Shores JH, Gamber RG, et al: Improving functional ability in the elderly via the Spencer technique, an osteopathic manipulative treatment: A randomized controlled trial. J Am Osteopath Assoc 102:387-396, 2002.

SUGGESTED READING

Badcock LJ, Lewis M, Hay EM, et al: Consultation and the outcome of shoulder-neck pain: A cohort study in the population. J Rheumatol 30:2694-2699, 2003.
Bergman GJ, Winters JC, van der Heijden GJ, et al: Groningen Manipulation Study. The effect of manipulation of the structures of the shoulder girdle as additional treatment for symptom relief and for prevention of chronicity or recurrence of shoulder symptoms. Design of a randomized controlled trial within a comprehensive prognostic cohort study. J Manipulative Physiol Ther 25:543-549, 2002.
Boix F, Roe C, Rosenborg L, et al: Kinin peptides in human trapezius muscle during sustained isometric contraction and their relation to pain. J Appl Physiol 98:534-540, 2005.
Bongers PM: The cost of shoulder pain. BMJ 322:64-65, 2001.
Borg K, Hensing G, Alexanderson K: Risk factors for disability pension over 11 years in a cohort of young persons initially sick-listed with low back, neck, or shoulder diagnoses. Scand J Public Health 32:272-278, 2004.
Ginn KA, Cohen ML: Conservative treatment for shoulder pain: Prognostic indicators of outcome. Arch Phys Med Rehabil 85:1231-1235, 2004.
Grooten WJ, Wiktorin C, Norrman L, et al: Seeking care for neck/shoulder pain: A prospective study of work-related risk factors in a healthy population. J Occup Environ Med 46:138-146, 2004.
Ijzelenberg W, Burdorf A: Impact of musculoskeletal co-morbidity of neck and upper extremities on healthcare utilization and sickness absence for low back pain. Occup Environ Med 61:806-810, 2004.
Kuijpers T, van der Windt DA, van der Heijden GJ, et al: Systematic review of prognostic cohort studies on shoulder disorders. Pain 109:420-431, 2004.
Miranda H, Viikari-Juntura E, Heistaro S, et al: A population study on differences in the determinants of a specific shoulder disorder versus nonspecific shoulder pain without clinical findings. Am J Epidemiol 161:847-855, 2005.
Mitchell C, Adebajo A, Hay E, et al: Shoulder pain: Diagnosis and management in primary care. BMJ 331:1124-1128, 2005.
Prescher A: Anatomical basics, variations, and degenerative changes of the shoulder joint and shoulder girdle. Eur J Radiol 35:88-102, 2000.
Rekola KE, Levoska S, Takala J, et al: Patients with neck and shoulder complaints and multisite musculoskeletal symptoms-a prospective study. J Rheumatol 24:2424-2428, 1997.
Sallay PI, Hunker PJ, Brown L: Measurement of baseline shoulder function in subjects receiving workers' compensation versus noncompensated subjects. J Shoulder Elbow Surg 14:286-297, 2005.
Sobel JS, Winters JC, Groenier K, et al: Physical examination of the cervical spine and shoulder girdle in patients with shoulder complaints. J Manipulative Physiol Ther 20:257-262, 1997.
van der Heijden GJ, van der Windt DA, de Winter AF: Physiotherapy for patients with soft tissue shoulder disorders: A systematic review of randomized clinical trials. BMJ 315:25-30, 1997.
van der Windt DA, Bouter LM: Physiotherapy or corticosteroid injection for shoulder pain? Ann Rheum Dis 62:385-387, 2003.
van der Windt DA, Koes BW, de Jong BA, et al: Shoulder disorders in general practice: Incidence, patient characteristics, and management. Ann Rheum Dis 54:959-964, 1995.
Vogt MT, Simonsick EM, Harris TB, et al: Neck and shoulder pain in 70- to 79-year-old men and women: Findings from the Health, Aging and Body Composition Study. Spine J 3:435-441, 2003.
Walker-Bone K, Reading I, Coggon D, et al: The anatomical pattern and determinants of pain in the neck and upper limbs: An epidemiologic study. Pain 109:45-51, 2004.
Wilson JJ, Best TM: Common overuse tendon problems: A review and recommendations for treatment. Am Fam Physician 72:811-818, 2005.

CHAPTER 10

Carpal Tunnel Syndrome

DEFINITION

- Carpal tunnel syndrome (CTS) is a clinical disorder resulting from compression of the median nerve at the wrist.[1]
- It is diagnosed by a constellation of symptoms and signs related to an entrapment (i.e., compression) neuropathy of the median nerve as it crosses the wrist underneath the transverse carpal ligament, which is contiguous with the flexor retinaculum.
- Classically, one or more of the following clinical presentations indicate the presence of the syndrome[2]:
  1. Paresthesias (e.g., tingling, burning, numbness) or pain may involve the first three digits of the hand along the distribution of the median nerve; the pain also may radiate to the palm or proximal to the wrist.
  2. Loss of manual dexterity or thenar weakness in the affected hand is not related to neck or arm pathology.
  3. Symptoms can be reproduced by tapping or direct pressure over the median nerve at the wrist (i.e., positive Tinel's sign) (Fig. 10.1).
  4. Symptoms can be reproduced by sustained compression of the carpal canal by means of forced flexion or extension for 1 minute (i.e., positive Phalen's sign).
- More specific diagnostic criteria were developed in 1993 by an expert panel on review of the scientific literature.[3]
- Symptoms include the following:
  1. Dull, aching discomfort in the hand, forearm, or upper arm
  2. Paresthesias in the hand
  3. Weakness or clumsiness of the hand
  4. Dry skin, swelling, or color changes in the hand
  5. Occurrences of any of these symptoms in the median nerve distribution
  6. Symptoms provoked or worsened by sleep, sustained hand or arm position, or repetitive action of the hand or wrist
  7. Symptoms mitigated by changes in hand posture or by shaking the hand
- Signs include the following:
  1. May be normal
  2. Positive Tinel's sign or Phalen's sign
  3. Sensory deficits in the median innervated region of the hand
  4. Motor deficit or hypotrophy of the median innervated thenar muscles
  5. Dry skin on the thumb and index and middle fingers

EPIDEMIOLOGY

Age

- CTS occurs in people of all ages.
- Most people in the general population afflicted with CTS are between the ages of 30 and 80 years, with a peak incidence occurring in the sixth decade.[4,5]
- The highest incidence of CTS among workers in the United States is in patients between 35 and 54 years old.[6,7]
- CTS is uncommon in patients younger than 30 years, but it is increasingly being reported in the elderly between 70 and 84 years old, with increased severity of symptoms in men.[8]
- CTS in children is most often the result of congenital anomalies or trauma.

Gender

- Females more often have CTS than males at all ages and in all countries.
- In the United States, 70% of workers with CTS are female.[9]
- In some countries, females are 10 to 30 times more likely to have CTS.

Prevalence

- CTS is one of the most common peripheral nerve entrapment syndromes.
- The estimated population lifetime cumulative incidence rate is 8%.[1]
- Prevalence in the general population is estimated in several ways. An example of the differences in prevalence estimation based on the method by which the information is gathered is provided by a study in Sweden[4]:
  1. By self-report, the rate is 14%.
  2. By abnormal electrophysiologic criteria for median neuropathy, it is 4.9%.
  3. By clinical examination, it is 3.8%.
  4. By clinical and electrophysiologic criteria combined, it is 2.7%.

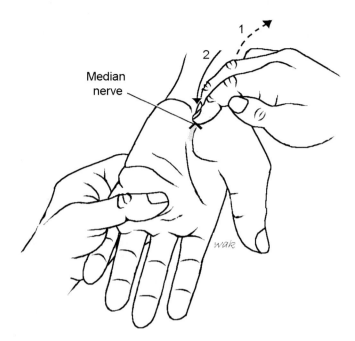

Figure 10.1 Tinel's sign is present (i.e., positive) if tapping (1) or direct pressure (2) over the median nerve elicits tingling or pain in the sensory distribution area of the median nerve (i.e., palmar and distal volar aspects of the thumb, index, middle fingers, or radial aspect of the fourth finger).

- In the United States, the estimate of CTS prevalence in the general population is between 3.7% and 16.3%.[10]
- In a selected high-risk population and using more general criteria, prevalence estimates are considerably higher. For example, 31.9% of industrial workers surveyed answered they had "abnormal feelings in the hands" in the past 4 weeks.[11]
- Rural and industrial areas have higher incidences than urban areas.[5]
- The incidence of CTS has increased dramatically since the 1980s due to changing work-related conditions (e.g., high-force, repetitive movements, bending of the wrist), personal characteristics (e.g., obesity, gender, age), compensation and financial gain, and epidemiologic and psychological factors due to the increased awareness of the syndrome.[10]

Natural Clinical Course

- About one (25%) in four of normal, asymptomatic workers with evidence of abnormal median nerve function as measured by electrodiagnostic (EDX) studies are likely to develop symptoms of CTS within 6 to 11 years.[12]
- After a person develops symptoms of CTS, the disorder tends to progress, with weekly fluctuations, unless changes in provocative factors are identified and removed. Although many patients recover spontaneously over a 6-month period, those who do not and are not treated can develop permanent median nerve damage.

- Up to 90% of patients with mild to moderate CTS respond to conservative management.
- Patients with CTS resulting from underlying pathology (e.g., diabetes, wrist fracture) tend to have a less favorable prognosis than those with no apparent underlying cause.
- CTS patients with normal EDX studies consistently have much less favorable operative outcomes and more complications than those with abnormalities on EDX studies, although axonal loss on EDX examination indicates a less favorable prognosis.
- A 15-month multicenter study of the natural course of CTS in Italy[13,14] reported the following:
  1. Younger patients improved more frequently than older ones.
  2. Prognosis was related to the duration of symptoms. The shorter the duration of symptoms, the better the prognosis, but patients with baseline bilateral symptoms and a positive Phalen's sign had a worse prognosis.
  3. Functional assessment correlated with age and neurophysiologic severity as assessed by EDX studies; elderly patients had poor functional abilities and abnormal EDX results.
  4. Symptoms did not correlate with age or severity assessment using EDX studies. Young patients had severe symptoms without sensory or motor impairment, and elderly patients with mild discomfort displayed severe sensory and motor functional impairment.
  5. In most cases, the evolution of symptoms and hand dysfunction was concordant (i.e., worsening, improvement, or no change in symptoms was mirrored in hand functional status). Neurophysiologic assessment also demonstrated concordance with functional status.[15]

Effect on Society

- Several effects were described in the 2003 U.S. Bureau of Labor Statistics report of nonfatal injuries and illnesses in the workplace.[9,16]
  1. CTS accounts for more lost work days (median, 25 days per year in 2001) than any other nonfatal injury or illness (median, 6 days).
  2. CTS is responsible for most injuries that caused workers to miss more than 31 days per year.
  3. The workers most affected are female (70%), non-Hispanic white (75%), and between 25 and 54 years old (84%).
  4. Two groups of occupations—(1) operators, fabricators and laborers and (2) technical, sales, and administrative support—together account for 70% of all work-related CTS. Precision production, craft, and repair workers account for 16%.
  5. Among industries, the manufacturing industry has the greatest incidence of CTS, followed by the finance, insurance, and real estate industries.
  6. Computing activities (i.e., data entry) accounted for one half of the CTS cases in California in 2001.
- Other affected occupations are office and business machinery workers, hand tool workers, meatpackers, electronic parts assemblers, frozen food processors, musicians, dental hygienists, and others engaged in repetitive motion activities.[17]
- The average lifetime cost of CTS, including medical bills and lost time from work, is estimated to be about $30,000 for each injured worker.[18]

- Surgery may not relieve symptoms or improve function. In one cohort, 75% of workers had surgery for CTS and, on average, returned to work 3 months later. Four years after treatment, 46% still experienced moderate to severe pain, 47% had moderate to severe numbness, and 40% had difficulty grasping and using small objects. Only 14% were symptom free.[19]

Risk Factors

- The risk of development of CTS appears to be multifactorial, including genetic, medical, social, demographic, and work-related and non–work-related factors.
- Repetitive wrist and hand motions are the most common risk factor.
- Forceful work with the hands, hand-wrist vibration, and force plus repetition and force plus posture combinations are also risk factors.[7]
- Diabetes (i.e., peripheral neuropathy), hypothyroidism, rheumatoid arthritis,[20] and pregnancy[21,22] may predispose a person to CTS.
- Independent risk factors include female gender, obesity,[4,23,24] and genetic predisposition in females (e.g., hand size, wrist size).[24,25]
- Prolonged gripping, prolonged bending of the neck forward, working with arms at or above shoulder height, low job control, many changes in tasks, and low job support are independently associated with hand paresthesias.[11]
- Elevated serum levels of low-density lipoprotein (LDL) cholesterol may be a risk factor.[26]

FUNCTIONAL ANATOMY

- The wrist's eight bones, called carpal bones, form the floor of a tunnel-like structure through which the median nerve passes. The roof of the tunnel is the transverse carpal ligament (Fig. 10.2).
- The flexor digitorum tendons run alongside the median nerve within the tunnel (see Fig. 10.2).
- After passing through the carpal tunnel, the median nerve divides into sensory and motor branches.
- The sensory component of the median nerve innervates the palmar aspects and the posterior distal phalanges of the first three fingers and the lateral (radial) half of the fourth finger.
- The motor component innervates the first and second lumbricals, opponens pollicis, abductor pollicis brevis, and flexor pollicis brevis muscles. Only the abductor pollicis muscle relies solely on the median innervation; the other muscles also receive innervation from the radial nerve.
- The autonomic component carries sympathetic efferents to most of the hand and is involved with the regulation of sweat gland and blood flow activity and thermoregulation.
- Like other peripheral nerves, the median nerve has a loosely adherent outer connective tissue sheath known as the epineurium. The epineurium and associated blood vessels, along with intraneural gliding surfaces of the fascicles, permit

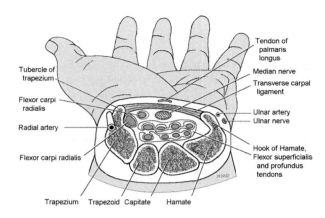

Figure 10.2 Anatomy of the carpal tunnel. Notice the proximity of the median nerve to the roof of the tunnel, which is the transverse carpal ligament.

the nerve to move about 1 cm during the wrist flexion and extension and finger movements.[27] This reduces stretch to the nerve during movement.

- The wrist joint is composed of the radius, three carpal bones, and the attached cartilage. Its primary motions are flexion (range, 90 degrees) and extension (range, 70 degrees) and abduction (range, 20 degrees) and adduction (range, 50 degrees). Combining these motions results in circumduction.[28]
- Carpometacarpal joints are synovial joints that share a common joint cavity with the intercarpal joints. They are more likely to have restriction of motion in anterior (ventral) glide. The first carpometacarpal joint (the thumb) is a separate saddle-type joint with a concave and a convex articular surface; although axial rotation is limited, motions in all other planes are permitted.

PATHOPHYSIOLOGY

Causes of Carpal Tunnel Syndrome

- The cause of most cases of CTS is unknown (idiopathic).
- Less common causes of CTS
  1. Trauma or overuse can cause localized edema or tenosynovitis of carpal tunnel tendons.
  2. Space-occupying lesions or structures (i.e., hypertrophic lumbrical muscles, tumors or cysts) can compress the median nerve.[27]
  3. Rheumatoid arthritis and other connective tissue diseases cause edema and thickening of the synovium of the carpal joints and the surrounding connective tissues within the carpal canal.
  4. Congestive heart failure, renal dialysis, and pregnancy can cause peripheral edema that can lead to increased swelling of structures and pressure within the carpal canal.[27]
  5. Myxedema hypothyroidism, acromegaly, and mucopolysaccharidosis can cause an accumulation of extracellular matrix in the carpal tunnel.[27]

Increased Carpal Tunnel Interstitial Fluid Pressure

- Median nerve compression in the carpal tunnel is thought to be caused by increased pressure against the nerve caused by an increase in the contents of the canal or decrease in the cross-sectional area of the canal.
- Abnormally high carpal tunnel pressures exist in patients with CTS. The increased pressure likely causes obstruction to venous outflow, backpressure, tissue congestion, edema formation, and ultimately, ischemia in the nerve. The median nerve initially undergoes demyelination, followed by axonal degeneration. Sensory fibers often are affected first, followed by motor fibers. Autonomic nerve fibers carried in the median nerve also may be affected.[29]
- Increasing wrist extension or flexion, forearm supination, finger-pinching maneuvers, holding and gripping tasks, and increasing metacarpophalangeal flexion greater than 45 degrees lead to increasing extraneural pressure in the carpal tunnel.[27]
- In animal models, low-magnitude, short-duration extraneural pressure can initiate the process of nerve injury and repair and can cause structural tissue changes that persist for at least 1 month. This entails endoneurial edema, demyelination, inflammation, distal axonal degeneration, fibrosis, growth of new axons, remyelination, and thickening of the perineurium and endothelium. The degree of axonal degeneration is associated with the amount of endoneurial edema.[27]

Histopathology

- The typical pathologic findings in the flexor tendon subsynovial connective tissue of idiopathic CTS patients include vascular proliferation, vascular hypertrophy, and vascular obstruction with wall thickening. There is also a decreased amount of elastin in and around the blood vessel walls, enabling fibroblast proliferation.[30]
- Noninflammatory fibrosis of the subsynovial connective tissue surrounds the flexor tendons.[31]
- There is an increase in synovial tissue edema and vascular sclerosis (i.e., endothelial thickening of the vascular walls). Increased numbers of lymphocytes and histiocytes (i.e., inflammatory cells) occur in only 10% of CTS patients.[27]

Biochemistry

- Biochemical studies of surgical specimens suggest that a variety of regulatory molecules may induce fibrous and vascular proliferation and that this may be a response to mechanical stresses.[31]
- Intermittent compression produces ischemia of the median nerve. Reperfusion injury may occur during periods of recovery. Intermittent perfusion of the cellular tissue after ischemia releases free oxygen radicals. With continued oxidative stress, the normal antioxidant system is overwhelmed, and cellular injury ensues, affecting nerve and synovium cells. Cellular damage leads to extravasation of fluid, which is rapidly absorbed by the synovium, producing edema and compression of the nerve. Nerve compression produces hypoxic endoneurial blood flow, resulting in neuronal edema and intraneural fibrosis.[32]
- Anoxic capillary damage leads to increased vascular permeability, exudation of fluid, and synovial edema, progressing to fibrosis in the synovium.
- High levels of interleukin-6 in the flexor tenosynovium of CTS patients stimulate the production of acute-phase proteins and can induce cellular proliferation, angiogenesis, and differentiation in fibroblastic and nerve cell types. Conversely, there are normal levels of interleukin-1, which is associated with activation of the inflammatory response. Idiopathic CTS pathogenesis is a result of a tendinosis rather than a tendonitis.[32,33]
- Cells within the vessels and tenosynovium in the carpal tunnel during the intermediate phase of CTS, when the histology of the tenosynovium changes from edematous to fibrotic, have increased levels of prostaglandins (e.g., PGE_2) and vascular endothelial growth factor (VEGF). These molecules induce edema by increasing vascular permeability. VEGF also induces angiogenesis, which occurs in the intermediate stage of CTS. However, angiogenesis appears to take place as a part of a regenerative reaction that fails and results in fibrosis instead.[34]
- The extracellular matrix in surgical specimens displays a greater density of keratin sulfate, a proteoglycan whose production, unlike other proteoglycans, does not rely on oxidative metabolism and therefore persists in anoxic or ischemic environments. The increase in keratin over chondroitin sulfate levels, for example, can alter the hydration status of the proteoglycan matrix and render the tissues less able to withstand the compressive forces within the canal.[35]
- PGE_2 activates adenylate cyclase, which increases intracellular cyclic adenosine monophosphate (cAMP). This increase in cAMP levels can inhibit functional responses to other inflammatory stimuli.[36]
- Increases in PGE_2 can also cause sensitization of the nerve endings so that a normal stimulus that would not necessarily cause pain becomes painful.[36]

Median Nerve Response to Mechanical Stimulation or Stress

- In addition to compression and excessive use of the wrist and fingers, *persistent vibration* induces intraneural edema, demyelination, and axonal degeneration. Interstitial and perineural fibrosis also occurs.[27]
- Schwann cells change their gene and protein expression in response to mechanical stimuli; shear stress decreases the expression of myelin-associated glycoprotein and myelin basic protein mRNA. The local downregulation of myelin-associated glycoprotein creates an environment allowing axonal sprouting. Schwann cell proliferation begins 2 to 4 weeks after injury and leads to a twofold to threefold increase in cell numbers by 8 months. Concomitant Schwann cell apoptosis also occurs.[37]
- After tissue injury and inflammation, macrophages express inducible nitric oxide synthetase (iNOS), which generates localized increases in nitric oxide (NO). NO is also involved

in the neural regeneration process after compression injury to the median nerve. It inhibits neurotoxic enzymes and produces reactive oxidative species that alter the neurons' proangiogenic pathways.[37]

- Within minutes to hours, elevated extraneural pressure can inhibit intraneural microvascular blood flow, axonal transport (i.e., axoplasmic flow), and nerve function, and within 7 to 10 days, it can cause endoneurial edema with increased intrafascicular pressure and displacement of myelin in a dose-response manner. Remyelination begins 14 to 28 days after injury. Epineural and perineural fibrosis along with an increased expression of type I collagen form a neural scar.[37]
- Swelling of the nerve trunk proximal to the compression site is caused by an increase in the amount of endoneurial connective tissue, edema in the epineurium and endoneurial space, and obstruction of axoplasmic flow.[38]
- Ultrasonographic measurements of the median nerve's cross-sectional area in CTS patients confirm expansion of the nerve.[31]
- Magnetic resonance imaging (MRI) of the carpal tunnel in symptomatic patients in advanced stages of CTS shows palmar bowing of the transverse carpal ligament, swelling of the median nerve at the level of the pisiform, flattening of the median nerve at the level of the hook of the hamate, and increased signal intensity within the median nerve on T2-weighted images. Synovial swelling may surround the flexor tendons within the carpal canal.[38,39]

Neck Muscle Imbalance

- Increased flexor or extensor motor activity is an expression of dysfunctional sternocleidomastoid and cervical paraspinal muscle activity (as measured by asymmetric active range of neck motion and electromyographic [EMG] tracings).
- Active neck motion exercises restore the symmetry of neck muscle activity and reduce CTS signs (as measured by EDX studies) and symptoms.[40,41]

Pathogenesis of Carpal Tunnel Syndrome Progression

- Stage I
  1. Intermittent paresthesias and deficits of sensation that occur primarily at night are likely caused by changes in intraneural microcirculation that are associated with some edema, which disappears during the day.[27]
- Stage II
  1. Progressive compression of the median nerve leads to more severe and constant symptoms that do not disappear during the day.
  2. Paresthesias, numbness, impaired dexterity, and possibly, thenar muscle weaknesses are likely the result of persistent edema that alters the microcirculation and morphology of the median nerve.
  3. Segmental demyelination may also occur during this stage.

- Stage III
  1. In this final stage, constant pain with atrophy of the thenar muscles and permanent sensory dysfunction is caused by axonal degeneration of the median nerve.

Acute versus Chronic Carpal Tunnel Syndrome

- Compression of the median nerve in CTS can be classified as acute or chronic.
- Acute CTS occurs when there is a rapid accumulation of fluid causing elevated pressure within the carpal canal. This is observed in scenarios such as an acute distal fracture of the radius.
- Factors involved in the pathogenesis of chronic CTS can be divided into idiopathic, intrinsic (i.e., pregnancy, hemodialysis, hypothyroidism, rheumatoid arthritis, and gout), extrinsic (i.e., conditions that alter the size of the carpal arch such as scaphoid nonunion or rotary subluxation of the scaphoid), and associated disease states (i.e., diabetes, hemophilia, and myeloma).[42]

Nerve Motion Restriction

- Nerve excursion during flexion and extension of the wrist or flexion of the fingers results in strain on the nerve fibers and is restricted in patients with CTS.[27]
- Restriction is possibly caused by the adhesions of adjacent tissues and resultant traction, which can cause local regions of limited microvascular flow.

DIFFERENTIAL DIAGNOSIS

- Paresthesias that predominantly affect the fifth finger or extend to the thenar eminence or dorsum of the hand should suggest other diagnoses.
- Pain in the epicondylar region of the elbow, upper arm, shoulder, or neck is more likely to be due to other musculoskeletal diagnoses (e.g., epicondylitis) with which CTS commonly is associated. This more proximal pain also should prompt a careful search for other neurologic diagnoses (e.g., cervical radiculopathy).[29]
- Differential diagnoses are listed in Table 10.1.

HISTORY

- Intensity: can be mild or severe, waxing and waning[29]
- Precipitating factors: most commonly repetitive motion, prolonged wrist flexion or twisting
- Location: the distal palm, palmar aspect of the thumb (first), index (second), middle (third), and medial half of the ring (fourth) digits, as well as the posterior aspect of the distal phalanges of these digits (i.e., the sensory distribution of the median nerve)
- Radiation: The pain can radiate distally to the palm and fingers or extend proximally along the anterior forearm.

Table 10.1 Differential diagnosis of carpal tunnel syndrome

Pathophysiology*	Condition
Vascular	Raynaud's syndrome
	Cerebral vascular accident (CVA)
Inflammatory	Lateral epicondylitis
	Medial epicondylitis
	Mononeuritis multiplex
	Rheumatoid arthritis
Trauma	Reflex sympathetic dystrophy
	Compartment syndrome
	Fracture or dislocations of wrist bones
	Post-traumatic syringomyelia
	Radiation or trauma induced brachial plexopathy
Anatomic	Small wrists
	Bony deformities of carpal bones
Metabolic	Diabetic neuropathy
	Hypothyroidism
	Renal failure on dialysis
	Pregnancy
	Acromegaly
	Gout
	Hypercholesterolemia
Iatrogenic	Ischemic monomelic neuropathy after tourniquet use or arteriovenous fistula surgery
Neoplastic	Local or central tumor
	Neoplastic brachial plexopathy
Autoimmune/idiopathic	Amyloidosis
	Multiple sclerosis
Biomechanical	Myofascial pain
	Thoracic outlet syndrome
	Pronator teres syndrome
	Cervical disc disease
	Cervical myofascial pain
	Cervical spondylosis
Congenital/hereditary	Congenital anomalies of wrist or hand
	Hereditary neuropathy with liability to pressure palsies
	Mucolipidosis or mucopolysaccharidosis
Degenerative	Osteoarthritis
Environmental/infectious	Lyme disease
	Leprosy

*Using the VITAMIN ABCDE mnemonic.

- Clinical characteristics
  1. Numbness and tingling in the distribution of the median nerve is the most common complaint.
  2. Symptoms are often worse while sleeping,[10] and they awaken patients sometimes because patients have a tendency to flex the wrist when asleep, which increases pressure in the carpal tunnel.
  3. During the daytime, patients complain that the hands fall asleep or things slip from the fingers due to a loss of grip strength or an awareness of the object (i.e., proprioception deficit) and the numbness and tingling.
  4. Symptoms are usually intermittent and are associated with repetitive wrist motion or stationery wrist flexion activities (e.g., driving, reading the newspaper, crocheting, painting).
  5. Bilateral CTS is common, although the dominant hand is usually affected first and more severely than the other hand.
- Associated symptoms
  1. The sensory symptoms previously described commonly are accompanied by an aching sensation over the anterior aspect of the wrist.
  2. There can be a tight or swollen feeling in the hands or temperature changes (e.g., hands being cold or hot all of the time), sensitivity to changes in temperature (particularly cold), and a difference in skin color.
  3. Rarely, there are changes in palmar sweating (i.e., anhidrosis).
  4. Weakness or clumsiness and loss of power and dexterity in the hand (particularly for precision grips involving the thumb) are more likely caused by the loss of sensory feedback and pain than the loss of motor power.

PHYSICAL FINDINGS

Sensory Examination

- Pinprick sensation or 2-point discrimination (<5 mm) tests can be abnormal on the palmar aspect of the first three digits and radial one half of the fourth digit, although this is not an accurate test for CTS because of low sensitivity and specificity.
- The skin overlying the thenar eminence, hypothenar eminence, and dorsum of first web space should have normal sensation.

Motor Examination

- Wasting and weakness of the median-innervated hand muscles (i.e., LOAF muscles) may be detectable.
- LOAF is a mnemonic for the hand muscles: first and second *l*umbricals, *o*pponens pollicis, *a*bductor pollicis brevis, *f*lexor pollicis brevis.

Special Tests

- No standard test exists for defining the presence or absence of CTS.[1]
- A diagnostic test is considered accurate if it has a sensitivity of more than 85% and a specificity of more than 95%. In estimating the accuracy of a diagnostic test, calculating sensitivity and specificity is performed in relation to a reference or gold standard test. If an EDX test such as nerve conduction velocity is the reference or gold standard, no physical examination test is very accurate.[43,44] However, because electrodiagnosis is in

itself not a perfect standard, because it gives false-positive and false-negative results, other statistical tests need to be used to estimate the accuracy of a diagnostic test, such as latent class analysis (LCA).[45] The accuracy of tests using electrodiagnosis as a reference standard given later is derived from a systematic review by Massy-Westropp and colleagues.[44] The sensitivity and specificity calculations using LCA were derived from Lajoie and associates.[45]

- The Tinel test is performed by gently tapping over the median nerve in the carpal tunnel region (see Fig. 10.1). A positive test, also called the Hoffmann-Tinel sign, is when the maneuver elicits tingling sensation in the median nerve's distribution. Sensitivity ranges from 45% to 75% (compared with EDX testing) and 97% (using LCA). Specificity ranges from 40% to 67% (EDX) and 91% (LCA).

- The Phalen test is performed by having the patient place his or her hands back to back with the fingers pointing toward the floor and the elbows raised such that the forearms and arms are parallel to the floor and at the level of the patient's sternum. Tingling in the median nerve distribution induced by full flexion of the wrists for up to 60 seconds is designated a positive Phalen test result, or Phalen's sign. The sensitivity ranges from 43% to 86% for EDX testing and is 92% for LCA. Specificity ranges from 48% to 67% for EDX testing and is 88% for LCA. Having the patient hold the hands palm to palm to induce full extension is called the reverse Phalen test. It is not very sensitive (55% with EDX testing), but it is specific (100% with EDX testing).

- The carpal compression test is performed by applying firm pressure directly over the carpal tunnel, usually with the thumbs, for up to 30 seconds to reproduce symptoms. The sensitivity ranges from 49% to 89% (EDX testing), and specificity ranges from 54% to 96% (EDX testing).

Palpatory Examination

- Palpatory diagnosis for wrist somatic dysfunction involves examining the wrist for evidence of *t*issue texture abnormalities, *a*symmetry of structural landmarks, *r*ange of motion abnormalities, and *t*enderness (TART), including the soft tissues directly overlying the median nerve at the wrist. Using EDX testing as the gold standard, the sensitivity is 92%, and the specificity is 75%.[46] The lower specificity may indicate incidences of somatic dysfunction that do not cause CTS as diagnosed by EDX studies, which in itself is unable to detect 100% of CTS cases or milder cases of CTS that have not risen to the level of EDX detection.

- Assessment of the compliance and resistance of the forearm and wrist fascia by traction, compression, and twisting forces can display directions of restricted or resistant motion. Most commonly, restriction is observed for wrist extension, carpal canal transverse extension, thenar abduction with extension, wrist radial deviation, and forearm or wrist supination.[47]

- Associated primary or secondary somatic dysfunction is often found in the proximal limb, including the shoulder, ribs, upper back, and neck regions.[48-50]

LABORATORY AND RADIOGRAPHIC FINDINGS

- Nerve conduction studies and EMG are EDX studies that are often used as the reference standards in the diagnosis of CTS. EDX studies are often used to confirm the diagnosis of CTS, but they cannot exclude it, because the test results do not always correlate with symptoms or function.[2,51] For example, many patients with CTS have normal EDX study results (i.e., false negatives); in one study, 18% of asymptomatic controls had abnormal EDX results (i.e., false positives)[4]; in another study, asymptomatic people with median neuropathy identified by EDX testing did not develop CTS after 11 years follow-up (i.e., false positives).[51]

- EDX testing has an estimated sensitivity ranging from 4% (for measurement of sympathetic skin response) to 85% (for median sensory and mixed nerve conduction, wrist and palm segment compared with forearm or digit segment, and comparison of median and ulnar sensory conduction between wrist and ring finger). The specificity, however, is greater than 95%.[52]

- Using LCA (i.e., statistical analysis applied to diagnostic tests to estimate sensitivity and specificity when no standard test exists) with a prevalence of CTS at 60%, nerve conduction velocity has a sensitivity of 93% and specificity of 87%.[45]

- The sensitivity and specificity of diagnostic high-resolution ultrasound is comparable to those of nerve conduction studies, although their prognostic value remains unknown.[53]

- Dynamic MRI contributes to the diagnosis of CTS when clinical signs are confusing and results of EDX studies are negative.[39]

- MRI is useful to rule out space-occupying lesions and to visualize the anatomy before endoscopic surgery.

- There is insufficient evidence for routine laboratory screening for concurrent conditions in all newly diagnosed CTS patients.[20]

- CTS usually can be classified by EDX testing as follows[29]:
  1. Mild: sensory abnormalities alone
  2. Moderate: sensory plus motor abnormalities
  3. Severe: any evidence of axonal loss

MANUAL MEDICINE

Best Evidence

- Osteopathic manipulative treatment of the thoracic outlet, upper ribs, upper back, and lower cervical spine and tender points in the forearm improve symptoms and signs of CTS[48,50] (grade B evidence, small case series) (Table 10.2).

- Myofascial release of the carpal tunnel improves symptoms and signs of CTS[47,54] (grade B evidence, small case series).

- Wrist mobilization improves symptoms and signs of CTS[55] (grade A evidence, randomized, controlled trial [RCT]).

- Chiropractic manipulation of the upper extremities and spine is as effective as conservative medical care in improving symptoms and signs of CTS[56] (grade A evidence, RCT).

Risks

- Risks for manual treatments for CTS include further harm to the already compromised median nerve by increasing

Table 10.2   Evidence-based medicine of manual medicine for carpal tunnel syndrome

Evidence Level*	Recommendation	Studies
A	Manipulation of the upper extremities and spine is effective as conservative medical care in improving symptoms and signs of carpal tunnel syndrome (CTS).	Davis et al, 1998[56]
A	Wrist mobilization improves symptoms and signs of CTS.	Tak-Akabi and Rushton, 2000[55]
B	Manual treatment of the thoracic outlet, upper ribs, upper back and lower cervical spine, and tender points in the forearm improve symptoms and signs of CTS.	Ramey et al, 1999[50] Sucher, 1995[48]
B	Myofascial release combined with exercise of the carpal tunnel improves symptoms and signs of CTS.	Sucher, 1993[54] Sucher, 1994[47]

*Evidence levels: A, randomized, controlled trials, meta-analyses, and systematic reviews; B, case-control or cohort studies, retrospective studies, and certain uncontrolled studies; C, consensus statements, expert guidelines, usual practice, and opinion.

pressure within the carpal canal, increasing carpal tunnel edema, or pressing directly on the nerve.

- If abnormal anatomy, space-occupying lesions, or congenital anomalies are present, caution should be used in employing articulatory procedures.
- Avoid direct pressure on the median nerve by working along the edges (i.e., medial and lateral rows of carpal bones) of the carpal tunnel and staying clear of the central canal.[46]
- In the patient with osteoarthritis, the first carpometacarpal joint may be involved and may render it difficult to restore normal motion. The patient may not be able to tolerate manual forces due to pain or decreased available range of motion.
- The practitioner needs to be aware of the presence of bone spurs, synovitis, or contracture, which limits the compliance and range available in the joints, necessitating caution in the amount of force applied and the range of motion sought during treatment.[46]
- The practitioner needs to respect the patient's tolerance to pain and should maintain patient comfort and compliance by adjusting the degree or intensity of treatment while striving for effective treatment results.[46]

Benefits

- Improved biomechanical functions of the spine, costal cage, shoulder, and forearm from manipulation decrease swelling of the carpal tunnel and median nerve most likely by improving venous and lymphatic drainage and help to relieve symptoms and improve function.[49,50]
- Stretching the carpal tunnel with manipulation can reduce symptoms and improve neural conductivity of the median nerve.[47,54]
- Mobilization and neurodynamic manual therapy may postpone surgery in severe cases.[55]
- Therapy improves perceived comfort and function, nerve conduction, and finger sensation and decreases medication use and the concomitant potential side effects and complications in patients with mild to moderate CTS.[56]

Practice Recommendations

- Because of the paucity of specific evidence regarding efficacy of treatment of CTS in the worker population, the U.S. government's guidelines are heavily based on expert opinion.[57]
- Although surgical literature highlights the success of surgery over conservative treatments, trials of conservative treatment for mild to moderate CTS have shown efficacy and effectiveness. A trial of manual treatments and exercises, along with modifications or removal of provocative factors, is therefore reasonable for the first 2 to 3 months of treatment.
- If there is no improvement with conservative measures, surgical evaluation is indicated after 3 to 6 months.
- A combination of history, physical findings, and neurodiagnostic studies helps to confirm the diagnosis.[1]
- If results of testing for Phalen's sign and Tinel's sign are concordant (i.e., both positive or both negative), there is little gain from nerve conduction studies because the probability of a correct diagnosis based on these tests is fairly accurate. However, if there is discordance (i.e., one is positive and the other negative), the nerve conduction study can help to confirm the diagnosis.[45]
- The practitioner should consult the American Association of Electrodiagnostic Medicine, American Academy of Neurology, and the American Academy of Physical Medicine and Rehabilitation guidelines for EDX studies used in the diagnosis of CTS if EDX testing is employed as part of the diagnostic regimen or for follow-up assessment after treatment.[52]
- Osteopathic manipulative treatments for CTS can be applied as a conservative treatment[47,54] (grade B evidence, small case series) or after surgery to help alleviate pain and contractures (grade C evidence, expert experience or opinion).[46,58,59]
- Osteopathic manipulative treatments of somatic dysfunctions in the neck, upper back, rib cage, and upper extremity, including the thoracic outlet, are effective in treating CTS (grade B evidence, small case series[48-50]; grade C evidence, expert opinion[48,58])
- Self-stretching exercises coupled with myofascial release manual treatments are effective in treating CTS[60] (grade B evidence, small case series).

DIAGNOSTIC PROCEDURES

- The ICD-9 diagnostic code for upper extremity somatic dysfunction is 739.7.
- Although other codes are used, they are not specific as indicators for manual treatment.
- Physical evaluation procedures for CTS should begin with a general screening examination of the musculoskeletal system (see Chapter 3), followed by a regional examination of the affected limb and then a segmental examination of the affected wrist. Asymmetry of musculoskeletal structural landmarks, altered quantity or quality of active or passive neck, upper back or upper extremity motion (including the thoracic outlet), and tissue texture abnormalities (including tenderness and temperature variations) at the anterior (volar) wrist lead the practitioner to consider mechanical factors in the cause of CTS.
- Evaluation for evidence of cervical, ipsilateral shoulder, upper ribs, elbow, or wrist somatic dysfunction is necessary to determine whether manual treatment of these areas is indicated.
- A neurosensory and muscle strength examination of the upper extremities and provocative special tests, such as Tinel's, Phalen's, and carpal compression tests, should be performed. Spurling's maneuver (i.e., cervical extension and sidebending at C7 followed by axial head compression with the patient seated) is used for assessing cervical radiculopathy.
- Adson's test for possible vascular occlusion of the subclavian artery is performed by having the patient abduct the arm of the affected wrist with ipsilateral elbow extension coupled with ipsilateral head rotation while inhaling. If there is no change in radial pulse at the wrist, the vascular supply is not compromised by thoracic outlet syndrome.[28]
- Assessment of the compliance and resistance of the forearm and wrist bony and soft tissue components, especially the fascia, by wrist flexion, extension, translation, traction, compression, and twisting forces can display directions of restricted or resistant motion.
- Tender point assessment along the carpal bones and first metacarpophalangeal joint can identify possible points to treat with counterstrain.

TREATMENT PROCEDURES

- Manual medicine approaches to the patient with CTS entail addressing somatic dysfunction in the upper thoracic and cervical spine, shoulder, upper ribs, and elbow regions and addressing the pathophysiology at the carpal tunnel itself.
- The practitioner should strive to improve motion of dysfunctional spinal and costal joints, restore normal muscle tone in the affected paraspinal and limb muscles, and improve venous and lymphatic drainage from the wrist and axoplasmic flow along the median nerve.
- The sections on treatment procedures provide instruction in a few basic and effective techniques directed at mobilizing the carpal bones, stretching the transverse carpal ligament, and reducing wrist tender points associated with CTS.

Articulatory Treatment

Articulatory Treatment Procedure for Restricted Motions of Dorsiflexion

- The procedure is performed as follows:
  1. The patient is seated with the elbow of the affected wrist extended, the forearm pronated, and the palm facing the floor (Fig. 10.3).
  2. The practitioner stands in front of the patient.
  3. The practitioner grasps the patient's thenar and hypothenar eminences with his or her fingers (see Fig. 10.3A and B).
  4. The practitioner uses his or her thumbs to create a fulcrum on the dorsal surface of the patient's wrist (see Fig. 10.3C and D).
  5. The practitioner lifts the patient's thenar and hypothenar eminences while pressing downward on the patient's dorsal wrist distal to the radius and ulna to engage the restrictive barrier in dorsiflexion (see Fig. 10.3E).
  6. The practitioner rhythmically moves the patient's wrist within an arc of motion that repeatedly engages the restrictive barrier in dorsiflexion, being careful not to cause pain.
  7. This rhythmic motion is continued until as much range of motion as possible can be restored.

Articulatory Treatment Procedure for Restricted Motions of Palmar Flexion

- The procedure is performed as follows:
  1. The patient is seated with elbow of the affected wrist extended, the forearm pronated, and the palm facing the floor (Fig. 10.4).
  2. The practitioner stands in front of the patient.
  3. The practitioner grasps the patient's thenar and hypothenar eminences with his or her fingers (see Fig. 10.4A).
  4. The practitioner places his or her thumbs on the dorsal surface of the patient's wrist.
  5. The practitioner palmar flexes the patient's wrist, using his or her forefingers as the fulcrum just distal to the radius and ulna to engage the restrictive barrier in palmar flexion (see Fig. 10.4B).
  6. The practitioner rhythmically moves the patient's wrist within an arc of motion that repeatedly engages the restrictive barrier in palmar flexion, being careful not to cause pain.
  7. This rhythmic motion is continued until as much range of motion as possible can be restored.

Articulatory Treatment Procedure for Restricted Motions of Radial or Ulnar Deviation

- The procedure is performed as follows:
  1. The patient is seated (Fig. 10.5).
  2. The practitioner stands to the side of the patient.
  3. The practitioner uses one hand to grasp the patient's distal forearm just proximal to the wrist (see Fig. 10.5A).
  4. The practitioner uses his or her other hand to grasp the patient's hand just distal to the wrist.
  5. The practitioner rhythmically moves the patient's wrist within an arc of motion that repeatedly engages the restrictive barrier in radial or ulnar deviation, being careful not to cause pain.

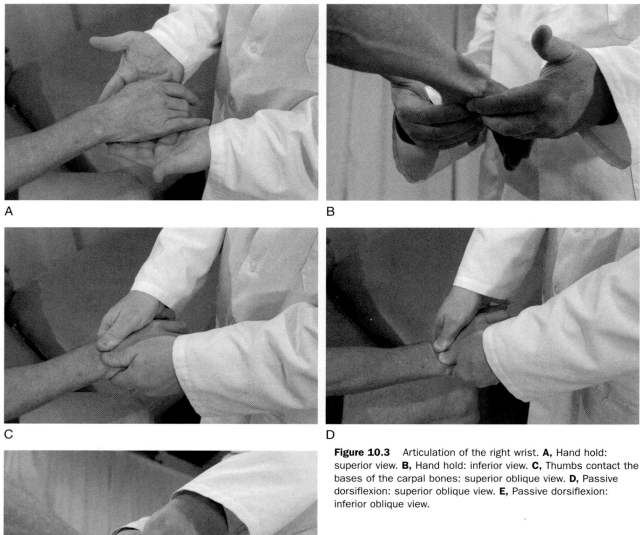

A

B

C

D

Figure 10.3   Articulation of the right wrist. **A,** Hand hold: superior view. **B,** Hand hold: inferior view. **C,** Thumbs contact the bases of the carpal bones: superior oblique view. **D,** Passive dorsiflexion: superior oblique view. **E,** Passive dorsiflexion: inferior oblique view.

E

6. This rhythmic motion is continued until as much range of motion as possible can be restored.

Myofascial Release

Myofascial Release Technique to Open the Carpal Canal
- The procedure is performed as follows:
  1. The patient is seated (Figs. 10.6 to 10.8).

2. The practitioner stands in front of the patient.
3. The patient's forearm on the affected side is positioned with the elbow flexed to 90 degrees, and the hand supinated.
4. The practitioner places his or her thumbs on ventral aspect of the patient's wrist at the margins of the attachments of the transverse carpal ligament. The hook of the hamate and the tubercle of the trapezium serve as the attachments for this ligament and are easily identifiable landmarks because they are the most prominent bones at the bases of

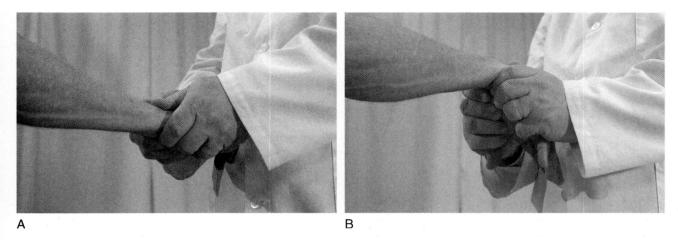

Figure 10.4   Articulation of the right wrist. **A,** Passive palmar flexion starting hand hold: inferior oblique view. **B,** Passive palmar flexion: inferior oblique view.

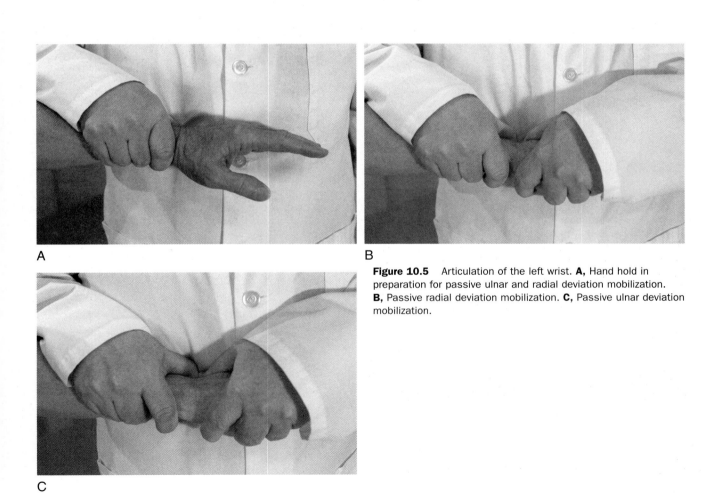

Figure 10.5   Articulation of the left wrist. **A,** Hand hold in preparation for passive ulnar and radial deviation mobilization. **B,** Passive radial deviation mobilization. **C,** Passive ulnar deviation mobilization.

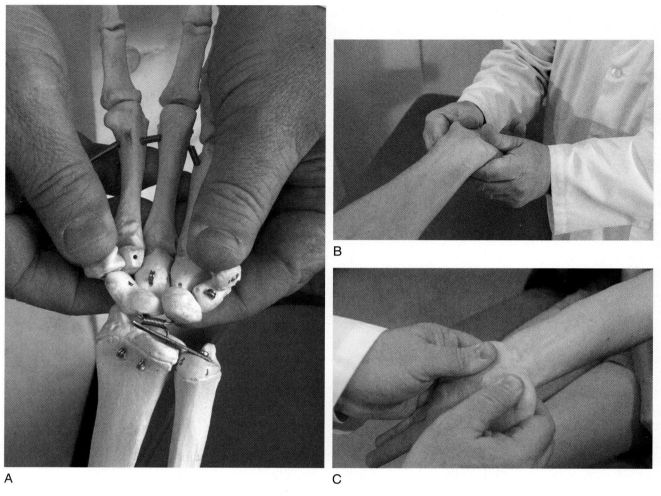

Figure 10.6   Myofascial release of the left wrist. **A,** The focus is on the trapezium and hamate transverse carpal ligament attachments. The hand hold is shown on a skeleton model. **B,** The focus is on the transverse carpal ligament: view from patient's perspective. **C,** The focus is on the transverse carpal ligament: superior oblique view.

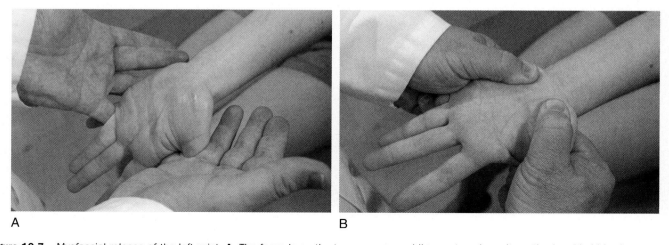

Figure 10.7   Myofascial release of the left wrist. **A,** The focus is on the transverse carpal ligament, and an alternative hand hold is shown: superior oblique view. **B,** The focus is the transverse carpal ligament, and an alternative hand hold is shown, with the thumbs contacting the trapezium and hamate bones: superior oblique view.

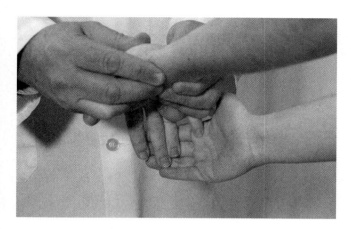

Figure 10.8 Myofascial release of the left wrist, focusing on the transverse carpal ligament with patient assisting by extending the fingers on the affected hand: inferior oblique view.

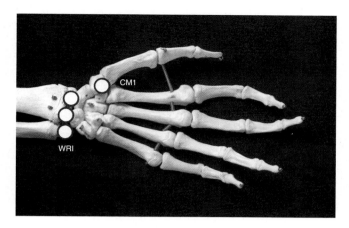

Figure 10.9 The locations of common counterstrain tender points found on patients with carpal tunnel syndrome are shown on left wrist of skeleton model. CM1, first metacarpal joint; WRI, wrist.

the thenar and hypothenar eminences, respectively (see Fig. 10.6A and B).

5. The practitioner's other fingers are placed on the dorsal surface of the patient's wrist.

6. The practitioner applies pressure centrally from the dorsal surface of the carpal bones simultaneously with pressure applied from the ventral edges of the carpal bones with the thumbs (see Fig. 10.6C).

7. A variation of this hand position may be used, with the practitioner contacting the web space between the patient's first and second digits and fourth and fifth digits with the web space between the fourth and fifth digits of the practitioner's hands (see Fig. 10.7A and B).

8. The practitioner applies pressure to the dorsal surface of the wrist with his or her fingers while simultaneously applying pressure to the ventral surface with his or her thumbs.

9. The practitioner, while maintaining this pressure, moves the thumbs laterally, stretching the underlying myofascial tissues.

10. Steps 6 and 7 are repeated until as much myofascial stretching as possible is achieved.

11. The patient may assist during the procedure by using his or her free hand to passively dorsiflex the wrist of the affected hand (see Fig. 10.8).

Counterstrain

Although several tender points related to CTS can be found, the two most commonly encountered are the first metacarpal joint (CM1) and the wrist (WRI) points (Fig. 10.9).

First Metacarpal Joint

• Location: The first metacarpal joint (CM1) counterstrain point is found on the lateral or palmar aspect of the base of the proximal first metacarpal (Fig. 10.10).

• The procedure is performed as follows:
1. The practitioner fully palmar flexes the patient's wrist, adducts the thumb toward the elbow, and adds radial or ulnar deviation of the wrist as needed until the position of maximum comfort is achieved (Fig. 10.11).
2. This position is maintained for 90 seconds.
3. The patient's wrist and hand are slowly and passively returned to the neutral position.
4. The practitioner then retests the counterstrain point for tenderness.

Wrist

• Location: Multiple counterstrain points are found on the volar surface of the wrist (Fig. 10.12A) at the bases of the carpal bones. A central point is demonstrated in Figure 10.12B.

• The procedure is performed as follows:
1. The operator flexes the patient's wrist and deviates it toward the tender point, adding pronation or supination as

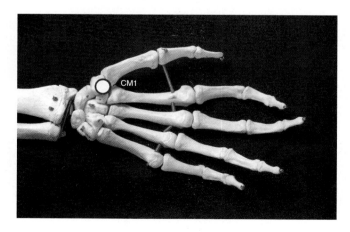

Figure 10.10 First metacarpal joint (CM1) tender point location on the left wrist of a skeleton model.

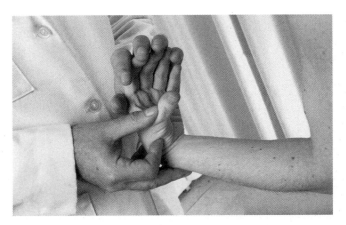

Figure 10.11   Treatment position for the first metacarpal joint tender point on the left wrist.

needed, until the position of maximum comfort is achieved (Fig. 10.13).
2. This position is maintained for 90 seconds.
3. The patient's wrist and hand are slowly and passively returned to the neutral position.
4. The practitioner then retests the counterstrain point for tenderness.

ADJUNCT TREATMENTS

Results of RCTs have provided evidence about the benefits and lack of benefits for various adjunct treatments.
- Beneficial (at least limited evidence)
  1. Carpal bone mobilization[61] (grade A evidence)
  2. Surgery[62]
  3. Corticosteroid injection[63]
  4. Short-term benefit from oral steroids[61]
  5. Splinting[61]

6. Yoga[61]
7. Therapeutic ultrasound possibly effective for up to 6 months[64]
8. Ergonomic computer keyboards with alternative force displacement of the keys or an alternative geometry[65] (grade A evidence)
- No benefit (compared with placebo or control)
  1. Magnet therapy[61]
  2. Laser acupuncture[61]
  3. Exercise[61]
  4. Nonsteroidal anti-inflammatory drugs[64]
  5. Vitamins[64]
  6. Diuretics[64]
  7. A systematic review of RCTs of conservative treatment options for CTS concluded no clear recommendations could be made based on the literature.[66]

EDUCATION

- Reassure the patient that recurrence of CTS following treatment is rare and that the majority of patients recover completely.
- To prevent workplace-related CTS, workers can do on-the-job conditioning, perform stretching exercises, take frequent rest breaks, wear splints to keep wrists straight, and use correct posture and wrist position. Wearing fingerless gloves can help keep hands warm and flexible.[18]
- Increasing individual control over work and the working environment may also be of benefit.

EXERCISES

- On-the-job exercises have proved to be cost saving and beneficial.[67]
- Home exercises are beneficial for treating CTS.

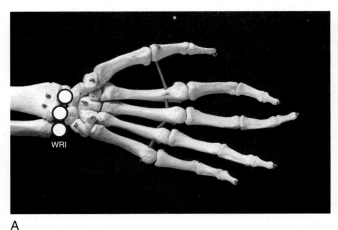

A

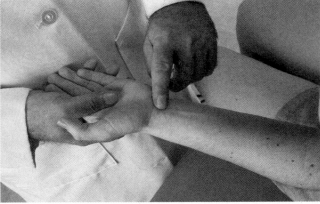

B

Figure 10.12   **A,** Location of the wrist (WRI) tender points on the left wrist of skeleton model. **B,** Location of one central WRI tender point on the left wrist as an example.

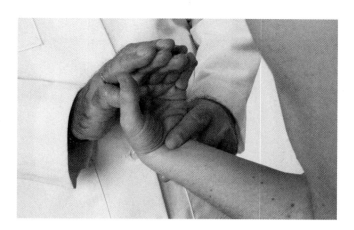

Figure 10.13 Treatment position for the wrist tender point on the center of the left wrist.

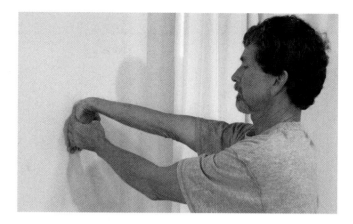

Figure 10.15 Right wrist dorsiflexion stretch using a wall and the left hand to further extend the fingers.

Exercise 1

- The exercise is performed as follows:
  1. Stand facing a wall (Fig. 10.14).
  2. With your elbow straight, reach forward and place the palm of your hand against the wall, with your fingers toward the floor.
  3. Lean slightly toward the wall until you feel the tissues at your wrist stretching.
  4. Hold this position for 30 seconds, and then relax your wrist.
  5. Repeat this exercise until you can comfortably do 3 sets of 10 repetitions.
- For added stretching, you can add the following variations to this exercise:
  1. Use your other hand to gently pull the fingers of your affected hand away from the wall (Fig. 10.15).
  2. Use your other hand to gently pull the thumb of your affected hand away from the wall (stretches the abductor

pollicis brevis muscle and fascia that is contiguous with the transverse carpal ligament) (Fig. 10.16).

Exercise 2

- The exercise is performed as follows:
  1. Starting position: Stand with your arm outstretched and your elbow straight, with the palm of your hand facing toward the ceiling. Bend your wrist so that your fingers face toward the floor (Fig. 10.17).
  2. Use your other hand to gently pull the fingers of your affected hand toward yourself.
  3. Hold this position for 30 seconds, and then relax your wrist.
  4. Return to the starting position, and this time, use your other hand to gently pull the thumb of your affected hand toward yourself (Fig. 10.18).

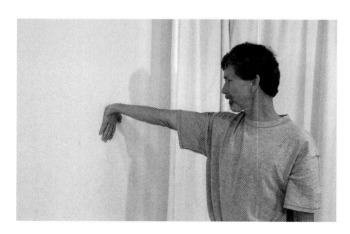

Figure 10.14 Right wrist dorsiflexion stretch using a wall.

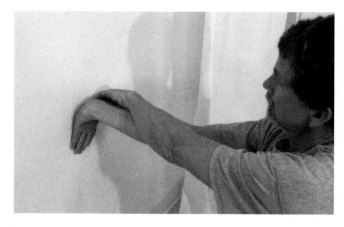

Figure 10.16 Right wrist dorsiflexion stretch using a wall and the left hand to further extend the thumb.

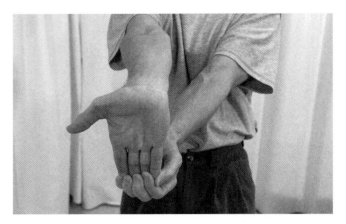

Figure 10.17   Right transverse carpal ligament stretch using the left hand to extend the fingers.

5. Hold this position for 30 seconds, and then relax your wrist.
6. Repeat this exercise until you can comfortably do 3 sets of 10 repetitions.

Exercise 3

- The exercise is performed as follows:
  1. Sit comfortably on a table, and place your affected hand flat on the table with your fingers facing behind you (Fig. 10.19). Make sure your elbow is straight.
  2. Lean on your affected hand slightly until you can feel the stretch at your wrist.
  3. Reach across with your other hand, grasp the thumb of your affected hand, and gently pull it away from the table (Fig. 10.20).
  4. Hold this position for 30 seconds, and then relax your hand.
  5. Repeat this exercise until you can comfortably do 3 sets of 10 repetitions.

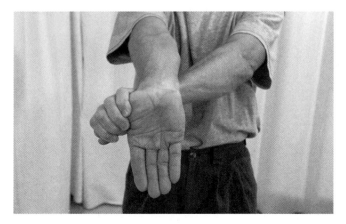

Figure 10.18   Right transverse carpal ligament stretch using the left hand to extend the thumb.

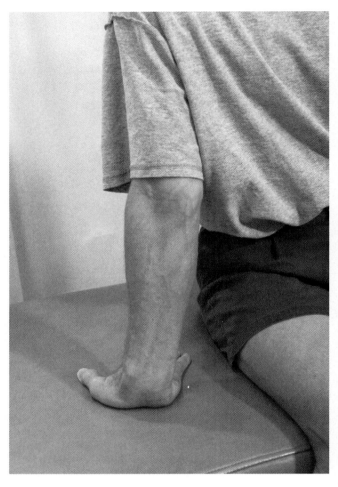

Figure 10.19   Seated passive right wrist dorsiflexion stretch with fingers pointing backward and the elbow extended.

CONTROVERSIES

- Diagnosis by EDX, clinical presentation alone, or ultrasound is still debated in the literature, although insurance companies often favor EDX testing for reimbursement of claims.
- The use of manipulative procedures as described by Sucher[47,48] have yet to be studied or reproduced in an RCT, although one is being conducted by the National Osteopathic Research Center in Fort Worth, Texas.
- Because no one test can diagnose CTS, researchers are developing a clinical prediction rule (CPR) based on five components of history, physical examination, and diagnostic tests. The CPR identified in this study consisted of one question (i.e., history of shaking the hand for symptom relief), wrist-ratio index greater than 0.67, Symptom Severity Scale score greater than 1.9, reduced median sensory field of digit 1, and age older than 45 years. The likelihood ratio for the CPR was 18.3 when results of all five tests were positive. The CPR identified was more useful for the diagnosis of CTS than any single test item and resulted in post-test probability changes of up to 56%. The CPR may alter the diagnostic and prognostic

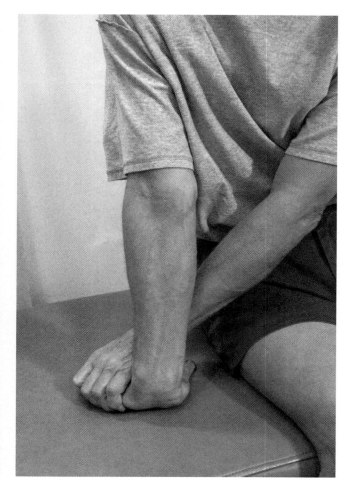

Figure 10.20 Seated passive right wrist dorsiflexion stretch using the left hand to further extend the right thumb to localize the stretch to the transverse carpal ligament.

criteria for CTS in the future if it proves to be applicable in all clinical settings.[68]

- Because there are no placebo- or sham-controlled studies used in surgical intervention clinical trials, the degree to which surgery is truly efficacious has not been determined with the highest of probabilities. Because decompression of the carpal tunnel by release of the flexor retinaculum is not always effective in relieving symptoms and restoring function, the theory that pressure against the median nerve as the primary cause of CTS is incomplete.

OPPORTUNITIES FOR RESEARCH

- The diagnosis of CTS is made by the patient's history and clinical signs alone, by the addition of EDX studies, or by EDX testing alone. Ultrasound is also being investigated as a potential reference standard. RCTs should include the use of the various diagnostic strategies and tests to discern which are most predictive of successful outcomes.[69]

- More RCTs are needed to compare treatments and to ascertain the duration of benefit.
- RCTs for CTS using manipulation of the carpal tunnel itself and somatic dysfunction found in the ipsilateral upper extremity, neck, ribs, and upper back need to be done.
- RCTs should combine patient-oriented evaluation and neurophysiologic evaluation with a focus on the effects of conservative therapies.[14]
- Investigations of metabolic changes in the cells of the subsynovial connective tissue (SSCT); the activity of matrix metalloproteinases, intracellular organelles, and other extracellular matrix macromolecules in the SSCT; and changes in mechanical properties and permeability of the SSCT should be undertaken. Animal models attempting to create median nerve compression by inducing pathology in the tenosynovium should be developed.[30]

REFERENCES

1. Rempel D, Evanoff B, Amadio PC, et al: Consensus criteria for the classification of carpal tunnel syndrome in epidemiological studies. Am J Pub Health 88:1447-1451, 1998.
2. D'Arcy CA, McGee S: Does this patient have carpal tunnel syndrome? JAMA 283:3110-3117, 2000.
3. Quality Standards Subcommittee of the American Academy of Neurology: Practice parameter for carpal tunnel syndrome (summary statement). Neurology 43:2406-2409, 1993.
4. Atroshi I, Gummesson C, Johnson R, et al: Prevalence of carpal tunnel syndrome in a general population. JAMA 282:153-158, 1999.
5. Mondelli M, Giannini F, Giacchi M: Carpal tunnel syndrome incidence in a general population. Neurology 58:289-294, 2002.
6. U.S. Department of Labor: Survey of Occupational Injuries and Illnesses. Nonfatal (OSHA Recordable) Injuries and Illnesses. Industry Incidence Rates and Counts. Washington, DC, U.S. Department of Labor, Bureau of Labor Statistics, Safety and Health Statistics Program, 2002. Available at www.bls.gov/iif/oshsum.htm/ Accessed December 28, 2005.
7. National Institute for Occupational Safety and Health Worker Health Chartbook 2004 (NIOSH Publication no. 2004-146) Chapter 2. Carpal Tunnel Syndrome. Available at http://www2.cdc.gov/NIOSH-chartbook/ch2/ch2-6-1.asp accessed February 3, 2007.
8. Bland JDP, Rudolfer SM: Clinical surveillance of carpal tunnel syndrome in two areas of the United Kingdom, 1991-2001. J Neurol Neurosurg Psychiatry 74:1674-1679, 2003.
9. U.S. Department of Labor: Survey of Occupational Injuries and Illnesses. Nonfatal (OSHA Recordable) Injuries and Illnesses. Case and Demographic Characteristics. Washington, DC, U.S. Department of Labor, Bureau of Labor Statistics, Safety and Health Statistics Program, 2003. Available at www.bls.gov/iif/oshcdnew.htm/ Accessed December 28, 2005.
10. Papanicolaou GD, McCabe SJ, Firrell J, et al: The prevalence and characteristics of nerve compression symptoms in the general population. J Hand Surg Am 26:460-466, 2001.
11. Lacey RJ, Lewis M, Sim J: The relationship between hand paresthesia and occupational factors: Results from a population study. Rheumatology 44:1287-1293, 2005.
12. Werner RA, Andary M: Carpal tunnel syndrome: Pathophysiology and clinical neurophysiology. Clin Neurophysiol 113:1373-1381, 2002.
13. Padua L, Padua R, Monaco ML, et al: Multiperspective assessment of carpal tunnel syndrome: A multicenter study. Neurology 53:1654-1659, 1999.
14. Padua L, Padua R, Aprile L, et al: Multiperspective follow-up of untreated carpal tunnel syndrome: A multicenter study. Neurology 56:1459-1466, 2001.
15. Padua L, Mondelli M: Evolution of hand dysfunction and symptoms in untreated carpal tunnel syndrome. Muscle Nerve 32:545-547, 2005.
16. National Institute for Occupational Safety and Health: Fatal and nonfatal injuries, and selected illnesses and conditions. Carpal tunnel syndrome. *In* Worker Health Chartbook 2004. NIOSH publication no. 2004-146. Available at http://www2a.cdc.gov/niosh-Chartbook/ch2/ch2-6-1.asp/ Accessed December 28, 2005.
17. Wellman H, Davis L, Punnett L, et al: Work-related carpal tunnel syndrome (WR-CTS) in Massachusetts, 1992-1997: Source of WR-CTS, outcomes, and employer intervention practices. Am J Ind Med 45:139-152, 2004.

18. National Institute of Neurological Diseases and Stroke (NINDS): Carpal Tunnel Syndrome Fact Sheet, November 2002. Updated October 13, 2005. NIH publication no. 03-4898. Available at http://www.ninds.nih.gov/disorders/carpal_tunnel/carpal_tunnel.htm/ Accessed December 28, 2005.

19. Manktelow RT, Binhammer P, Tomat LR, et al: Carpal tunnel syndrome: Cross-sectional and outcome study in Ontario workers. J Hand Surg Am 29:307-317, 2004.

20. van Dijk MA, Reitsma JB, Fischer JC: Indications for requesting laboratory tests for concurrent diseases in patients with carpal tunnel syndrome: A systematic review. Clin Chem 49:1437-1444, 2003.

21. Bahrami MH, Ravegani SM, Fereidouni M, et al: Prevalence and severity of carpal tunnel syndrome (CTS) during pregnancy. Electromyogr Clin Neurophysiol 45:123-125, 2005.

22. Pazzaglia C, Caliandro P, Aprile I, et al: Multicenter study on carpal tunnel syndrome and pregnancy incidence and natural course. Acta Neurochir Suppl 92:35-39, 2005.

23. Nathan PA, Istvan JA; Meadows KD: A longitudinal study of predictors of research-defined carpal tunnel syndrome in industrial workers: Findings at 17 years. J Hand Surg Br 30:593-598, 2005.

24. Boz C, Osmenoglu M, Altunayoglu V, et al: Individual risk factors for carpal tunnel syndrome: An evaluation of body mass index, wrist index and hand anthropometric measurements. Clin Neurol Neurosurg 106:294-299, 2004.

25. Nakamichi K, Tachibana S: Small hand as a risk factor for idiopathic carpal tunnel syndrome. Muscle Nerve 18:664-666, 1995.

26. Nakamichi K, Tachibana S: Hypercholesterolemia as a risk factor for idiopathic carpal tunnel syndrome. Muscle Nerve 32:364-367, 2005.

27. Rempel D, Dahlin L, Lundborg G: Pathophysiology of nerve compression syndromes: Response of peripheral nerves to loading. J Bone Joint Surg Am 81:1600-1610, 1999.

28. Kappler RE, Ramey KA: Upper extremities. In RC Ward (ed): Foundations for Osteopathic Medicine. Philadelphia, Lippincott Williams & Wilkins. 2003, pp 690-704.

29. Ashworth NL: Carpal tunnel syndrome. eMedicine April 8, 2005. Available at http://www.emedicine.com/pmr/topic21.htm#top/ Accessed December 28, 2005.

30. Jinrok O, Zhao C, Amadio PC, et al: Vascular pathologic changes in the flexor tenosynovium (subsynovial connective tissue) in idiopathic carpal tunnel syndrome. J Orthop Res 22:1310-1315, 2004.

31. Bland JD: Carpal tunnel syndrome. Curr Opin Neurol 18:581-585, 2005.

32. Sud V, Freeland AE: Biochemistry of carpal tunnel syndrome. Microsurgery 25:44-46, 2005.

33. Freeland AE, Tucci MA, Barbieri RA, et al: Biochemical evaluation of serum and flexor tenosynovium in carpal tunnel syndrome. Microsurgery 22:378-385, 2002.

34. Hirata H, Nagakura T, Tsujii M, et al: The relationship of VEGF and PGE_2 expression to extracellular matrix remodeling of the tenosynovium in the carpal tunnel syndrome. J Pathol 204:605-612, 2004.

35. Tucci M, Freeland A, Mohamed A, et al: The role of proteoglycans in idiopathic carpal tunnel syndrome. Biomed Sci Instrum 41:141-146, 2005.

36. Tucci MA, Barbieri RA, Freeland AE: Biochemical and histological analysis of the flexor tenosynovium in patients with carpal tunnel syndrome. Biomed Sci Instrum 33:246-251, 1997.

37. Gupta R, Rummler L, Steward O: Understanding the biology of compressive neuropathies. Clin Orthop 436:251-260, 2005.

38. Uchiyama S, Itsubo T, Yasutomi T, et al: Quantitative MRI of the wrist and nerve conduction studies in patients with idiopathic carpal tunnel syndrome. J Neur Neurosurg Psychiatry 76:1103-1108, 2005.

39. Brahme SK, Hodler J, Braun RM, et al: Dynamic MR imaging of carpal tunnel syndrome. Skeletal Radiol 26:482-487, 1997.

40. Skubick DL, Clasby R, Donaldson CCS, et al: Carpal tunnel syndrome as an expression of muscular dysfunction in the neck. J Occup Rehabil 3:31-44, 1993.

41. Donaldson CCS, Nelson DV, Skubiak DL, et al: Potential contributions of neck muscle dysfunctions to initiation and maintenance of carpal tunnel syndrome. Appl Psychophysiol Biofeed 23:59-72, 1998.

42. Kerwin G, Williams CS, Seiller JG III: The pathophysiology of carpal tunnel syndrome. Hand Clin 12:243-250, 1996.

43. Buch-Jaeger N, Foucher G: Correlation of clinical signs with nerve conduction tests in the diagnosis of carpal tunnel syndrome. J Hand Surg Br 19:720-724, 1994.

44. Massy-Westropp N, Grimmer K, Bain G: A systematic review of the clinical diagnostic tests for carpal tunnel syndrome. J Hand Surg Am 25:120-127, 2000.

45. LaJoie AS, McCabe SJ, Thomas B, et al: Determining the sensitivity and specificity of common diagnostic tests for carpal tunnel syndrome using latent class analysis. Plast Reconst Surg 116:502-507, 2005.

46. Sucher BM, Glassman JH: Upper extremity syndromes. In Stanton DF, Mein EA (eds): Manual Medicine. Physical Medicine and Rehabilitation Clinics of North America. Philadelphia, WB Saunders, 1996, pp 787-810.

47. Sucher BM: Palpatory diagnosis and manipulative management of carpal tunnel syndrome. J Am Osteopath Assoc 94:647-663, 1994.

48. Sucher BM: Palpatory diagnosis and manipulative management of carpal tunnel syndrome: Part 2. "Double crush" and thoracic outlet syndrome. J Am Osteopath Assoc 95:471-479, 1995.

49. Ramey KA, Kappler RE, Martin T: The effects of osteopathic manipulation in the treatment of carpal tunnel syndrome [abstract]. J Am Osteopath Assoc 94:755, 1994.

50. Ramey KA, Kappler RE, Chimata M, et al: MRI assessment of changes in swelling of wrist structures following OMT in patients with carpal tunnel syndrome. Am Acad Osteopath J 9:25-32, 1999.

51. Nathan PA, Keniston RC, Myers LD, et al: Natural history of median nerve sensory conduction in industry: Relationship to symptoms and carpal tunnel syndrome in 558 hands over 11 years. Muscle Nerve 21:711-721, 1998.

52. Jablecki CK, Andary MT, Floeter MK, et al: Practice parameter: Electrodiagnostic studies in carpal tunnel syndrome. Report of the American Association of Electrodiagnostic Medicine, American Academy of Neurology, and the American Academy of Physical Medicine and Rehabilitation. Neurology 58:1589-1592, 2002.

53. Ziswiler HR, Reichenbach S, Vogelin E, et al: Diagnostic value of sonography in patients with suspected carpal tunnel syndrome: A prospective study. Arthritis Rheum 52:304-311, 2005.

54. Sucher BM: Myofascial manipulative release of carpal tunnel syndrome: Documentation with magnetic resonance imaging. J Am Osteopath Assoc 93:1273-1278, 1993.

55. Tal-Akabi A, Rushton A: An investigation to compare the effectiveness of carpal bone mobilization and neurodynamic mobilization as methods of treatment for carpal tunnel syndrome. Man Ther 5:214-222, 2000.

56. Davis PT, Hulbert JR, Kassak KM, et al: Comparative efficacy of conservative medical and chiropractic treatments for carpal tunnel syndrome: A randomized clinical trial. J Manipulative Physiol Ther 21:317-326, 1998.

57. National Guideline Clearinghouse: Diagnosis and treatment of work-related carpal tunnel syndrome (OCTS). Available at http://www.guideline.gov/summary/summary.aspx?doc_id=4212&mode=full&ss=15/ Accessed December 28, 2005.

58. Elkiss ML, Rentz LE: Neurology. In RC Ward (ed): Foundations for Osteopathic Medicine. Philadelphia, Lippincott Williams & Wilkins. 2003, pp 435-449.

59. Wieting JM, Lipton JA: Osteopathic physical medicine and rehabilitation. In RC Ward (ed): Foundations for Osteopathic Medicine. Philadelphia, Lippincott Williams & Wilkins, 2003, pp 516-525.

60. Sucher BM: Myofascial release of carpal tunnel syndrome. J Am Osteopath Assoc 93:92-101, 1993.

61. O'Connor D, Marshall S, Massy-Westropp N: Non-surgical treatment (other than steroid injection) for carpal tunnel syndrome. Cochrane Database Syst Rev (1):CD003219, 2003.

62. Verdugo RJ, Salinas RS, Castillo J, et al: Surgical versus non-surgical treatment for carpal tunnel syndrome. Cochrane Database Syst Rev (3):CD001552, 2003.

63. Marshall S, Tardif G, Ashworth N: Local corticosteroid injection for carpal tunnel syndrome. Cochrane Database Syst Rev (4):CD001554, 2002.

64. Goodyear-Smith F, Arroll B: What can family physicians offer patients with carpal tunnel syndrome other than surgery? A systematic review of nonsurgical management. Ann Fam Med 2:267-273, 2004.

65. Verhagen AP, Bierma-Zeinstra SM, Feleus A, et al: Ergonomic and physiotherapeutic interventions for treating upper extremity work related disorders in adults. Cochrane Database Syst Rev (1):CD003471, 2004.

66. Gerritsen AAM, de Krom MCTFM, Struijs MA, et al: Conservative treatment options for carpal tunnel syndrome: A systematic review of randomized controlled trials. J Neurol 249:272-280, 2002.

67. Seradge H, Bear C, Bithell D: Preventing carpal tunnel syndrome and cumulative trauma disorder: Effect of carpal tunnel decompression exercises: An Oklahoma experience. J Okla State Med Assoc 93:150-153, 2000.

68. Wainner RS, Fritz JM, Irrgang JJ, et al: Development of a clinical prediction rule for the diagnosis of carpal tunnel syndrome. Arch Phys Med Rehabil 86:609-618, 2005.

69. Bachmann LM, Juni P, Reichenbach S; et al: Consequences of different diagnostic 'gold standards' in test accuracy research: Carpal Tunnel Syndrome as an example. Int J Epidemiol 34:953-955, 2005.

CHAPTER 11

Ankle Sprain

DEFINITION

- Ankle sprain may be defined as injury to the ligaments of the ankle joint, most commonly the lateral ligaments.
- Ankle sprains are classified according to severity (Table 11.1).

EPIDEMIOLOGY

- The ankle is the most commonly injured joint among athletes.
- Ankle sprain is a frequent cause of morbidity in the general population.

Age

- No specific age group appears to be affected, although most ankle sprains tend to occur in younger people and among athletically inclined individuals.
- Individuals who are older or physically inactive are more at risk for ankle injury.

Gender

- Both sexes are affected.
- Significant gender differences have not been reported.

Prevalence

- Sprains account for about 85% of ankle injuries.
- It is estimated that acute ankle injury accounts for about 10% to 30% of sports-related injuries.
- Annually, an estimated 1 million patients present to physicians with acute ankle trauma.
- More than 40% of ankle sprains are severe enough to potentially become chronic problems.[2-5]

Natural Clinical Course

- Most ankle injuries are mild and are thought to be self-treated.[6]
- More severe injuries respond well to conservative treatment. Typical conservative treatment consists of *p*rotection, *r*est, *i*ce, *c*ompression, and *e*levation (PRICE).[7]
- The most severe ankle injuries (grade III) may require casting or surgery.

Effect on Society

- No reliable data have been provided regarding societal effects such as taxpayer liability, disability claims compensation, or work loss.

Risk Factors

- Lack of physical conditioning or sedentary lifestyle
- Failure to stretch or warm up properly before physical activity
- Improper or inadequate footwear
- Performing physical activities on uneven ground or other surfaces
- History of previous ankle sprain
- Certain sports activities, such as basketball, cross-country running, and football, which are associated with a higher risk for ankle injury[1,6]

PATHOPHYSIOLOGY

- Ankle sprains have been characterized as grade I, grade II, or grade III (see Table 11.1).
- The most commonly injured ligament is the anterior talofibular, followed by the calcaneofibular ligament. The posterior talofibular ligament is rarely injured.
- The most common mechanism of injury in ankle sprains is a combination of plantar flexion and inversion.

Table 11.1   Grading system for ankle sprains

Grade	Characteristics
I	Mild sprain, mild pain, little swelling, and joint stiffness may be apparent
	Stretch or minor tear of the ligament without laxity (i.e., loosening)
	Usually affects the anterior talofibular ligament
	Minimal or no loss of function
	Can return to activity within a few days of the injury (with a brace or taping)
II	Moderate to severe pain, swelling, and joint stiffness are present
	Partial tear of one or more lateral ligaments
	Moderate loss of function with difficulty on toe raises and walking
	Takes up to 2 to 3 months before regaining close to full strength and stability in the joint
III	Severe pain may be present initially, followed by little or no pain due to total disruption of the nerve fibers.
	Swelling may be profuse and joint becomes stiff some hours after the injury
	Complete rupture of the ligaments of the lateral complex (i.e., severe laxity)
	Usually requires some form of immobilization lasting several weeks
	Complete loss of function (i.e., functional disability) and necessity for crutches
	Usually managed conservatively with rehabilitation exercises, but a small percentage may require surgery
	Recovery can be as long as 4 months

Adapted from Wexler RK: The injured ankle. Am Fam Physician 57:474-480, 1998.

- Excessive external rotation of the ankle results in a syndesmotic, or high, ankle sprain. These injuries are much less common than inversion injuries; however, they tend to be more disabling, and the recovery period from such an injury is longer.

DIFFERENTIAL DIAGNOSIS

- Ankle sprain should be differentiated from other serious clinical conditions.
- Table 11.2 lists items for consideration in the differential diagnosis of ankle injury.

HISTORY

- The patient may have a history of trauma, fall, or twisting injury.[6]
- Pain may be felt over the anterolateral part of the ankle (with inversion injury) on weight bearing
- The ankle itself feels weak.
- Ankle instability may be experienced.

Table 11.2   Differential diagnosis of acute ankle injury

Ankle fracture
Avulsion fracture of the fibula
Peroneal tendon subluxation
Achilles tendon rupture
Interosseous membrane tear

Adapted from Wexler RK: The injured ankle. Am Fam Physician 57:474-480, 1998.

PHYSICAL FINDINGS

- Physical examination findings may include the following:
  1. Bruising
  2. Edema
  3. Inability to bear weight on the affected foot
  4. Tenderness on palpation
  5. Normal ankle and subtalar movement (grade I)
  6. Avulsion or hairline fractures of the fibula, tibia, calcaneus, fifth metatarsal, cuboid, or talus
- The anterior drawer test is useful for assessing the integrity of the anterior talofibular ligament. The practitioner stabilizes the distal tibia and fibula with one hand and grasps the heel of the affected ankle with the other hand and then attempts to move the ankle anteriorly relative to the rest of the leg. A movement of 4 mm or more is considered a positive indication for anterior talofibular ligament rupture.[6,7]

LABORATORY AND RADIOGRAPHIC FINDINGS

- No laboratory studies are indicated for isolated ankle sprains.
- The Ottawa ankle rules can be used to determine when radiographic studies are indicated in the patient with ankle trauma (Table 11.3).
- Stress radiographs of the ankle are useful in determining the extent of ligamentous injury.
- Magnetic resonance imaging (MRI) can determine the integrity of the collateral ligaments of the ankle. MRI is usually not indicated unless unusual features (e.g. extensive swelling, ecchymosis, pain) are present.
- Arthrography of the ankle is useful in determining the exact site and extent of ligamentous injury. It is indicated only when contemplating surgical correction of a ruptured ligament.

MANUAL MEDICINE

Best Evidence

- Various forms of manual therapies have been shown to be useful in the treatment and rehabilitation of ankle sprains. Physical therapy modalities are commonly used as part of the treatment of ankle sprains. Chiropractic manipulation has also been efficacious in the treatment of ankle injuries.[9]

Table 11.3   Ottawa rules for use of radiographs for patients with acute ankle injuries

Radiographic Series	Symptoms and Signs
Ankle series—required only if the patient has pain in the malleolar zone and any one of these findings	Bone tenderness at the posterior edge or tip of the lateral malleolus
	Bone tenderness at the posterior edge or tip of the medial malleolus
	Inability to bear weight immediately and in the emergency department
Foot series—required only if the patient has pain in the midfoot zone and any one of these findings	Bone tenderness at the base of the fifth metatarsal
	Bone tenderness at the navicular
	Inability to bear weight immediately and in the emergency department

Adapted from Wolfe MW, Uhl TL, Mattacola CG, et al: Management of ankle sprains. Am Fam Physician 63:93-104, 2001; Stiell IG, McKnight RD, Greenberg GH, et al: Implementation of the Ottawa ankle rules. JAMA 271:827-832, 1994.

Osteopathic manipulative treatment has been recommended as a useful treatment for ankle sprains in particular.

- Blood[10] showed a relationship between ankle sprain and somatic dysfunctions in other body regions, such as the rib cage and thoracic spine. He recommended osteopathic manipulative treatment of these regions and of the foot and ankle, and he described specific exercises for the rehabilitation of ankle sprain. A clinical trial[11] showed that a single osteopathic manipulative treatment performed in the emergency room on patients resulted in less edema and perceived pain and increased the range of motion.

Risks

- No specific studies have addressed the risks of manual treatment for sprained ankle.
- Expert consensus supports avoiding high-velocity, low-amplitude (HVLA) techniques in treating the acutely injured, edematous, or inflamed ankle and when fracture is present or highly suspected.
- Nonforceful techniques may be used with caution in these situations. No reports have been published on significant contraindications or adverse effects using nonforceful techniques.[12]

Benefits

- Reported benefits of manual treatment for sprained ankle include the following:
  1. Reduced edema
  2. Reduction in perceived pain
  3. Less need for pain medication
  4. Earlier restoration of functional ability and range of motion
  5. Increased patient satisfaction

Practice Recommendations

- The Institute for Clinical Systems Improvement[13] published a set of recommended guidelines for the diagnosis and treatment of acute ankle injuries. Table 11.4 provides a summary of these guidelines.

Table 11.4   Guidelines for the diagnosis and treatment of acute ankle injuries

Management Approach*	Clinical Circumstances and Comments
Same-day visits should be scheduled for patients experiencing these symptoms, signs, or circumstances	Sudden, intense pain with rapid onset of swelling; cold or numbness in the foot; presence of gross deformity; complicating conditions (e.g., diabetes, neuropathy); a work-related injury or the inability to bear any weight
Treatment of the non-emergent and nonclinical patient should follow the PRICE principle	P, protection; R, relative rest; I, ice; C, compression/support; E, elevation
An ankle radiograph series (anteroposterior, lateral, and mortis views) should be obtained for this patient	Patient with pain in the malleolar zone and bone. *Caution:* A Salter Harris type I fracture of the distal fibula may be present even with normal radiographic findings
A foot radiographic series is required for this patient	Patient with pain in the navicular region, including bone tenderness at the base of the fifth metatarsal or base of the navicular bone, or an inability to bear weight at the time of the evaluation
Rehabilitation of confirmed ankle sprains	Flexibility, strengthening, and balance exercises and following a reasonable progression for return to work
Following a plan that has significantly reduced the recurrence of ankle sprain	An effective rehabilitation program for the person with the ankle injury combined with a prophylactic ankle bracing

*Scope and target population for these recommendations: Patients were 5 years old or older and presented with acute lateral ankle pain caused by inversion of the ankle.

Adapted from Institute for Clinical Systems Improvement: Guidelines for the Treatment of Ankle Sprains. Bloomington, MN, Institute for Clinical Systems Improvement, July 2001.

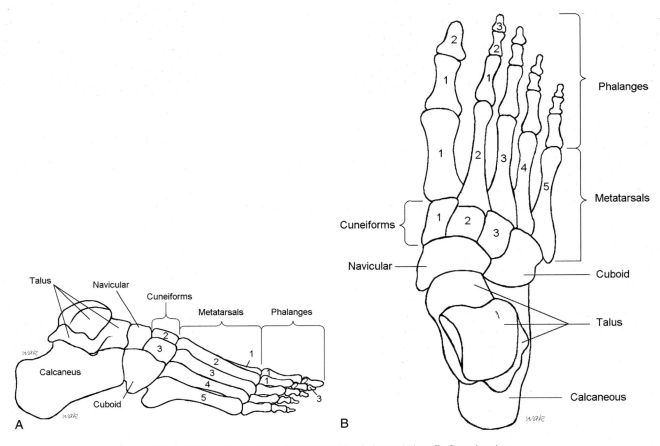

Figure 11.1   Bones of the foot and ankle. **A,** Lateral view. **B,** Superior view.

FUNCTIONAL ANATOMY

- The skeletal structure of the foot consists of 26 bones: 7 tarsal bones (i.e., talus, calcaneus, navicular, cuboid, medial cuneiform, intermediate cuneiform, and lateral cuneiform), 5 metatarsal bones, and 14 phalanges (Fig. 11.1). Sesamoid bones may be found on either side of the plantar surface of the first metatarsal.
- The bones are arranged to produce three arches: two longitudinal arches (medial and lateral) and one transverse arch.

The arches act as shock absorbers in balancing the body. The medial longitudinal arch transmits the force of body weight to the ground in the standing position and to the great toe when walking or running.[14]
- The longitudinal arches consist of tarsal and metatarsal bones arranged to form arches running from anterior to posterior. The medial longitudinal arch consists of the calcaneus, the talus, the navicular, the three cuneiforms, and the first, second, and third metatarsals (Fig. 11.2). The lateral longitudinal arch includes the calcaneus, the cuboid, and the fourth and fifth metatarsals. The transverse arch is made up of the

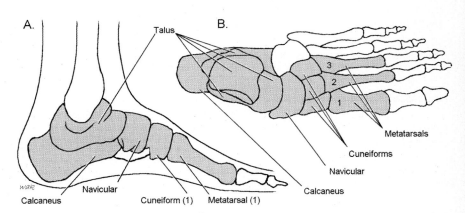

Figure 11.2   The median longitudinal arch of the foot. **A,** Medial view. **B,** Superior view.

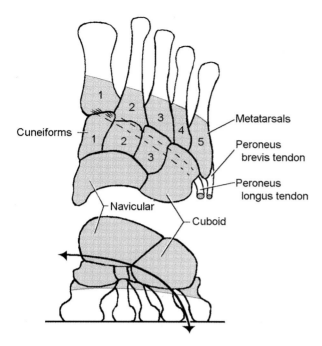

Figure 11.3   The transverse arch of the foot.

cuboid, navicular, the three cuneiforms, and proximal parts of all five metatarsals (Fig. 11.3).

- An articular capsule surrounds the joint and extends from the tibia and malleoli to the talus. The major ligaments of the ankle joint are the medial (deltoid) ligament and the lateral ligament, which includes three separate parts: the anterior talofibular ligament, the posterior talofibular ligament, and the calcaneofibular ligament (Fig. 11.4).
- The major muscles of the foot and ankle include the gastrocnemius, soleus, and the peroneal muscles, the extensor hallucis brevis and the extensor digitorum brevis.
- The major tendons of the foot and ankle include the tendons of the tibialis anterior, the extensor hallucis longus, the extensor digitorum longus, and the peroneus tertius.[15]

MANUAL DIAGNOSTIC PROCEDURES

Evaluations for Somatic Dysfunctions of the Ankle

Evaluation for Anterior or Posterior Fibular Head Restriction

- The procedure is performed as follows:
  1. The patient is seated.
  2. The practitioner sits on the side of the involved ankle.
  3. The practitioner stabilizes the patient's lower leg with one hand (Fig. 11.5).

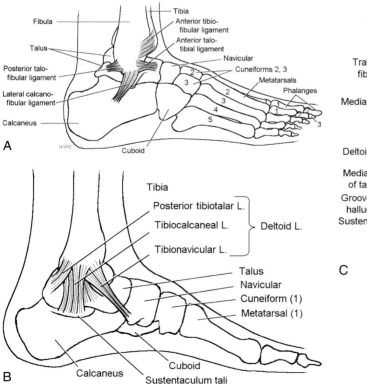

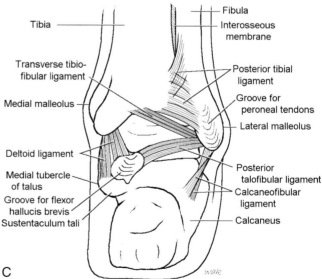

Figure 11.4   The ligaments of the ankle joint. **A,** Lateral view. **B,** Medial view. **C,** Posterior view.

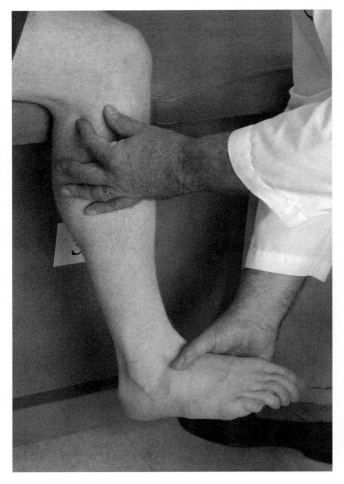

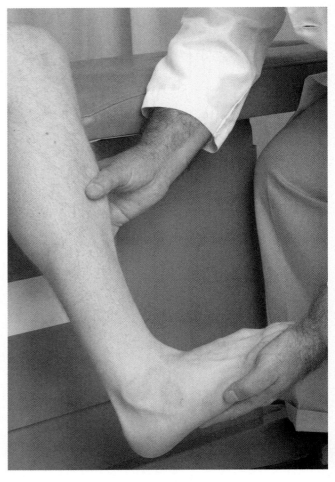

Figure 11.5 Evaluation for anterior or posterior fibular head somatic dysfunction.

Figure 11.6 Evaluation for restricted dorsiflexion of the ankle joint.

4. With his or her other hand, the practitioner grasps the fibular head, placing the thumb on the anterior part of the fibular head and the pad of the index finger on the posterior aspect.

5. The practitioner passively moves the proximal fibular head anteriorly and posteriorly in the plane of the joint, observing the range and quality of the movement.

6. The practitioner compares the degree of anterior and posterior movement of the involved leg with that of the opposite leg.

7. A proximal fibular head that resists anterior movement is described as a posterior fibular head; one that resists posterior movement is described as an anterior fibular head.

Evaluation for Talotibial Joint Somatic Dysfunction

Restricted Dorsiflexion or Plantar Flexion

• The procedure is performed as follows:
1. The patient is seated on the examination table with the feet dangling.
2. The practitioner sits facing the patient.

3. The practitioner grasps the patient's involved foot, placing his or her hand under the plantar surface of the foot (Figs. 11.6 and 11.7).

4. The practitioner dorsiflexes the foot, observing the range and quality of movement.

5. The practitioner compares the dorsiflexion of the involved foot with that of the opposite one.

6. The practitioner then places his or her hand on the dorsal surface of the involved foot.

7. The practitioner plantar flexes the foot, observing the range and quality of movement.

8. The practitioner compares the plantar flexion of the involved foot with that of the opposite one.

9. A talotibial joint that resists dorsiflexion is described as being plantar flexed; one that resists plantar flexion is described as being dorsiflexed.

Restricted Inversion or Eversion

• The procedure is performed as follows:
1. The patient is seated on the examination table with the feet dangling.
2. The practitioner sits facing the patient.

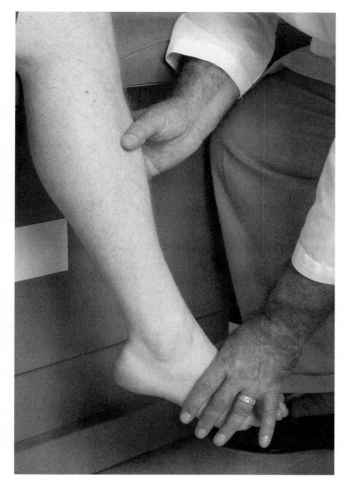

Figure 11.7   Evaluation for restricted plantar flexion of the ankle joint.

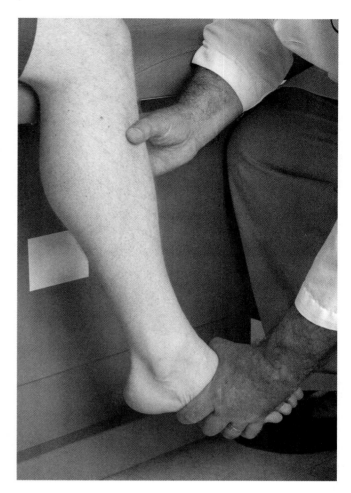

Figure 11.8   Evaluation for restricted inversion of the ankle joint.

3. The practitioner grasps the patient's involved foot, placing his or her hand on the dorsal surface of the foot (Figs. 11.8 and 11.9).
4. The practitioner inverts the foot, observing the range and quality of movement.
5. The practitioner compares the inversion of the involved foot with that of the opposite foot.
6. The practitioner then everts the involved foot, observing the range and quality of movement.
7. The practitioner compares the eversion of the involved foot with that of the opposite foot.
8. A talotibial joint that resists inversion is described as being everted; one that resists eversion is described as being inverted.
• The practitioner should examine the involved ankle for the following counterstrain points (Fig. 11.10): flexion ankle (FAN), extension ankle (EXA), medial ankle (MAN), lateral ankle (LAN), and talus (TAL).

Myofascial Restriction of the Ankle Region
• The procedure is performed as follows:
  1. The patient is supine.
  2. The practitioner stands at the end of the table facing the patient.

3. The practitioner grasps the ankle to be treated by interlacing his or her fingers over the dorsal aspect of the forefoot and placing his or her thumbs against the plantar surface of the foot (Fig. 11.11).
4. The practitioner passively moves the ankle in each of three planes of motion: dorsiflexion and plantar flexion, inversion and eversion, and compression and distraction. For each motion, the practitioner determines whether there is symmetry in the range of motion or there is more ease of movement in one direction or the other.

MANUAL TREATMENT PROCEDURES

Muscle Energy Techniques

Treatment of Posterior Fibular Head Somatic Dysfunction
• Example: posterior right fibular head
• The procedure is performed as follows:
  1. The patient is seated on the table with the legs dangling freely.
  2. The practitioner is seated in front of the patient.

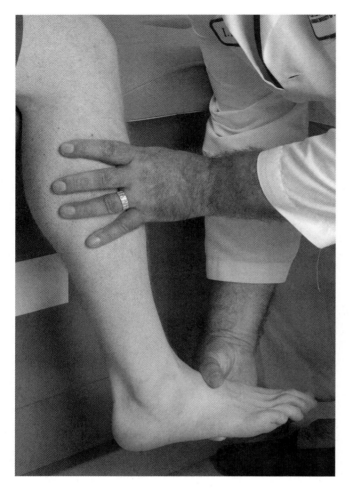

Figure 11.9 Evaluation for restricted eversion of the ankle joint.

3. The practitioner grasps the right proximal fibular head with the thumb and forefinger of his or her left hand (Fig. 11.12).
4. With the right hand, the practitioner grasps the patient's right forefoot.
5. The practitioner inverts and internally rotates the patient's forefoot and simultaneously moves the proximal fibular head anteriorly until the restrictive motion barrier is engaged.
6. The patient attempts to evert and dorsiflex the foot against the practitioner's unyielding resistance. This position is held for 3 to 5 seconds, and the patient then relaxes the foot.
7. The practitioner engages the next restrictive motion barrier by further inverting and internally rotating the foot and moving the proximal fibular head further anteriorly.
8. Steps 6 and 7 are repeated three to five times.
9. The practitioner retests the patient.

Treatment of Anterior Fibular Head Somatic Dysfunction
- Example: anterior right fibular head
- The procedure is performed as follows:
  1. The patient is seated on the table with the legs dangling freely.

2. The practitioner is seated in front of the patient.
3. The practitioner grasps the right proximal fibular head with the thumb and forefinger of his or her left hand (Fig. 11.13).
4. With the right hand, the practitioner grasps the patient's right forefoot.
5. The practitioner inverts and externally rotates the patient's forefoot and simultaneously moves the proximal fibular head posteriorly until the restrictive motion barrier is engaged.
6. The patient attempts to evert and plantar flex the foot against the practitioner's unyielding resistance. This position is held for 3 to 5 seconds, and the patient then relaxes the foot.
7. The practitioner engages the next restrictive motion barrier by further inverting and externally rotating the foot and moving the proximal fibular head further posteriorly.
8. Steps 6 and 7 are repeated three to five times.
9. The practitioner retests the patient.

Treatment of Talotibial Joint Somatic Dysfunction

Treatment of Restricted Dorsiflexion
- The procedure is performed as follows:
  1. The patient is seated on the examination table with the feet dangling.
  2. The practitioner sits facing the patient.
  3. The practitioner places the palm of one hand on the plantar surface of the forefoot to be treated and dorsiflexes the foot until the restrictive motion barrier is engaged. The practitioner uses his or her other hand to stabilize the patient's lower extremity (Fig. 11.14).
  4. The patient plantar flexes the foot against the practitioner's unyielding resistance. This position is held for 3 to 5 seconds, and the patient then relaxes the foot.
  5. The practitioner further dorsiflexes the foot to engage the next restrictive motion barrier.
  6. Steps 4 and 5 are repeated three to five times.
  7. The practitioner retests the patient.

Treatment of Restricted Plantar Flexion
- The procedure is performed as follows:
  1. The patient is seated on the examination table with the feet dangling.
  2. The practitioner sits facing the patient.
  3. The practitioner places the palm of one hand on the dorsal surface of the forefoot to be treated and plantar flexes the foot until the restrictive motion barrier is engaged. The practitioner uses his or her other hand to stabilize the patient's lower extremity (Fig. 11.15).
  4. The patient dorsiflexes the foot against the practitioner's unyielding resistance. This position is held for 3 to 5 seconds, and the patient then relaxes the foot.
  5. The practitioner further plantar flexes the foot to engage the next restrictive motion barrier.
  6. Steps 4 and 5 are repeated three to five times.
  7. The practitioner retests the patient.

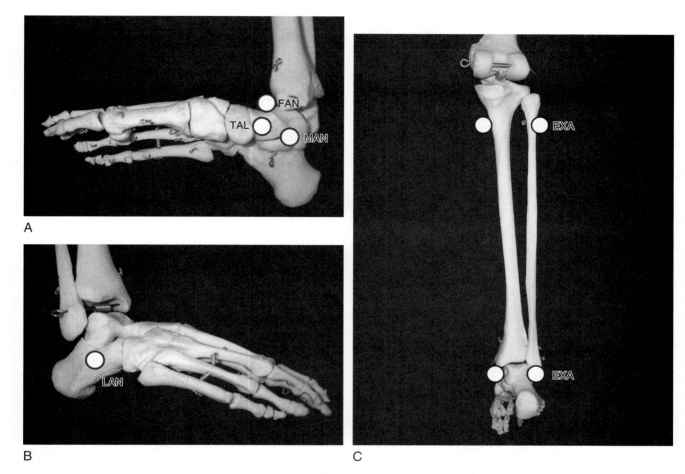

Figure 11.10 Locations of the ankle counterstrain points. **A**, Medial view. **B**, Lateral view. **C**, Posterior view. EXA, extension ankle; FAN, flexion ankle; MAN, medial ankle; TAL, talus.

Treatment of Restricted Inversion

- The procedure is performed as follows:
  1. The patient is seated on the examination table with the feet dangling.
  2. The practitioner sits facing the patient.
  3. The practitioner uses one hand to grasp the lower leg on the affected side and stabilize it. With his or her other hand, the practitioner inverts the foot until the restrictive motion barrier is engaged (Fig. 11.16).
  4. The patient everts the foot against the practitioner's unyielding resistance. This position is held for 3 to 5 seconds, and the patient then relaxes the foot.
  5. The practitioner further inverts the foot to engage the next restrictive motion barrier.
  6. Steps 4 and 5 are repeated three to five times.
  7. The practitioner retests the patient.

Treatment of Restricted Eversion

- The procedure is performed as follows:
  1. The patient is seated on the examination table with the feet dangling.

2. The practitioner sits facing the patient.
3. The practitioner uses one hand to grasp the lower leg on the affected side and stabilize it. With his or her other hand the practitioner everts the foot until the restrictive motion barrier is engaged (Fig. 11.17).
4. The patient then inverts the foot against the practitioner's unyielding resistance. This position is held for 3 to 5 seconds and then the patient relaxes the foot.
5. The practitioner further everts the foot to engage the next restrictive motion barrier.
6. Steps 4 and 5 are repeated three to five times.
7. The practitioner retests the patient.

Counterstrain Techniques

Flexion Ankle
- Location: The flexion ankle (FAN) counterstrain point is immediately medial to tendon of extensor digitorum longus as it crosses the ankle joint (Fig. 11.18).
- The procedure is performed as follows (Fig. 11.19):
  1. The patient is prone on the examination table with the knee on the affected side flexed to 90 degrees.

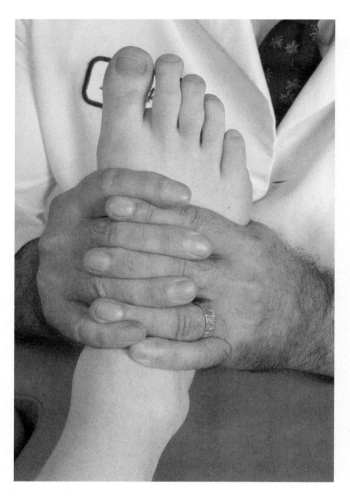

Figure 11.11 Evaluation for myofascial restriction of the ankle region.

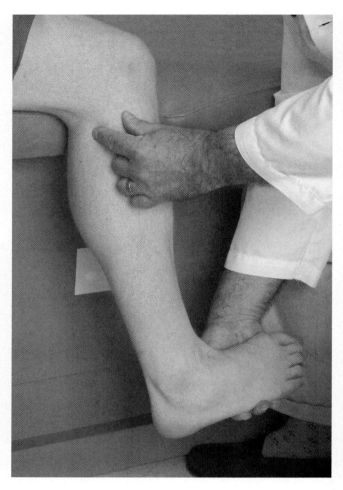

Figure 11.12 Muscle energy treatment for posterior fibular head somatic dysfunction.

2. The practitioner monitors the counterstrain point with the index finger of one hand.
3. The practitioner uses his or her other hand to dorsiflex the patient's foot until the optimal position of comfort is obtained. This position is maintained for 90 seconds.
4. The patient's foot is then slowly returned to the neutral position.
5. The practitioner retests the counterstrain point.

Extension Ankle
- Locations:
  1. Two extension ankle (EXA) points are located on the medial and lateral heads of the gastrocnemius muscle, in the inferolateral portion of the popliteal fossa (Fig. 11.20A).
  2. Two points are located on the medial and lateral aspects of the Achilles tendon, at its insertion on the calcaneus (Fig. 11.21A).
- The procedure is performed as follows (see Figs. 11.20B and 11.21B):
  1. The patient is prone on the examination table.
  2. The practitioner stands on the side of the lower extremity to be treated.

3. The practitioner places one foot on the table and rests the dorsal aspect of the patient's foot on his or her thigh.
4. The more tender set of counterstrain points is treated first. The practitioner monitors the points with the index and middle fingers of one hand.
5. With his or her other hand, the practitioner induces marked plantar flexion of the patient's foot until the position of optimal comfort is achieved.
6. This position is maintained for 90 seconds.
7. The patient's foot is then slowly returned to the neutral position.
8. The practitioner retests the counterstrain points.

Medial Ankle
- Location: The medial ankle (MAN) counterstrain point is approximately 2 cm inferior to the medial malleolus (Fig. 11.22).
- The procedure is performed as follows (Fig. 11.23):
  1. The patient is prone on the examination table, with the knee on the affected side flexed to 90 degrees.
  2. The practitioner monitors the counterstrain point with the index finger of one hand.

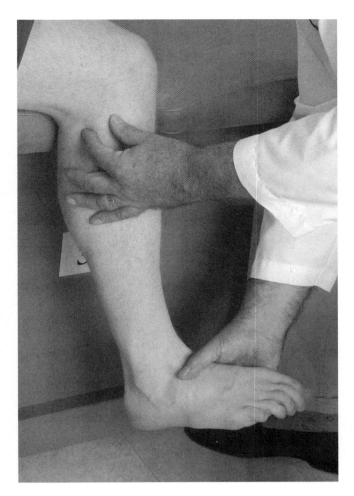

Figure 11.13 Muscle energy treatment for anterior fibular head somatic dysfunction.

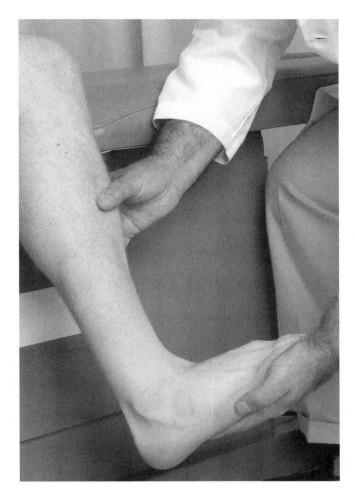

Figure 11.14 Muscle energy treatment for restricted dorsiflexion of the ankle joint.

3. The practitioner uses his or her other hand to invert the patient's foot until the optimal position of comfort is obtained. Some internal rotation of the forefoot may also be required. This position is maintained for 90 seconds.
4. The patient's foot is then slowly returned to the neutral position.
5. The practitioner retests the counterstrain point.

Lateral Ankle
- Location: The lateral ankle (LAN) counterstrain point is just inferior and 3 cm anterior to the lateral malleolus (Fig. 11.24).
- The procedure is performed as follows (Fig. 11.25).
  1. The patient is prone on the examination table, with the knee on the affected side flexed to 90 degrees.
  2. The practitioner monitors the counterstrain point with the index finger of one hand.
  3. The practitioner uses his or her other hand to evert the patient's foot until the optimal position of comfort is obtained. This position is maintained for 90 seconds.
  4. The patient's foot is then slowly returned to the neutral position.
  5. The practitioner retests the counterstrain point.

Talus
- Location: The talus counterstrain point is 2 cm anterior to the medial malleolus (Fig. 11.26).
- The procedure is performed as follows (Fig. 11.27):
  1. The patient is prone on the examination table, with the knee on the affected side flexed to 90 degrees.
  2. The practitioner monitors the counterstrain point with the index finger of one hand.
  3. The practitioner uses his or her other hand to invert the patient's foot until the optimal position of comfort is obtained. Some internal rotation of the forefoot may also be required. This position is maintained for 90 seconds.
  4. The patient's foot is then slowly returned to the neutral position.
  5. The practitioner retests the counterstrain point.

Myofascial Release Technique

Myofascial Release of the Ankle Region
- The procedure is performed as follows:
  1. The patient is supine.

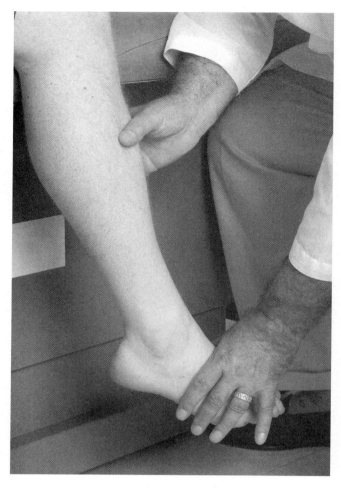

Figure 11.15   Muscle energy treatment for restricted plantar flexion of the ankle joint.

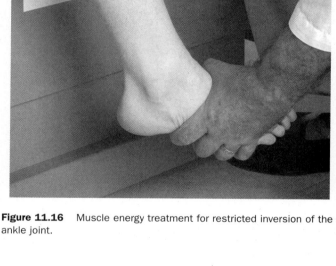

Figure 11.16   Muscle energy treatment for restricted inversion of the ankle joint.

2. The practitioner stands at the end of the table and faces the patient.
3. The practitioner grasps the ankle to be treated by interlacing his or her fingers over the dorsal aspect of the forefoot and placing his or her thumbs against the plantar surface of the foot (Fig. 11.28).
4. The practitioner moves the ankle comfortably into all directions of ease observed during the evaluation process.
5. The ankle is maintained in this position until the myofascial tissues soften and relaxation of the tissues takes place.
6. The practitioner retests the patient.

ADJUNCT TREATMENTS

- *R*est, *i*ce, *c*ompression, and *e*levation (RICE) are used for acute injuries.
- Heat therapy is used for later recovery stages.
- Exercises and proprioceptive retraining are used to restore functional ability and reduce the risk of recurrent ankle sprain.

- Supportive devices, such as taping or air casts, are used to enhance healing and recovery.
- Balance boards and similar devices help to increase the range of motion, improve ankle strength, and restore proprioception.
- Nonsteroidal anti-inflammatory medications are used for control of inflammation and pain relief.[1,2]

EDUCATION

- Prevention of future ankle sprains depends on the type of activity engaged in. Certain sports (e.g., soccer, basketball, volleyball) have high incidence of ankle sprains.
- Adequate training and conditioning helps to prevent future injury or minimize injury severity.
- An adequate warm-up period and gradual transition into the activity can help the patient.
- Patients should wear shoes with good stability.
- Patients should exercise on even surfaces if possible.

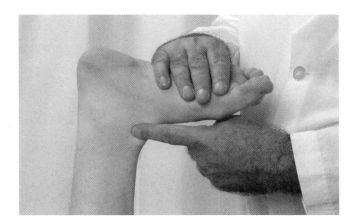

Figure 11.19 Treatment position for the flexion ankle counterstrain point.

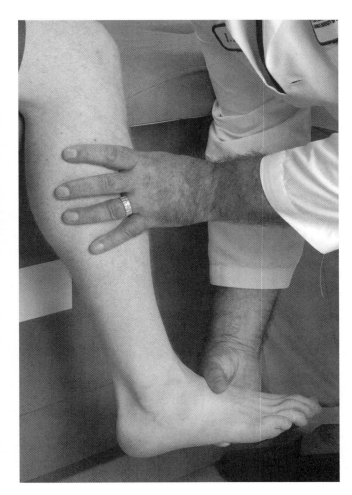

Figure 11.17 Muscle energy treatment for restricted eversion of the ankle joint.

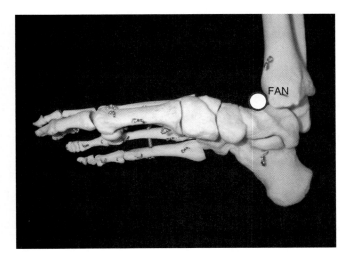

Figure 11.18 Location of the flexion ankle (FAN) counterstrain point: medial view.

- Patients should use of supportive devices such as high-top shoes, lace-up ankle braces, or Velcro ankle braces, and ankle taping may be helpful during activities to prevent further injury.[2,6,16]

EXERCISES

Exercise 1

- The exercise is performed as follows:
  1. Stand behind a chair (Figs. 11.29 and 11.30).
  2. Place your hands on the back of the chair for support.
  3. Lift your healthy foot off the floor.
  4. Raise your injured foot so that you are standing on your toes on that foot.
  5. Hold this position for 3 to 5 seconds, and then slowly lower this foot.
  6. Repeat steps 4 and 5 until you can comfortably perform 10 repetitions of this exercise.

Exercise 2

- The exercise is performed as follows:
  1. Stand behind a chair (Figs. 11.31 and 11.32).
  2. Place your hands on the back of the chair for support.
  3. Raise both feet so that you are standing on your heels.
  4. Hold this position for 3 to 5 seconds, and then slowly lower your feet.
  5. Repeat steps 3 and 4 until you can comfortably perform 10 repetitions of this exercise.

Exercise 3

- The exercise is performed as follows:
  1. Stand behind a chair (Figs. 11.33 and 11.34).
  2. Place your hands on the back of the chair for support.

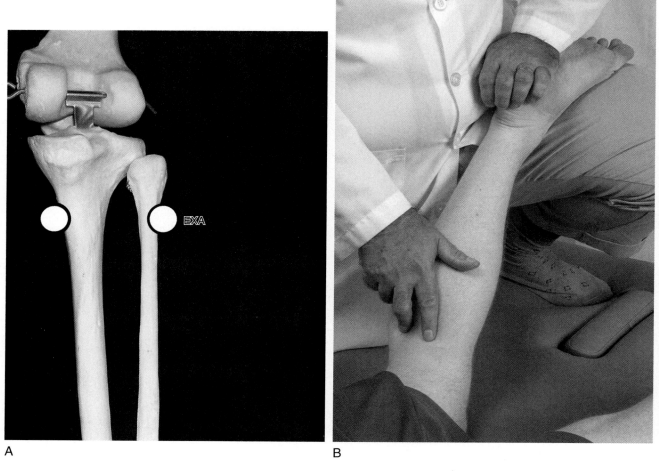

A   B

Figure 11.20   A, Location of the proximal extension ankle (EXA) counterstrain points: posterior view. **B,** Treatment position for the proximal EXA counterstrain points.

3. Place your healthy foot slightly forward on the floor and your injured foot slightly behind.
4. Lean your body forward, keeping your injured foot flat on the floor. Lean forward until you feel the muscles in your calf begin to stretch.
5. Hold this position for 3 to 5 seconds and then relax your leg.
6. Repeat steps 4 and 5 until you can comfortably perform 10 repetitions of this exercise.
7. Repeat the entire exercise with the opposite leg.

Exercise 4

• The exercise is performed as follows:
1. Sit comfortably in a chair (Figs. 11.35 and 11.36).
2. Roll up a towel lengthwise and place it under your injured foot, grasping both ends of the towel with your hands.
3. Lift your injured foot off the floor so it is resting on its heel.
4. Push your foot toward the floor while you use the towel to resist this movement at the same time.
5. Hold this position for 3 to 5 seconds.
6. Repeat steps 4 and 5 until you can comfortably perform 10 repetitions of this exercise.

Exercise 5

• The exercise is performed as follows:
1. Sit comfortably in a chair (Fig. 11.37 and 11.38).
2. Lift your injured foot off the floor, and straighten your leg on that side.
3. Roll up a towel lengthwise, and place it under your injured foot, grasping both ends of the towel with your hands.
4. Push your foot toward the floor while you use the towel to resist this movement at the same time.
5. Hold this position for 3 to 5 seconds.
6. Repeat steps 4 and 5 until you can comfortably perform 10 repetitions of this exercise.

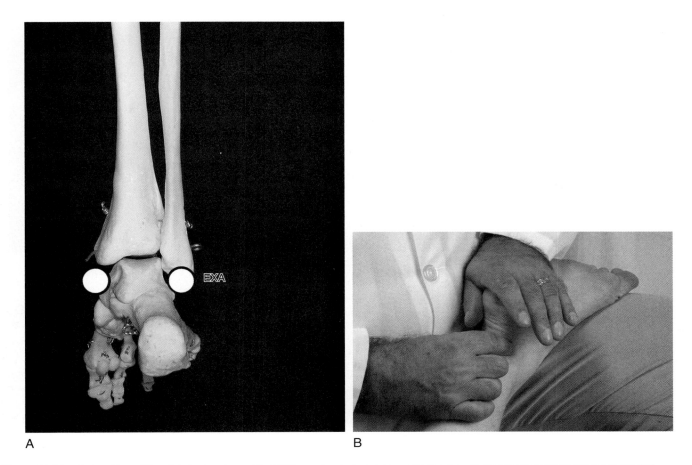

A   B

Figure 11.21   **A,** Location of the distal extension ankle (EXA) counterstrain points: posterior view. **B,** Treatment position for the distal EXA counterstrain points.

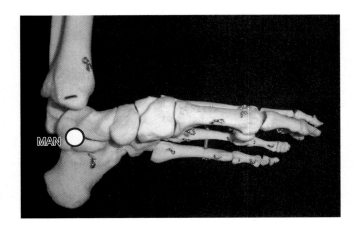

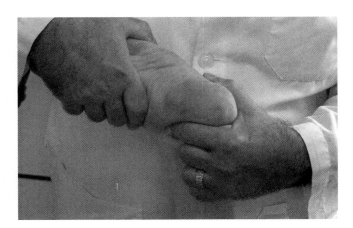

Figure 11.23   Treatment position for the medial ankle counterstrain point.

Figure 11.22   Location of the medial ankle (MAN) counterstrain point.

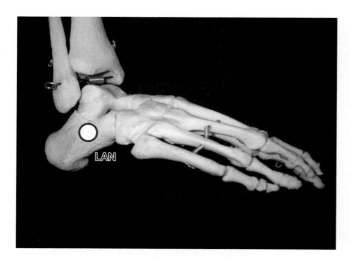

Figure 11.24 Location of the lateral ankle (LAN) counterstrain point.

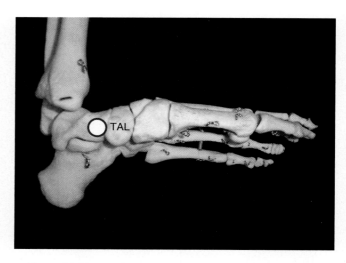

Figure 11.26 Location of the talus (TAL) counterstrain point.

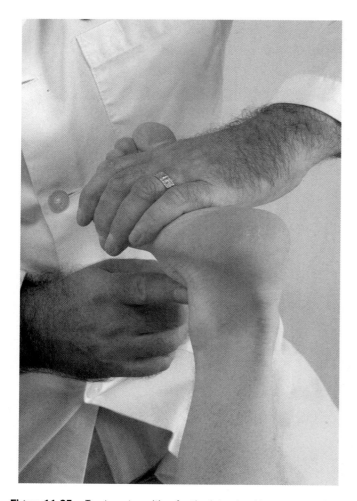

Figure 11.25 Treatment position for the lateral ankle counterstrain point.

CONTROVERSIES

- The use of arthroscopy in patients with known instability who require reconstruction is controversial.
- Some experts question the value of stress radiography in evaluating a sprained ankle. Opponents think that stress radiography does not consistently show a difference between injured and uninjured tissues. They also suggest that joint laxity does not always correlate with symptoms.
- Questions remain about advising patients who are returning to activities. Patients may need to modify certain activities to avoid the risk of recurrent injury. Some activities, such as high-risk sports, may need to be avoided altogether. Deciding what to advise patients in these situations is extremely difficult.

OPPORTUNITIES FOR RESEARCH

- Some areas for future research include the following:
  1. Gathering more precise epidemiologic data about acute and chronic ankle sprain

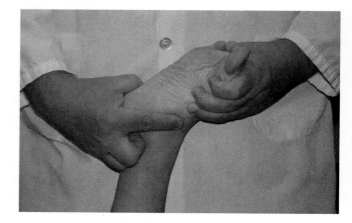

Figure 11.27 Treatment position for the talus counterstrain point.

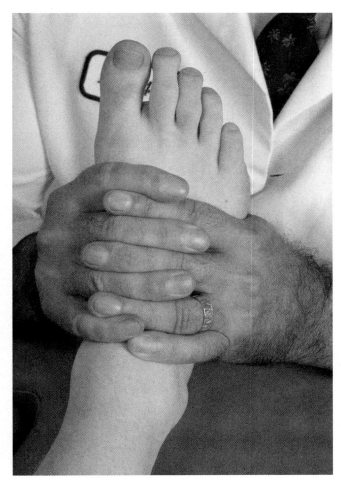

Figure 11.28 Treatment position for myofascial restriction of the ankle region.

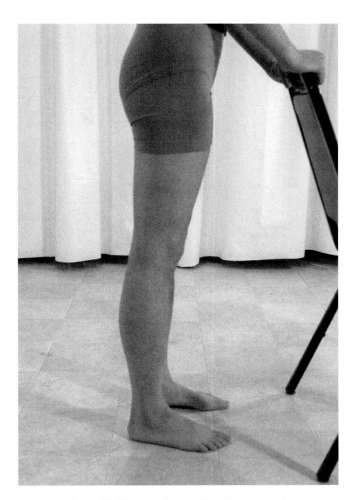

Figure 11.29 Starting position for exercise 1.

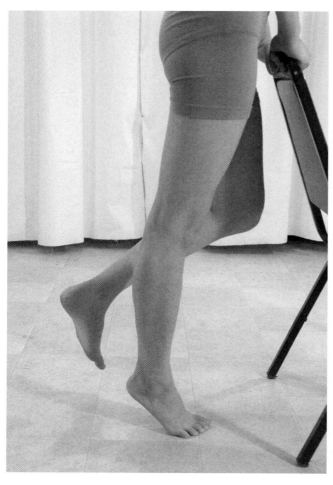

Figure 11.30   Exercise 1: standing on the toes of the injured foot.

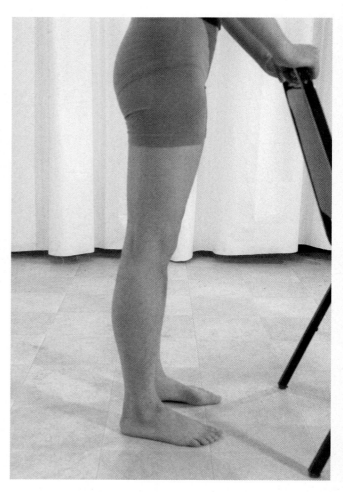

Figure 11.31   Starting position for exercise 2.

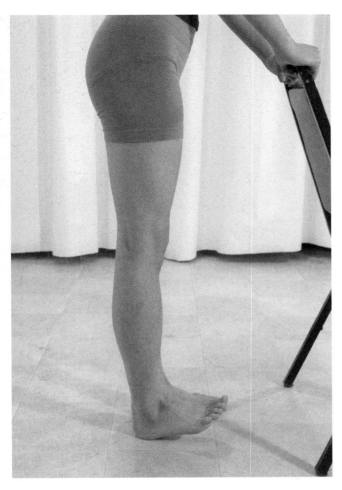

Figure 11.32 Exercise 2: standing on the heels of both feet.

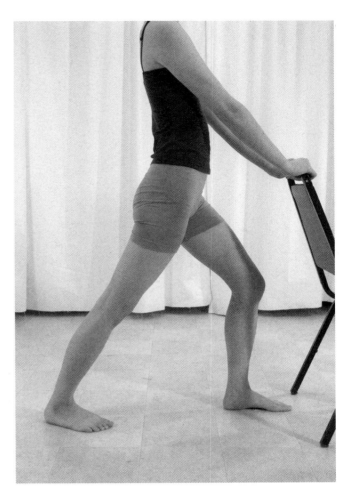

Figure 11.33 Starting position for exercise 3.

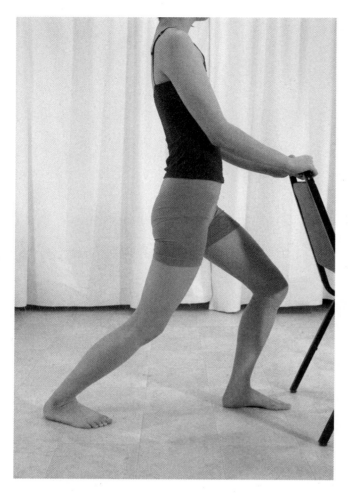

Figure 11.34   Exercise 3: stretching the calf muscles.

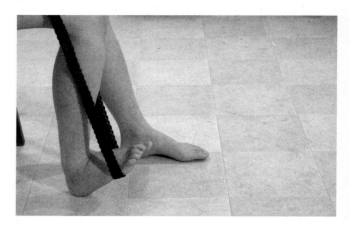

Figure 11.36   Exercise 4: plantar flexing the ankle against resistance.

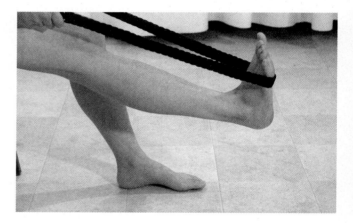

Figure 11.37   Starting position for exercise 5.

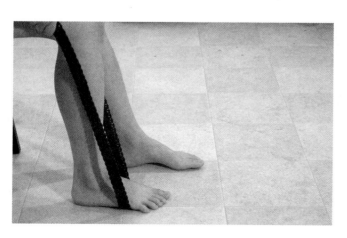

Figure 11.35   Starting position for exercise 4.

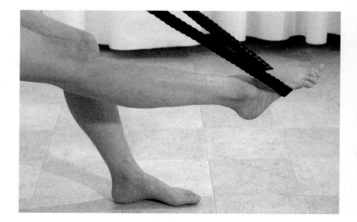

Figure 11.38   Exercise 5: plantar flexing the ankle against resistance.

2. Development of improved treatment methodologies to prevent recurrent ankle sprain

3. Development of methods for identifying patients at high risk for ankle injury, allowing them the opportunity to take measures to prevent ankle injury

4. Development of better ways to evaluate patients after recovery from ankle injury, enabling better advice about returning to high-risk activities

REFERENCES

1. Wexler RK: The injured ankle. Am Fam Physician 57:474-480, 1998.
2. Wolfe MW, Uhl TL, Mattacola CG, et al: Management of ankle sprains. Am Fam Physician 63:93-104, 2001.
3. Barker HB, Beynnon BD, Renstrom PA: Ankle injury risk factors in sports. Sports Med 23:69-74, 1997.
4. Bennett WF: Lateral ankle sprains. Part II. Acute and chronic treatment. Orthop Rev 23:504-510, 1994.
5. Safran MR, Benedetti RS, Bartolozzi AR 3rd, et al: Lateral ankle sprains: A comprehensive review. Part 1. Etiology, pathoanatomy, histopathogenesis, and diagnosis. Med Sci Sports Exerc 31(Suppl):S429-S437, 1999.
6. Foster R: Acute ankle sprains. Available at www.emedicine.com/ Accessed September 9, 2005.
7. Hockenbury RT, Sammarco GJ: Evaluation and treatment of ankle sprains. Physician Sports Med 29:57-64, 2001.
8. Stiell IG, McKnight RD, Greenberg GH, et al: Implementation of the Ottawa ankle rules. JAMA 271:827-832, 1994.
9. Pellow JE, Brantingham JW: The efficacy of adjusting the ankle in the treatment of subacute and chronic grade I and grade II ankle inversion sprains. J Manipulative Physiol Ther 24:17-24, 2001.
10. Blood SD: Treatment of the sprained ankle. J Am Osteopath Assoc 79:680-692, 1980.
11. Eisenhart AW, Gaeta TJ, Yens DP: Osteopathic manipulative treatment in the emergency department for patients with acute ankle injuries. J Am Osteopath Assoc 103:417-421, 2003.
12. Ward RC: Foundations for Osteopathic Medicine, 2nd ed. Philadelphia, Lippincott William & Wilkins, 2003.
13. Institute for Clinical Systems Improvement: Guidelines for the Treatment of Ankle Sprains. Bloomington, MN, Institute for Clinical Systems Improvement, July 2001.
14. Wadsworth CT: Manual Examination and Treatment of the Spine and Extremities. Baltimore, Williams & Wilkins, 1988.
15. Norkin CC, Levangie PK: Joint Structure and Function, 2nd ed. Philadelphia, FA Davis, 1992.
16. Kibler WB: Rehabilitation of the ankle and foot. In Kibler WB, Herring SA, Press JM, et al (eds): Functional Rehabilitation of Sports and Musculoskeletal Injuries. Gaithersburg, MD, Aspen Publishers, 1998, pp 273-279.

SUGGESTED READING

Beynnon BD, Renstrom PA, Alosa DM, et al: Ankle ligament injury risk factors: A prospective study of college athletes. J Orthop Res 19:213-220, 2001.
Birrer RB: Ankle injuries. In Birrer RB (ed): Sports Medicine for the Primary Care Physician, 2nd ed. Washington, DC, Library of Congress, 1994, pp 543-552.
Boyd PM, Bogdan RJ: Sports injuries. In Lorimer DL (ed): Neales' Common Foot Disorders: Diagnosis and Management: A General Clinical Guide, 4th ed. Edinburgh, Churchill Livingstone, 1993, pp 179-180.
Boytim MJ, Fischer DA, Neumann L: Syndesmotic ankle sprains. Am J Sports Med 19:294-298, 1991.
Bulucu C, Thomas KA, Halvorson TL, et al: Biomechanical evaluation of the anterior drawer test: The contribution of the lateral ankle ligaments. Foot Ankle 11:389-393, 1991.
Clanton TO, Schon LG: Athletic injuries to the soft tissues of the foot and ankle. In Mann RA, Coughlin MJ (ed): Surgery of the Foot and Ankle, vol II, 6th ed. St Louis, Mosby, 1993, pp 1121-1140.
Crichton KJ, Fricker PA, Purdam C, et al: Injuries to the pelvis and lower limb. In Bloomfield J, Fricker PA, Fitch KD (eds): Science and Medicine in Sport, 2nd ed. Victoria, Blackwell Science, 1995, pp 463-467.
Davis SG, Trevino PF: Ankle injuries. In Baxter DE (ed): The Foot and Ankle in Sport. St Louis, Mosby, 1995, pp 147-161.
DeLee JC, Drez D: Orthopaedic Sports Medicine: Principles and Practice, vol 2. Philadelphia, WB Saunders, 1994, pp 1718-1724.
Dettori JR, Pearson BD, Basmania CJ, et al: Early ankle mobilization. Part I. The immediate effect on acute, lateral ankle sprains (a randomized clinical trial). Mil Med 159:15-20, 1994.
Hopkinson WJ, St Pierre P, Ryan JB, et al: Syndesmosis sprains of the ankle. Foot Ankle 10:325-330, 1990.
Karlsson J, Lundin O, Lind K, et al: Early mobilization versus immobilization after ankle ligament stabilization. Scand J Med Sci Sports 9:299-303, 1999.
Labovitz JM, Schweitzer ME: Occult osseous injuries after ankle sprains: Incidence, location, pattern, and age. Foot Ankle Int 19:661-667, 1998.
Laing P: The painful foot. In Merriman LM, Tollafield DR (eds): Assessment of the Lower Limb. Edinburgh, Churchill Livingstone, 1995, p 379.
Lazarus ML: Imaging of the foot and ankle in the injured athlete. Med Sci Sports Exerc 31(Suppl):S412-S420, 1999.
LeBlanc KE: Ankle problems masquerading as sprains. Prim Care 31:1055-1067, 2004.
Mattacola CG, Lloyd JW: Effects of a 6-week strength and proprioception training program on measures of dynamic balance: A single-case design. J Athletic Train 32:127-135, 1997.
McCluskey LC, Black KP: Ankle injuries in sports. In Gould JS, et al (eds): Operative Foot Surgery. Philadelphia, WB Saunders, 1994, pp 901-936.
Perlman M, Leveille D, DeLeonibus J, et al: Inversion lateral ankle trauma: Differential diagnosis, review of the literature, and prospective study. J Foot Surg 26:95-135, 1987.
Robbins S, Waked E: Factors associated with ankle injuries. Preventative measures. Sports Med 25:63-72, 1998.
Shapiro MS, Kabo JM, Mitchell PW, et al: Ankle sprain prophylaxis: An analysis of the stabilizing effect of braces and tape. Am J Sports Med 22:78-82, 1994.
Simon RR, Koenigsknecht SJ: Emergency Orthopedics: The Extremities. Norwalk, CT, Appleton & Lange, 1995, pp 295-307.
Singer KM, Jones DC: Ligament injuries of the ankle and foot. In Nicholas JA, Hershmann EB (eds): The Lower Extremity and Spine in Sports Medicine, vol 2. St Louis, Mosby, 1995, pp 475-497.
Stiell IG, Greenberg GH, McKnight RD, et al: A study to develop clinical decision rules for the use of radiography in acute ankle injuries. Ann Emerg Med 21:384-390, 1992.
Thacker SB, Stroup DF, Branche CM, et al: The prevention of ankle sprains in sports. A systematic review of the literature. Am J Sports Med 27:753-760, 1999.
Turbutt I: Radiographic assessment. In Merriman LM, Tollafield DR (eds): Assessment of the Lower Limb. Edinburgh, Churchill Livingstone, 1995, pp 255-256.

CHAPTER 12

Manual Medicine Coding

CLASSIFICATION SYSTEMS

Two coding classification systems are required by third-party payers for reimbursement:
- ICD-9-CM: The International Classification of Diseases, 9th Revision, Clinical Modification
- CPT: Current Procedural Terminology

Within these coding systems, there is terminology of particular relevance to manual medicine. The term *somatic dysfunction* is used to designate impaired or altered function of related components of the somatic (body framework) system; skeletal, arthrodial, and myofascial structures, and related vascular, lymphatic, and neural elements. The term can be further amplified to denote the specific dysfunction (e.g., myositis, neuralgia, limited arthrodial motion) and associated visceral pathology (e.g., colitis, pneumonitis). An example is lumbar and sacral somatic dysfunction with lumbar myositis and right sciatic neuralgia.[1]

The term *osteopathic manipulative treatment* is defined as a form of manual treatment applied by a physician to eliminate or alleviate somatic dysfunction and related disorders. Because this treatment can be accomplished by a variety of techniques, this terminology can be amplified to indicate the specific technique employed (e.g., counterstrain, myofascial release) and the specific body regions treated.

ICD-9-CM

The ICD-9-CM classification system is used to report the diagnosis. The publication itself is broken up into parts:
- Volume 1: The tabular list has numeric codes with up to five digits for some diagnoses. For example, "739, nonallopathic lesions, not elsewhere classified" includes segmental dysfunction and somatic dysfunction. There also are specific fourth digits used to denote the specific body region involved.
  1. Examples include the cervical region (739.1) and the thoracic region (739.2).
  2. Others include the head region (739.0), lumbar region (739.3), sacral region (739.4), pelvic region (739.5), lower extremities (739.6), upper extremities (739.7), rib cage (739.8), and abdomen and other (739.9).
- Volume 2: The index to diseases is arranged alphabetically by presenting symptom or disease.
  1. An example is "Dysfunction, somatic."
  2. Various anatomic regions are listed with appropriate numbers.

The following diagnostic codes are examples of those used by osteopathic physicians to indicate application of osteopathic manipulative treatment.[2]
- 307.81, mental disorders: neurotic disorders, personality disorders, and other nonpsychotic mental disorders; special symptoms or syndromes, not elsewhere classified; tension headache
- 719 codes, arthropathies and related disorders: other and unspecified disorders of joint; pain in joint, mainly: pelvic region and thigh (719.45) and arthralgia (719.48)
- 723 codes, diseases of the musculoskeletal system and connective tissue: dorsopathies; other disorders of cervical region, mainly: cervicalgia (723.1) and cervicocranial syndrome (723.2)
- 724.2, diseases of the musculoskeletal system and connective tissue: dorsopathies; other and unspecified disorders of the back, lumbago
- 728.85, diseases of the musculoskeletal system and connective tissue: rheumatism, excluding the back; disorders of muscle, ligament, and fascia; spasm of muscle
- 729.1, diseases of the musculoskeletal system and connective tissue: rheumatism, excluding the back; other disorders of soft tissues; myalgia and myositis, unspecified
- 739 series, osteopathies, chondropathies, and acquired musculoskeletal deformities: nonallopathic lesions, not elsewhere classified: head region (739.0), cervical region (739.1), thoracic region (739.2), lumbar region (739.3), sacral region (739.4), pelvic region (739.5), lower extremities (739.6), upper extremities (739.7), rib cage (739.8), and abdomen and other (739.9)
- 847 codes, injury and poisoning: sprains and strains of joints and adjacent muscles. sprains and strains of other and unspecified parts of back, mainly: neck (847.0), thoracic region (847.1), lumbar region (847.2), and sacrum (847.3)

Researchers evaluating the cost of care of various practitioners in a randomized clinical trial in Southern California involving care for health maintenance organization patients with low back pain, who were randomized to care from a medical doctor (MD) alone or with the addition of a physical therapist (PT) or a doctor of chiropractic (DC), used the following ICD-9-CM codes to define low back pain[3]:

353.1, 353.4
715.0, 715.5, 715.90
719.4
720.0, 720.2
721.3, 721.4, 721,42, 721.8, 721.90, 721.91
722.1, 722.10, 722.3, 722.51, 722.52, 722.6, 722.7, 722.73, 722.8, 722.83, 722.9, 722.93
724.00, 724.02, 724.2, 724.3, 724.4, 724.5, 724.6, 724.7, 724.79, 724.8, 724.9
729.1
737.0, 737.30, 737.39
739.3, 739.4, 739.5
839.2, 839.20, 839.3, 839.30, 839.41, 839.42
846.0, 846.1, 846.2, 846.3, 846.8, 846.9
847.2, 847.3, 847.4, 847.9

PHYSICIANS' CURRENT PROCEDURAL TERMINOLOGY

The physicians' CPT states that osteopathic manipulative treatment is a form of manual treatment applied by a physician to eliminate or alleviate somatic dysfunction and related disorders. This treatment may be accomplished by a variety of techniques.

Evaluation and management (E/M) services may be reported separately if (using the modifier -25) the patient's condition requires a significant, separately identifiable E/M service, above and beyond the usual preservice and postservice work associated with the procedure. The E/M service may be caused or prompted by the same symptoms or condition for which the OMM service was provided. As such, different diagnoses are not required for reporting OMM and E/M service on the same date.

Body regions referred to are the head region; cervical region; thoracic region; lumbar region; sacral region; pelvic region; lower extremities; upper extremities; rib cage region; and abdomen and viscera region.

- 98925, osteopathic manipulative treatment (OMT), one to two body regions involved
- 98926, three to four body regions involved
- 98927, five to six body regions involved
- 98928, seven to eight body regions involved
- 98929, nine to ten body regions involved

The OMT codes (98925 through 98929) are structured by the number of body regions treated, not the body site or the techniques employed. These codes should be used for inpatient and outpatient treatment. An example is 98925, osteopathic manipulative treatment (OMT), one to two body regions involved.

There also are two-digit modifiers, which may be attached to the five-digit procedure code to indicate that a service or procedure that has been performed has been altered in some way from the code descriptor. For Medicare, the -25 modifier must be attached to the E/M code reported in conjunction with OMT.

APPROPRIATE USE OF OSTEOPATHIC MANIPULATIVE TREATMENT CODES

After the physician evaluates the patient and arrives at a diagnosis, it is allowable to use an E/M code in addition to the appropriate OMT code (98925 through 98929), provided the physician has documented in the patient's record the E/M service provided. The E/M service must be appropriately documented along with the OMT service provided. However, separate diagnoses are not required for the separate services.

Coding Case Study

A 35-year old man complains of pain in the neck and upper back after painting his house. He also complains of exacerbation of previous lumbar disc herniation with radiculitis after a motorcycle accident 3 years earlier. After evaluation of the patient, the diagnosis is as follows:
- Neck muscle strain
- Upper back muscle strain
- Lumbar radiculitis
- Somatic dysfunction of the cervical spine
- Somatic dysfunction of the thoracic spine
- Somatic dysfunction of the lumbar spine

The physician then uses osteopathic manipulative treatment to treat the patient's cervical, thoracic, and lumbar regions.

Diagnosis Coding
- Muscle strain: neck (847.0)
- Muscle strain: thoracic region (847.1)
- Lumbar radiculitis
- Somatic dysfunction, cervical (739.1)
- Somatic dysfunction, lumbar (739.3)
- Somatic dysfunction, thoracic (739.2)

Procedure Coding
- Osteopathic manipulative treatment (OMT); five to seven body regions involved: 98927
- Office or other outpatient visit for the evaluation and management of an established patient, which requires at least two of these three key components:
  1. A detailed history
  2. A detailed examination
  3. Medical decision-making of moderate complexity (99214-25)

Explanation of Code Selection
For the diagnosis coding of somatic dysfunction, it is necessary to code to the fourth digit (e.g., 739.1), and the practitioner should code to the most specific ICD-9 code. Not coding to the fourth digit could cause the payer to reject this claim. Code 98927 was selected for the OMT provided because five regions were treated. Because the patient had been seen by the physician within the past 3 years, this was an established patient, which should be reflected in selecting the E/M code. A detailed history and examination were performed, and medical decision-making of moderate complexity was provided; therefore, CPT code

99214 was selected. The -25 modifier was added because it indicates to the payer that a significant, separate identifiable E/M service was provided in addition to the OMT.

REVIEWING THE EXPLANATION OF BENEFITS

The explanation of benefits (EOB) provided by the payer should be reviewed. The EOB indicates what you billed and how it was recorded by the claims processor. Sometimes, errors are made by the claims processor in entering data, and an error could be a reason for rejection of the claim.

Make sure you have attached the -25 modifier to the E/M code reported, because not doing this will flag the E/M service for nonpayment. Be sure that the patient has met all insurance deductibles and co-payments. Ensure that OMT is covered under the patient's policy. A patient's insurance information should be updated each time the physician sees that patient to ensure that the patient has not changed payers or type of coverage.

Claims Appeal

When you are sure that all of the previous conditions have been satisfied and you feel that an error has been made in processing, you need to send an appeal letter to the payer. The letter should include the claim number (which is listed on the EOB), the patient's identification number, the provider (physician) identification number, and an explanation from the physician about why this claim is being appealed. Complete documentation should be attached, including a copy of the original claim filed and the EOB. If possible, you should address your appeal to a specific individual at the payer, such as the carrier medical director or claims manager. The claims processor who processed the original claim has little or no authority to adjust the claim.

The American Academy of Osteopathy (AAO) Louisa Burns Osteopathic Research Committee (LBORC) has developed and validated an osteopathic medical record and follow-up SOAP note form (i.e., *s*ubjective data, *o*bjective data, *a*ssessment, and *p*lan), which includes musculoskeletal examination findings, ratings of pain using a visual analog scale, rating of severity of somatic findings, and response to manipulative and adjunctive interventions. The LBORC has developed an electronic medical record and a national web-based database for gathering information about the incidence and characteristics of patients with somatic dysfunction and their response to osteopathic treatment, including manipulation. Both can be obtained by contacting the AAO (www.academyofosteopathy.org).

REFERENCES

1. American Osteopathic Association: Coding guide. Available at http://www.osteopathic.org or http://do-online.org or contact the American Osteopathic Association in Chicago, IL.
2. Sleszynski SL, Glonek T: Outpatient osteopathic SOAP note form: Preliminary results in osteopathic outcomes-based research. J Am Osteopath Assoc 105:181-205, 2005.
3. Kominski GF, Heslin KC, Morgenstern H, et al: Economic evaluation of four treatments for low back pain. Results from a randomized controlled trial. Med Care 43:428-435, 2005.

Index

Note: Page numbers in **boldface** refer to figures and tables

A

abdominal muscles, exercises to strengthen
        weak, 124–25
    Core Stability Basic Exercise, 125
    Curls, 125, **125**
    Curls for Weaker Abdominal Muscles,
        125, **125**
    Lateral Curls, 125, **125**
acupuncture, 120
adjunct treatments
    for ankle sprain, 302
    for carpal tunnel syndrome, 286
    for cervicogenic headache, 201–202
    for low back pain, 120
    for shoulder pain and dysfunction,
        266–67
    for temporomandibular joint
        dysfunction (TMJ), 217
    for upper back and neck pain, **174**,
        174–75
allodynia, 8
American Academy of Family Physicians,
    1, 84, 140–41
American Academy of Neurology,
    1, 280
American Academy of Osteopathy (AAO),
    1, 10, 84
    position paper on osteopathic
        manipulative treatment of the
        cervical spine, 140, 179–80,
        185–87
American Academy of Physical Medicine
    and Rehabilitation, 1, 280
American Association of Electrodiagnostic
    Medicine, 280
American Back Society, 84
American College of Rehabilitative
    Medicine, 84
American Osteopathic Association (AOA),
    10, 84
    position paper on osteopathic
        manipulative treatment of the
        cervical spine, 140, 179–80,
        185–87
American Society of Orthopedic
    Medicine, 1
anatomic position, 11
anatomic range of motion, 29
ankle sprain, 291–311
    adjunct treatments, 302
    age and, 291

ankle sprain—Cont'd
    controversies, 306
    definition, 291
    differential diagnosis, 292, **292**
    education, 302–303
    epidemiology, 291
    exercise, 303–304, **307–10**
    functional anatomy, 294–95,
        294–95
    gender and, 291
    history, 292
    laboratory and radiographic findings,
        292, **293**
    manual diagnostic procedures, 295–97,
        296–300
    manual medicine
        benefits, 293
        best evidence, 292–93
        practice recommendations,
            293, **293**
        risks, 293
    manual treatment procedures
        counterstrain techniques, 299–301,
            303–306
        muscle energy techniques, 297–99,
            300–303
        myofascial release technique,
            301–302, **307**
    natural clinical course of, 291
    pathophysiology, 291–92, **292**
    physical findings, 292
    prevalence of, 291
    references, 311
    research opportunities, 306, 311
    risk factors, 291
    societal effects, 291
    suggested reading, 311
antagonistic inhibition, see reciprocal
    inhibition
anterior superior iliac spines (ASIS)
    examination of, 92–94, **93**
antidromic transmission, 5
articulatory techniques, 63–64
    for carpal tunnel syndrome, 281–82,
        282–83
    for low back pain, 102–105, **102–105**
    shoulder treatment, 237–40, **238–39**
    thoracic (costal) cage, 255–56, **256**,
        258–59
    for upper back and neck pain, 157
atantoaxial (AA) joint, 18, **19**

B

back pain, mechanical
    low back pain, see low back pain,
        mechanical
    upper back pain, see upper back pain,
        mechanical neck and
Bergman, G. J. D., 233
bind and ease concept, 31, 32, 67
Both-Legs Hip Roll, 122, **123**
British Medical Journal, 141, 233
bucket-handle motion, 20, **21**

C

calcitonin gene-related peptide
    (CGRP), 5
caliper motion, 21, **21**
Canadian Institutes of Health Research
    (CIHR), 31
Cardone, Dennis, 1
carpal tunnel syndrome, 273–90
    adjunct treatments, 286
    age and, 273
    controversies, 288–89
    definition, 273, **274**
    diagnostic procedures, 281
    differential diagnosis, 277, **278**
    education, 286
    epidemiology, 273–75
    exercises, 286–88, **287–89**
    functional anatomy, 275, **275**
    gender and, 273
    history, 277–78
    laboratory and radiographic findings, 279
    manual medicine
        benefits, 280
        best evidence, 279
        practice recommendations, 280, **280**
        risks, 279–80
    natural clinical course of, 274
    pathophysiology, 275–77
        acute versus chronic carpal tunnel
            syndrome, 277
        biochemistry, 276
        causes, 275
        histopathology, 276
        increased carpal tunnel interstitial
            fluid pressure, 276
        median nerve response to mechanical
            stimulation or stress, 276–77
        neck muscle imbalance, 277
        nerve motion restriction, 277

carpal tunnel syndrome–Cont'd
   pathogenesis of carpal tunnel
      syndrome progression, 277
   physical findings, 278–79
      motor examination, 278
      palpatory examination, 279
      sensory examination, 278
      special tests, 278–79
   prevalence of, 273–74
   references, 289–90
   research opportunities, 289
   risk factors, 275
   societal effects of, 274–75
   treatment procedures, 281–86
      articulatory, 281–82, **282–83**
      counterstrain, 285–86, **285–87**
      myofascial release, 282–85, **284–85**
central nervous system, 192
cervical spine
   active and passive motion assessments,
      47, **48**
   headache, cervicogenic, *see* cervicogenic
      headache
   mechanics, 18–20
      atantoaxial (AA) joint, 18, **19**
      occipitoatlantal (OA) joint, 18, **19**
      typical cervical joints, 18, **20**
   see also upper back pain, mechanical
      neck and
cervicogenic headache, 189–205
   adjunct treatments, 201–202
   age and, 189
   associated symptoms, 195
   characteristics of, 194
   controversies, 202
   definition, 189, **190**
   diagnostic procedures, 197
   differential diagnosis, 193–94, **194–96**
      algorithm for acute or chronic
         headache evaluation, **196**
      characteristics of similar headache
         types, **194**
      red flag, **195**
   education, 202
   epidemiology, 189–90
   exercises, 202
   functional anatomy, 190–93
      muscles, 190–92, **191**
      the myodural bridge, **191**, 192
      nerves, 192–93, **193**
      see also upper back pain, mechanical
         neck and
   gender and, 189
   history, 194–95
   intensity of, 194
   laboratory and radiographic
      findings, 196
   location of, 194
   manual medicine, 196–97
      benefits, 197
      best evidence, 196
      practice recommendations, 197
      risks, 196–97
   natural clinical course of, 189
   pathophysiology, 193

cervicogenic headache–Cont'd
   physical findings, 195–96
   precipitating factors, 194
   prevalence of, 189
   radiation of, 194
   references, 204–205
   research opportunities, 202
   risk factors, 190
   societal effects of, 189–90
   treatment procedures, 197–201
      functional techniques, 200–201,
         201–204
      muscle energy techniques, 199–200,
         199–201
      myofascial release, 197–99,
         198–99
Cervicogenic Headache International
      Study Group, diagnostic criteria
      for cervicogenic headache of,
      189, **190**
Childs, J. D., 82
chiropractors, 1
   low back pain treatment by, 80
Clinical Evidence, 141
Cochrane Review, 81, 141
coding classification systems, 313–15
   appropriate use of osteopathic
      manipulative treatment codes,
      314–15
   claims appeal, 315
   CPT: Current Procedural
      Terminology, 314
   ICD-9-CM, 313–14
   overview, 313
   references, 315
   reviewing the explanation of benefits
      (EOB), 315
compliance (of joint motion), 29
complications, 60
   spinal manipulation procedures, 83, 180,
      185-86, 208-09
   shoulder manipulation procedures, 233
consent, patient, 60
contraindications, **60**, 60-61
   manual neck pain, for, 140, **140**
Core Stability Basic Exercise, 125
costal cage, *see* thoracic (costal) cage
counternutation, 18, **20**
counterstrain techniques, 68–70
   for ankle sprain, 299–301,
      303–306
   for carpal tunnel syndrome, 285–86,
      285–87
   determining locations of tender
      points, **69**
   keys to treat a tender point with, **69**
   for low back pain, 116–20, **116–21**
   quantifying the level of tenderness, **69**
   for shoulder pain and dysfunction
      rib counterstrain, 263–66, **264–66**
      shoulder treatment, *see* shoulder
         treatment procedures, counterstrain
   for temporomandibular joint
      dysfunction (TMJ), 214–16,
      214–17

counterstrain techniques–Cont'd
   for upper back and neck pain
      cervical spine treatment, 169–74,
         169–74
      upper thoracic treatment, 159–60,
         161–63
CPT: Current Procedural Terminology, 314
cranial (parasympathetic) nerves,
      192, **193**
Curls, 125, **125**
Curls for Weaker Abdominal Muscles,
      125, **125**

D

designing a management plan for somatic
      dysfunction, 61–70
   articulatory techniques, 63–64
   counterstrain techniques, 68–70
   functional technique, 67–68
   maintenance and prevention, 62
   the manipulative prescription
      dosage guidelines, 62
      duration of treatment, 62
      frequency of treatment, 62
      goals of manual treatment, 61–62
   methods of treatment, 62–70
   muscle energy techniques, 65–67
   myofascial release (MFR), 64–65
   soft tissue techniques, 62–63
diagnostic procedures, overview of manual,
      35–58
   documentation, 57–58
      ICD-9 diagnostic codes for somatic
         dysfunction by body region,
         58, **58**
   references, 58
   regional examination procedures,
      54–55, 55
   screening examination, *see* screening or
      general impression examination
   segmental examination, 55–56
   summary, 56, **57**
   validity and reliability of examination
      procedures, 56–57
Disorders of the Neck and Upper Back (Work
      Loss Data Institute), 139
differential diagnosis
   ankle sprain, 292, **292**
   carpal tunnel syndrome, 277, **278**
   cervicogenic headache, 193–94, **194–96**
   low back pain, mechanical, 78, **79-80**
   shoulder pain and dysfunction, **229-30**,
      230
   temporomandibular joint dysfunction,
      208
   upper back pain, mechanical neck and,
      137-38, **138**
Dombroski, R. Todd, 1
dominant eye, determining the, 35–36
Downward-Arched Back, 123, **123**
Dutch College of General
      Practitioners, 234

E

ease and bind concept, 31, **32**, 67

eccentric or isolytic muscle energy technique, 65, 66
education
    for ankle sprain, 302–303
    for carpal tunnel syndrome, 286
    for cervicogenic headache, 202
    for low back pain, 120–21
    for shoulder pain and dysfunction, 267
    for temporomandibular joint dysfunction (TMJ), 217–18
    for upper back and neck pain, 175
evidence-based medicine (EBM), 1–2
exercises for ankle sprain, 303–304, **307–10**
exercises for carpal tunnel syndrome, 286–88, **287–89**
exercises for cervicogenic headache, 202
exercises for low back pain, 121–26
    to improve mobility of the lumbar spine, 121–23
        Both-Legs Hip Roll, 122, **123**
        Downward-Arched Back, 123, **123**
        One-Leg Hip Roll, 122, **122**
        Pelvic Tilt with an Arched Back, 121, **122**
        Pelvic Tilt with a Flat Back, 121, **122**
        Scared Cat, 122–23, **123**
        Sphinx Pushup, 122, **123**
    overview, 121
    to strengthen low back muscles, 123–24
        Opposite Leg and Arm Raise, 124, **124**
        Single-Arm High Raise, 124, **124**
        Single-Arm Raise, 124, **124**
        Single-Leg Raise, 124, **124**
    to strengthen weak abdominal muscles, 124–25
        Core Stability Basic Exercise, 125
        Curls, 125, **125**
        Curls for Weaker Abdominal Muscles, 125, **125**
        Lateral Curls, 125, **125**
    to stretch the leg muscles, 125–26
        Hamstring Stretches, 125–26, **126**
        Piriformis Stretch, 126, **126**
exercises for shoulder pain and dysfunction, 267, **268–71**
exercises for temporomandibular joint dysfunction (TMJ), 218–19
    for an inability to fully open the jaw, 218
    for increasing side-to-side movement of the jaw, **218**, 218–19
    for increasing the forward and backward movement of the jaw, 219, **219**
exercises for upper back and neck pain, 175–79
    lateral neck and anterior chest muscle stretches
        Posterior Occipital Muscle Stretch, 179, **181**
        Scalene and Anterior Neck Muscle Stretches, 179, **180**
        Suboccipital Neck Muscle Stretch, 179, **181**

exercises for upper back and neck pain–Cont'd
    neck exercises to improve muscle tone, 176–79
        Isometric Contraction for Anterior Neck Muscles, 176–78, **178**
        Isometric Contraction of Lateral Neck Muscles, 178–79, **179**
        Isometric Contraction of Posterior Neck Muscles, 178, **179**
    neck exercises to improve range of motion
        Neck Extension Stretch, 175, **176**
        Neck Flexion Stretch, 175, **175**
        Neck Rotation Stretch, 176, **178**
        Neck Sidebending (Lateral Flexion) Stretch, 175–76, **177**
        starting or rest position for, 175, **175**
extension of a vertebral unit, **12**, 12

F
facilitation, **6**
FEBERE test, 52, **53–54**
flexed versus extended vertebral units, **13**, 13
flexion of a vertebral unit, **12**, 12
Friedman, Harry D., 1
Fryette, Harrison H., 14
functional technique, 67–68
    for cervicogenic headache, 200–201, **201–204**
    for shoulder pain and dysfunction, 247–49, **248–49**
    costal cage functional techniques, 263, **263**

G
gait analysis, 36–37, **37–38**
general impression examination, *see* screening or general impression examination
glycosaminoglycans (GAGs), 7–8, 63, 64
Golgi tendon apparatus, 3

H
hamstring muscle tension test, 51, **52**
Hamstring Stretches, 125–26, **126**
hamstring tension test, 97, **97**
Hay, E.M., 233
headache, cervicogenic, *see* cervicogenic headache
high-velocity, low-amplitude (HVLA) manual technique, 59, 60
    for temporomandibular joint dysfunction (TMJ), 208
    for upper cervical somatic dysfunction, controversies concerning, 179–81
hip drop test, **43**, 43–44
hip shift test, **42**, 42–43
Hruby, Ray, 1
hyperalgesia, 8
hypersensitivity, 8
hypertonic psoas muscle, 110
hypotonicity of antagonistic muscle, 6, **7**

I
ICD-9-CM classification system, 313–14
ilium, 74, **76**
ilosacral motion, 21
indications,
    lumbosacral somatic dysfunction, 113
inferior innominate shear, 22, **23**
inferior lateral angles of the sacrum, examination of, 94, **95**
inflare somatic dysfunction, 23, **24**
innominate bones, 74, **76**
    movement of the, 21–23, **22–24**
Institute for Clinical Systems Improvement, 81, 293, **293**
International Federation of Manual Medicine, 1, 84
International Headache Society, diagnostic criteria for cervicogenic headache of, 189, **190**
ischium, 74, **76**
isometric contraction
    for Anterior Neck Muscles, 176–78, **178**
    of Lateral Neck Muscles, 178–79, **179**
    of Posterior Neck Muscles, 178, **179**
isometric muscle energy technique, 65, 66
isotonic muscle energy technique, 65, 66

L
L5, 84, **85**, 94
Lateral Curls, 125, **125**
leg-length symmetry assessment, 53–55
leg muscles, exercises to stretch the, 125–26
    Hamstring Stretches, 125–26, **126**
    Piriformis Stretch, 126, **126**
lordotic curve of the cervical spine, 18
low back pain, mechanical, 71–128
    adjunct treatments, 120
    age and, 71
    controversies, 126–27
    definition, 71
    differential diagnosis, 78, **79–80**
    education, 120–21
    epidemiology, 71–72
    exercises, *see* exercises for low back pain
    functional anatomy, 72–77
        lumbar region, 72–74, **72–76**
        pelvic region, 74–77, **76–77**
    gender and, 71
    history, 78–80
    laboratory and radiographic findings, 80, **80**
    manual diagnostic procedures, 84–101
        lumbar somatic dysfunction diagnosis, *see* lumbar somatic dysfunction diagnosis
        lumbar spine anatomic landmarks, 84–85, **85**
        overview, 84
        pelvic anatomic landmarks, 92–94
        pelvic somatic dysfunction diagnosis, *see* pelvic somatic dysfunction diagnosis
    manual medicine, 80–84
        benefits, 83

low back pain, mechanical—Cont'd
  best evidence, 80–83
  practice recommendations, 83–84
  risks, 83
  manual treatment procedures, 101–20
    articulatory procedures: lumbar spine,
      102–105, **102–105**
    functional (indirect) technique for
      lumbosacral somatic dysfunction,
      113–15, 113–16
    lumbar and pelvic strain and
      counterstrain, 116–20,
      116–21
    muscle energy procedures: lumbar
      spine, 105–10, **106–109**
    muscle energy procedures: pelvis,
      110–12, 110–13
    soft tissue and myofascial release
      procedures: lumbar spine,
      101–102, **102**
  natural clinical course, 71
  pathophysiology, 77–78, **78–79**
  physical findings, 80
  prevalence of, 71
  references, 127–28
  research opportunities, 127
  risk factors, 71–72
  societal effects, 71
  suggested reading, 128
lower extremity mobility test (squat test),
  44, **45**
lumbar region, 72–74, **72–76**
  exercises to improve mobility of the
    lumbar spine, see exercises for low
    back pain, to improve mobility of
    the lumbar spine
lumbar somatic dysfunction diagnosis,
  86–92
  patient position, 86
  segmental motion examination, 86–92,
    87–88
    active, 87, **89**
    interpretation of findings, 89–92,
      91–92
    passive, 88, **90**
    prone, 88, **91**
  temperature variation, assessment of,
    86, **86**
  tissue texture change, assessment of,
    86, **86**

M
manual medicine coding, see coding
  classification systems
manual treatment by primary care
  physicians, overview of, 1–2
massage therapists, low back pain
  treatment by, 80
mechanical back pain
  low back pain, see low back pain,
    mechanical
  upper back pain, see upper back pain,
    mechanical neck and
medical training in osteopathic manual
  approaches, 1–2

Michigan State University, 1, 84
muscle energy techniques, 65–67
  for ankle sprain, 297–99, **300–303**
  for cervicogenic headache, 199–200,
    199–201
  for low back pain
    lumbar spine, 105–10, **106–109**
    pelvis, **110–12**, 110–13
  shoulder treatment procedures
    adduction and abduction, 246–47,
      246–47
    flexion, 245–46, **245–46**
    rotation, 243–45, **244**
  for temporomandibular joint
    dysfunction (TMJ), 213–14,
    213–14
  thoracic (costal) cage treatment, see
    thoracic (costal) cage treatment
    procedures, muscle energy
    techniques
  for upper back pain, 157–58, **158**
myodural bridge, **191**, 192
myofascial release (MFR), 64–65
  for ankle sprain, 301–302, **307**
  for carpal tunnel syndrome, 282–85,
    284–85
  for cervicogenic headache, 197–99,
    198–99
  for mechanical low back pain, 101–102,
    102
  shoulder treatment procedures
    with patient prone, **242–43**, 243
    scapular release, 240–41, **240–41**
    subscapularis release, **241**, 241–42
  for temporomandibular joint
    dysfunction (TMJ), 217, **218**
  thoracic (costal) cage treatment
    procedures, 254–55, **255–56**
  for upper back and neck pain
    cervical spine treatment, 164–67,
    164–67
    upper thoracic treatment procedures,
    157, **157**
myofascial tissues, defined, 64
myotatic reflex, 3–4, **5**

N
National Guidelines Clearinghouse, 139,
  141, 181
National Institutes of Health (NIH),
  U.S., 31
  spinal manipulative treatment and, 80
Neck Flexion Stretch, 175, **175**
neck pain, mechanical, see upper back pain,
  mechanical neck and
Neck Rotation Stretch, 176, **178**
Neck Sidebending (Lateral Flexion) Stretch,
  175–76, **177**
Nelson, C. R., 14
neurogenic inflammation, **6**
neuroimmune pathophysiology, 5–6,
  6, 7
neuropathic pain, 8, **9**
New England Journal of Medicine, 82
nutation, 18, **20**

O
One-Leg Hip Roll, 122, **122**
Opposite Leg and Arm Raise, 124, **124**
oriental medical doctors
  low back pain treatment, 80
osteopaths, 1
  low back pain treatment, 80
osteopathy in the cranial field (OCF)
  manual technique, 59
outflare innominate dysfunction, 23, **24**

P
patient walking: gait analysis, 36–37, **37–38**
pelvic and lower extremity symmetry tests,
  47–48, **49–50**
pelvic region, 74–77, **76–77**
pelvic somatic dysfunction diagnosis,
  95–101
  determination of specific somatic
    dysfunction diagnosis
    iliosacral somatic dysfunctions,
      100, **100**
    sacroiliac somatic dysfunctions,
      100–101, **101**
  hamstring tension test, 97, **97**
  interpretation of tests and
    examination of appropriate
    landmarks, 99
  leg length assessment, 97–99, **98**
  motion tests
    backward-bending test, 99, **99**
    lumber spring test, 99–100, **100**
  seated flexion test, 97, **97**
  standing flexion test, 95–96, **96**
  Trendelburg test or sacroiliac joint
    motion test, 96, **96**
Pelvic Tilt with an Arched Back,
  121, **122**
Pelvic Tilt with a Flat Back, 121, **122**
peripheral nerves, 192–93
physical therapists, 1
  low back pain treatment, 80
physiological range of motion, 29
Piriformis Stretch, 126, **126**
Posterior Occipital Muscle Stretch,
  179, **181**
posterior superior iliac spines (PSISs),
  84, **85**
  examination of, 94, **94**
postural assessment, patient standing,
  37–40, **39–40**
primary afferent nociceptors, 5
primary care physicians, overview of
  manual treatment by, 1–2
psoas tension test, 92, **92**
pubic symphysis, 23, **24**, 74, **76**
  examination of, 92–93, **93**
pump-handle motion, 20, **21**

R
RAND Corporation, 180–81, 208
randomized clinical trials, 2,
  carpel tunnel syndrome, 286, 289, 313
  cervicogenic headache, 203
  low back pain, mechanical, 81–83, 120

randomized clinical trials–Cont'd
  neck and upper back pain, mechanical, 180
  shoulder pain, 233, 266-67, 270
reciprocal inhibition, 4–5, 65, 66–67
  for temporomandibular joint dysfunction (TMJ), 216–17
restricted motion of a joint, 29
restrictive motion barrier, 29, **30**
rib cage motion screening, 48–50, **51**
rotation, vertebral, 12, **13**

S

sacral sulcus, examination of, 94, **95**
sacroiliac joint motion test or Trendelburg test, 96, **96**
sacrum, 23–29, 74–76, **76–77**
  sacral axes of motion, 23–24, **25–26**
    inferior transverse axis, 24, **26**
    left oblique axis, 24, **26**
    middle transverse axis, 23, **25**
    right oblique axis, 24, **26**
    superior sacral axis, 23, **25**
  sacral motions, 24–29, **27–29**
    backward sacral torsions, 28, **29**
    forward sacral torsions, 28, **29**
  variations in sacral anatomy, 76
Scalene and Anterior Neck Muscle Stretches, 179, **180**
Scared Cat, 122–23, **123**
scoliosis screening test, 40, **41**, 84, **84**
screening or general impression examination, 36–55
  FEBERE test, 52, **53–54**
  outline of, 36
  patient prone
    leg-length symmetry assessment, 53–55
    mobility assessment of Ribs 11 and 12, 53, **54**
  patient seated, 44–47
    active and passive spine mobility tests, 45–47, **46–47**
    cervical spine active and passive motion assessments, 47, **48**
    seated flexion test, 44–45, **45**
  patient standing, 37–44
    hip drop test, **43**, 43–44
    hip shift test, **42**, 42–43
    lower extremity mobility test (squat test), 44, **45**
    postural assessment, 37–40, **39–40**
    scoliosis screening test, 40, **41**
    standing flexion test, 40–42, **42**
    standing spine sidebending test, 43
    upper extremity mobility test, 44, **44**
  patient supine, 47–50, 47–53
    hamstring muscle tension test, 51, **52**
    pelvic and lower extremity symmetry tests, 47–48, **49–50**
    rib cage motion screening, 48–50, **51**
    upper extremity mobility test, 52–53

screening or general impression examination–Cont'd
  patient walking: gait analysis, 36–37, **37–38**
  seated flexion test, 44–45, **45**, 97, **97**
seated patient, screening or general impression examination with, *see* screening or general impression examination, patient seated
Seffinger, Michael, 1
shoulder pain and dysfunction, 221–72
  adjunct treatments, 266–67
  age and, 221
  controversies, 267
  defined, 221
  diagnostic procedures, 234–37
    active motion, 234–35
    neurologic evaluation, 234
    observation, 234
    palpation, 236, **237**
    passive motion, 235
    vascular evaluation, 234
  differential diagnosis, **229–30**, 230
  education, 267
  epidemiology, 221–22
  exercises, 267, **268–71**
  functional anatomy, 222–30
    costal articulations, 226–27, **227**
    costal muscles, 227–28, **227–28**
    scapulohumeral rhythm, 226
    shoulder bursae, 226
    shoulder joint and articulations, 222–23
    shoulder motions, 224–26, **226**
    shoulder muscles, 223–24, **223–25**
    thoracic cage motions, 228, **229**
  gender and, 221
  history, 230–31
  laboratory and radiographic findings, 232–33
  manual medicine
    benefits, 233
    best evidence, 233
    practice recommendations, 233–34, **234**
    risks, 233
  natural clinical course of, 221–22
  pathophysiology, 228–30
  physical findings and special tests, 231–32, **231–32**
  prevalence of, 221
  references, 271–72
  research opportunities, 267–70
  risk factors, 222
  societal effects of, 222
  suggested reading, 272
  treatment procedures
    shoulder treatment procedures, *see* shoulder treatment procedures
    thoracic (costal) cage, *see* thoracic (costal) cage treatment procedures
shoulder treatment procedures, 237–53
  articulatory technique, 237–40, **238–39**
  counterstrain
    lateral coracoid, 252–53, **253**

shoulder treatment procedures–Cont'd
    long head of the biceps, 251, **251–52**
    short head of the biceps, 252, **252**
    subscapularis, 251, **251**
    supraspinatus, 249, **250**
    teres minor, 249–51, **250**
  functional technique, 247–49, **248–49**
  muscle energy: isometric and isotonic techniques
    adduction and abduction, 246–47, **246–47**
    flexion, 245–46, **245–46**
    rotation, 243–45, **244**
  myofascial release
    with patient prone, **242–43**, 243
    scapular release, 240–41, **240–41**
    subscapularis release, **241**, 241–42
sidebending (lateral flexion), vertebral, 12, **13**
side effects, overview f, 61
Single-Arm High Raise, 124, **124**
Single-Arm Raise, 124, **124**
Single-Leg Raise, 124, **124**
soft tissue techniques, 62–63
somatic afferent spinal chord pathways, 3, **4**
somatic dysfunction mechanisms, 3–33
  associated pathophysiology, 8–10, **10**
  biomechanics, 11–31
  central-peripheral nervous system sensitization, 6, **7**
  cervical spine mechanics, 18–20
    atantoaxial (AA) joint, 18, **19**
    occipitoatlantal (OA) joint, 18, **19**
    typical cervical joints, 18, **20**
  characteristics of somatic-neural reflexes, 3–5
    myotatic reflex, 3–4, **5**
    reciprocal inhibition, 4–5
    somatic motor and sensory systems, 3, **4**
  clinical characteristics of somatic dysfunction, 10–11
  controversies, 31
  costal cage mechanics, 20–21, **21**
  definition of somatic dysfunction, 3
  diagnosis criteria, **4**
  ease and bind concept, 31, **32**
  local and distant effects of, 8
  motion barrier concept, 29–31, **30**
    anatomic barrier, **30**, 31
    physiologic barrier, 30, **30**
    restrictive barrier, **30**, 31
  myofascial adaptations, 7–8
  neuroimmune pathophysiology, 5–6, **6**, **7**
  neuropathic pain, 8, **9**
  nomenclature of spinal motion, 11–14
    facet orientations, 13–14, **13–14**
    principle motions, 12
    standard terminology, 11–12
    vertebral position, motion, and motion restriction, 12–13
  pathophysiology, 3–11

somatic dysfunction mechanisms—Cont'd
  pelvic mechanics
    innominates, 21–23, **22**–24
    pubic symphysis, 21–29, 23, **24**
    sacrum, *see* sacrum
  principles of spinal motion, 14–16,
    15–16
  references, 33
  research opportunities, 31–33
  reversal of the pathophysiology, 10
  somatic dysfunction, 16–18
    type I, 16–17, **17**, 19
    type II, 16, 17–18, **18**, **19**
somatosamtic reflex, 3, **4**
Sphinx Pushup, 122, **123**
spine mobility tests, active and passive,
  45–47, **46–47**
standards for manual evaluation and
  treatment, 1
standing flexion test, 40–42, **42**,
  95–96, **96**
standing patient, screening examination
  with, *see* screening or general
  impression examination, patient
  standing
Steele, Carl, 1
Strickland, 3, 82
Suboccipital Neck Muscle Stretch, 179, **181**
superior innominate shear, 22, **23**
supine patient, screening examination of,
  see screening or general impression
  examination, patient supine
surgical consultation, 120
sympathetic nerves, 192

T

TART (tissue texture changes, asymmetry
  of anatomic landmarks, range of
  motion abnormalities, and
  tenderness) changes, 10
temporomandibular joint dysfunction
  (TMJ), 207–20
  adjunct treatments, 217
  age and, 207
  controversies, 219
  definition, 207
  differential diagnosis, 208
  education, 217–18
  epidemiology, 207
  exercises, 218–19
    for an inability to fully open the
    jaw, 218
    for increasing side-to-side movement
    of the jaw, **218**, 218–19
    for increasing the forward and
    backward movement of the jaw,
    219, **219**
  functional anatomy, 209–10, **209–11**
  gender and, 207
  history, 208
  laboratory and radiographic
    findings, 208
  manual diagnostic procedures, 210–13,
    211–13
  manual medicine

temporomandibular joint dysfunction
  (TMJ)—Cont'd
  benefits, 209
  best evidence, 208
  practice recommendations, 209
  risk, 208–209
  manual medicine treatment procedures
    counterstrain techniques, 214–16,
    214–17
    muscle energy techniques, 213–14,
    213–14
    myofascial release technique, 217, **218**
    pterygoid muscle inhibition release,
    216–17
  natural clinical course of, 207
  pathophysiology of, 207–208
  physical findings, 208
  prevalence of, 207
  references, 220
  research opportunities, 219
  risk factors, 207, **208**
  societal effects of, 207
  suggested reading, 220
thoracic (costal) cage
  mechanics, 20–21, **21**
  shoulder pain and dysfunction
    functional anatomy, *see* shoulder pain
    and dysfunction, functional
    anatomy
    treatment procedures, *see* thoracic
    (costal) cage treatment procedures
thoracic (costal) cage treatment procedures,
  253–66
  articulatory techniques, 255–57, **256**,
    258–59
  diaphragm myofascial release technique,
    254–55, **255–56**
  functional techniques, 263, **263**
  muscle energy techniques, 257–63
    for rib exhalation somatic
    dysfunction: Rib 1, 260–61, **261**
    for rib exhalation somatic
    dysfunction: Rib 2, **261**, 261–62
    for rib exhalation somatic
    dysfunction: Ribs 3 to 5, 262, **262**
    for rib exhalation somatic
    dysfunction: Ribs 6 to 10, 262, **262**
    for rib exhalation somatic
    dysfunction: Ribs 11 to 12,
    262–63, **263**
    for rib inhalation somatic
    dysfunction: Rib 1, 257, **259**
    for rib inhalation somatic
    dysfunction: Ribs 11 and 12,
    259–60, **260**
    for rib inhalation somatic dysfunction:
    Ribs 2 to 5, 257–59, **260**
    for rib inhalation somatic dysfunction:
    Ribs 6 to 10, 259, **260**
    pectoralis minor direct myofascial
    release technique, 255, **256**
  rib counterstrain, 263–66, **264–266**
  thoracic spine soft tissue procedures
    lateral recumbent position,
    253–54, **254**

muscle energy techniques—Cont'd
  prone pressure soft tissue technique,
    253, **254**
thoracic spine, *see* upper back pain,
  mechanical neck and
TMJ, *see* temporomandibular joint
  dysfunction (TMJ)
treatment procedures overview, 59–70
  choice of procedure, 70
  classification of manipulative
    procedures, 59–60
    combined techniques, 59–60, **60**
    direct techniques, 59, **60**
    indirect techniques, 59, **60**
  clinical conditions covered, 59
  clinical wisdom, 70
  contraindications and precautions, 60–61
    direct techniques, 61
    general principles, 60
    indirect techniques, 61
  designing a management plan for
    somatic dysfunction, *see* designing a
    management plan for somatic
    dysfunction
  references, 70
  side effects, 61
  see also specific conditions
Trendelburg test or sacroiliac joint motion
  test, 96, **96**

U

uncinate process, 132–33, **133**
U.S. Department of Defense, guidelines
  for management of low back pain,
  81, 83
U.S. Department of Health Care Policy
  and Research, 1, 80
upper back pain, mechanical neck and,
  129–84
  adjunct treatments, **174**, 174–75
  age and, 129
  cervical spine treatment procedures,
    162–74
    counterstrain treatment, 169–74,
    169–74
    functional treatment, 167–69, **168**
    myofascial release treatment, 164–67,
    164–67
    soft tissue treatment, 161–64, **164**
  controversies, 179–81
  definition, 129
  differential diagnosis, 137–38, **138**
  education, 175
  epidemiology, 129–30
  exercises, *see* exercises for upper back and
    neck pain
  functional anatomy: cervical spine,
    130–34, **131–36**
    anterior, **131**
    anterior cervical muscles, **134**
    atlantoaxial (AA) joint, 130, **132**
    atlantoaxial (AA) rotation, **133**
    atlas: superior view, 130, **132**
    atlas and vertebral and basilar arteries,
    superior view of, **134**

upper back pain, mechanical neck and—Cont'd
  axis: superior view, 130, **132**
  cervical multifidi muscles, **136**
  cervical rotation muscles, 133–34, **136**
  lateral cervical spine view of facet angles, 132, **133**
  lateral head and neck and cervical spine anatomic relationships, **131**
  occipitoatlantal (OA) and anlantoaxial joints: coronal view section, 132, **133**
  occipitoatlantal (OA) joint in neutral, extension, and flexion, **132**
  posterior, **131**
  posterior cervical muscles, **135**
  scalene muscles, 133, **135**
  superficial posterior cervical muscles, **135**
  supoccipatal muscles, 133, **135**
  typical cervical vertebra: uncinate process illustrated, 132–33, **133**
  vertebral artery, 133, **134**
  functional anatomy: thoracic spine, 134–36, **136–37**
  gender and, 129
  history, 138
  laboratory and radiographic findings, 139, **139**
  manual diagnostic procedures, 141–53
    atlantoaxial segmental diagnosis, 151–52, **154**
    cervical somatic dysfunction diagnosis: segmental examination, 149, **149–50**
    cervical spine anatomic landmarks, 147–49, **148–49**

upper back pain, mechanical neck and—Cont'd
    C3 to C7 segmental diagnosis, 152–53, **155–56**
    occipitoatlantal segmental diagnosis, 149–51, **151–53**
    overview, 141
    thoracic somatic dysfunction diagnosis: segmental examination, 142–47, **142–47**
    thoracic spine anatomic landmarks, 141–42, **141–42**
  manual medicine
    benefits of, 140
    best evidence, 139–40, **140**
    practice recommendations, 140–41, 185–87
    risks of, 140, **140**
  manual treatment procedures, 153–74
    cervical spine treatment, *see* cervical spine treatment procedures
    upper thoracic treatment, *see* upper thoracic treatment procedures
  natural clinical course of, 129
  pathophysiology, 136–37, **137**
  physical findings, 138–39, **138–39**
  position paper on osteopathic manipulative treatment of the cervical spine, 140, 179–80, 185–87
  prevalence of, 129
  references, 182–83
  research opportunities, 181–82
  risk factors, 130, **130–31**
    comorbid conditions, **130**
    non-work, **131**

upper back pain, mechanical neck and—Cont'd
    radiating neck pain, associated with, **131**
    work environment-related, **130**
  societal effects of, 129–30
  suggested reading, 183–84
  upper thoracic treatment procedures, 153–60
    anterior thoracic counterstrain treatment, 159, **161–62**
    articulatory treatment, 157
    functional treatment, 158–59, **160**
    muscle energy treatment: Type I and Type II dysfunctions, 157–58, **158**
    myofascial release treatment, 157, **157**
    posterior thoracic counterstrain treatment, 160, **163**
    soft tissue treatment, 153–57, **156**
upper extremity mobility test, 44, **44**, 52–53

V

vertebral unit, structural foundation of, **13**, 13
Veterans Administration, guidelines for management of low back pain, **81**
visceral diseases, 8
viscerosomatic reflexes, 8, **10**

W

windup, 5
Winters, J.C., 233
Work Loss Data Institute, 139, 141
workshops on osteopathic manual approaches for physicians, 1–2